# HEALTH AND DISEASE:
# A READER

**Edited by**
**BASIRO DAVEY, ALASTAIR GRAY**
**AND CLIVE SEALE**

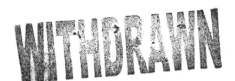

OPEN UNIVERSITY PRESS
Buckingham · Philadelphia

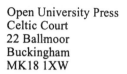

Open University Press
Celtic Court
22 Ballmoor
Buckingham
MK18 1XW

email: enquiries@openup.co.uk
world wide web: http://www.openup.co.uk

and
325 Chestnut Street
Philadelphia, 19106, USA

First edition published 1984
Reprinted 1986, 1988, 1989, 1990, 1992, 1993

First published in this second edition 1995
Reprinted in this edition 1995, 1996, 1999

A catalogue record of this book is available from the British Library

ISBN  0 335 19326 9 (hb)    0 335 19209 2 (pb)

**Library of Congress Cataloging-in-Publication Data**
Health and disease : a reader / edited by Basiro Davey, Alastair Gray,
 and Clive Seale. — Rev. ed.
    p.   cm.
  Includes bibliographical references and index.
  ISBN 0–335–19326–9   ISBN 0–335–19209–2 (pbk.)
  1. Public health.  2. Social medicine.  3. Medical care.
 I. Davey, Basiro.  II. Gray, Alastair, 1953– .  III. Seale, Clive.
 RA436.H43   1994
 362.1—dc20
                                              94–2470
                                                 CIP

Typeset by Graphicraft Typesetters Ltd, Hong Kong
Printed in Great Britain by Redwood Books

# Contents

# Acknowledgements

1   Abridged selections from *Mirage of Health* by René Dubos published by Harper Colophan, New York, 1979. Published by permission of the estate of the late René Dubos.
2   Original article by Irvine Loudon © The Open University 1984, by permission of the Open University.
3   Reprinted from *Culture, Medicine and Psychiatry* 2, 1978, pp. 107–137, copyright © 1978 by D. Reidel Publishing Company, Dordrecht, Holland, by permission of D. Reidel Co. Reprinted by permission of Kluwer Academic Publishers. Reprinted from *New Society*, 5 November 1981, by permission of *New Society*.
4   Reprinted from Mildred Blaxter, *Health and Lifestyles*, 1990, Tavistock Publications, by permission of Routledge.
5   Reprinted from Susan Sontag, *Illness as Metaphor*, Chapter 4, 1978. Reproduced by permission of Penguin Books Ltd.
6   Reprinted from Ursula Sharma, 'Using alternative therapies: marginal medicine and central concerns' in Abbott, P. and Payne, G. (eds) *New Directions in the Sociology of Health*, Falmer Press, 1990, pp. 140–152.
7   Reprinted from David Armstrong, 'The problem of the whole-person in holistic medicine', in *Holistic Medicine*, 1, pp. 27–36, 1986.
8   Reprinted from R. Littlewood and M. Lipsedge, *Aliens and Alienists*, revised edition, Routledge (Unwin Hyman) 1989. Reproduced by permission of Routledge.
9   Original article by Mary James © The Open University 1995, by permission of the Open University.
10   Reprinted from Sarah Nettleton, 'Protecting the vulnerable margin: towards an analysis of how the mouth came to be separated from the body', *Sociology of Health and Illness*, 1988 **10** (2), pp. 156–169, by permission of Blackwell Publishers.
11   Reprinted from Erving Goffman, 'The insanity of place', *Relations in Public: Microstudies of the Public Order*, Allen Lane, The Penguin Press, 1971. Reproduced by permission of Penguin Books Ltd.

12   Reprinted from Julia Burton-Jones, *Caring for the Carers*, used by permission of Scripture Union.

13   Reprinted from Andrew Nocon and Tim Booth, *The Social Impact of Asthma* published by Joint Unit for Social Services Research, The University, Sheffield.

14   Reprinted from Sally Macintyre and David Oldman, 'Coping with migraine' in Davies, A. and Horobin, G. (eds) *Medical Encounters*, Croom Helm, 1977. Reproduced by permission of Routledge.

15   Reprinted from David Kelleher, 'Coming to terms with diabetes' in Anderson, R. and Bury, M. (eds) *Living with Chronic Illness*, Routledge, 1988.

16   Original article by Neil Small © The Open University 1995, by permission of the Open University.

17   The extract from *Pride Against Prejudice: Transforming Attitudes to Disability* by Jenny Morris, first published by The Women's Press Ltd, 1991, 34 Great Sutton Street, London EC1V 0DX, reprinted on pages 107–110 is used by permission of The Women's Press Ltd.

18   Reprinted from Naomi Pfeffer, 'The stigma of infertility' in Stanworth, M. (ed.) *Reproductive Technologies: Gender, Motherhood and Medicine*, Polity Press, Cambridge, 1987.

19   Reprinted from Jocelyn Cornwell, *Hard-earned Lives*, Chapter 7, 1984, Tavistock Publications, by permission of Routledge.

20   Reprinted from Tony Parker, *The People of Providence*, 1985, Hutchinson, London. Reproduced by permission of Rogers, Coleridge & White Ltd.

21   Reprinted from F. Engels, *The Condition of the Working Class in England*, translated by the Institute of Marxism-Leninism, Moscow, Panther Books, 1969, by permission of Panther Books and Lawrence and Wishart.

22   Reprinted from J. N. Morris, 'Inequalities in health: ten years and little further on' in *The Lancet*, Vol. 336, pp. 491–493, 25th August 1990, © by The Lancet Ltd.

23   Reprinted from George Brown, 'Depression: a sociological view' in Tuckett, D. and Kaufert, J. M. (eds) *Basic Readings in Medical Sociology*, Tavistock Publications, 1978, by permission of Routledge.

24   Reprinted from J. Drèze and A. Sen, *Hunger and Public Action*, Chapter 3, 1989, Clarendon Press, Oxford.

25   Reprinted from the Royal College of Physicians Medical Services Study Group, '*Deaths under 50*' in *British Medical Journal*, 2, pp. 1061–1062, by permission of the *British Medical Journal*.

26   Reprinted from Richard Asher, *Talking Sense*, Pitman, 1972, by permission of Pitman Publishing Ltd., London.

27   Reprinted from Barry Bogin, 'Why must I be a teenager at all?' in *New Scientist*, 6 March 1993.

28   Reprinted from P. Laslett, *A Fresh Map of Life*, Chapter 1, 1989, Weidenfeld and Nicolson, London.

29   Reprinted from Helen Roberts, Susan Smith and Carol Bryce, 'Prevention is better . . .' in *Sociology of Health and Illness*, 15 (1993), pp. 447–463. Blackwell Publishers.

30   Reprinted from T. McKeown, *The Modern Rise of Population*, Edward Arnold, 1976, by permission of Edward Arnold Publishers Ltd.

31   Reprinted from Simon Szreter, (1988) *The Society for the Social History of Medicine*, pp. 1–37.

32  Reprinted from *Effectiveness and Efficiency: Random Reflections on Health Services* by A. L. Cochrane, Nuffield Provincial Hospitals Trust, 1971.

33  Reprinted from *The Lancet* 16 February 1980, *The Guardian* and the *British Medical Journal* by permission.

34  Reprinted from C. La Vecchia, 'Assessment of screening for cancer', *International Journal of Technology Assessment in Health Care*, 1991 Vol. 7, pp. 275–285, © Cambridge University Press.

35  Reprinted from Marc Strassburg, 'The global eradication of smallpox' in *American Journal of Infection Control*, **19**, pp. 220–225, with permission from Mosby-Year Book, Inc.

36  Reprinted from I. Illich, *Limits to Medicine*, Marion Boyars, 1976, by permission of Marion Boyars Publishers Ltd.

37  Reprinted from V. Navarro, *Medicine under Capitalism*, Prodist, 1976, by permission of the author.

38  Original article by Alan Williams © The Open University 1995, by permission of the Open University.

39  Reprinted from Rosemary Stevens, *The Evolution of the Health-care Systems in the US and the UK*, by permission of the author.

40  Reprinted from P. Day and R. Klein 'Britain's health care experiment' in *Health Affairs*, 1991, Fall issue, pp. 40–59, published by People to People Health Foundation, Millward, USA.

41  Original article by Fedelma Winkler © The Open University 1995, by permission of the Open University.

42  Reprinted from David Werner, 'The village health-worker: lackey or liberator?' in Skeet, M. and Elliott, K. (eds) *Health Auxilliaries and the Health Team*, Croom Helm, 1978, by permission of Croom Helm Ltd.

43  A. Ramesh and B. Hyma, 'Traditional Indian medicine in practice in an Indian metropolitan city', reprinted with permission from *Social Science and Medicine*, **15**, pp. 69–81, by permission of Elsevier Science Ltd., Pergamon Imprint, Oxford, England.

44  Extract from *A short cut to better services: day surgery in England and Wales*, Audit Commission (1990), published by HMSO, London.

45  Reprinted from A. Bowling and A. Cartwright, *Life After Death: a study of elderly widowed*, Tavistock Publications, 1982, by permission of Routledge.

46  Reprinted from David Field, 'We didn't want him to die on his own' in *Journal of Advanced Nursing*, 9, 1984, pp. 59–70.

47  Reprinted from Thurstan B. Brewin, 'Truth, trust and paternalism' in *The Lancet*, **31**, 31 August 1985 pp. 490–492 © by The Lancet Ltd.

48  Reprinted from A. Oakley, *Women Confined*, Martin Robertson, 1980, by permission of Blackwell Publishers, Oxford.

49  Reprinted from Second report on maternity services (the 'Winterton Report') House of Commons Health Committee (1992), published by HMSO, London.

50  Reprinted from Roger Jeffery, 'Normal rubbish: deviant patients in casualty departments' in *Sociology of Health and Illness*, 1, 1979, pp. 90–108. By permission of Blackwell Publishers, Oxford.

51  Reprinted from E. Paterson, 'Food-work' in Atkinson, P. and Heath, C. (eds) *Medical Work*, Gower, 1981, by permission of Gower Publishing Co. Ltd.

52  Reprinted from J. Desmond Bernal, *The World, The Flesh and The Devil*, 1929, Jonathan Cape. Reproduced by permission of Routledge.

53   Reprinted from Margaret Whitehead and Göran Dahlgren, 'What can be done about inequalities in health?' in *The Lancet*, **338**, 26 October 1991, pp. 1059–1063.
54   Reprinted from L. Breslow, 'A health promotion primer for the 1990s' in *Health Affairs*, 1990, Summer issue, pp. 6–21, published by People to People Health Foundation, Millward, USA.
55   Reprinted from Paula Whitty and Ian Jones, 'Public health heresy: a challenge to the purchasing orthodoxy' in *The British Medical Journal*, **304**, 18 April 1992, pp. 1039–1041.
56   Original article by Patrick C. Pietroni © The Open University 1995, by permission of the Open University.
57   Reprinted from Alexander Leaf, 'Potential health effects of global climatic and environmental changes' in *The New England Journal of Medicine*, **321**, No. 23, 7 December 1989, pp. 1577–1583.
58   Reprinted from Chris Beckett, 'The welfare man' in *Interzone*, August 1993, pp. 48–56.
59   Reprinted from Sally Vincent, 'Exits', *The Guardian Weekend*, 19 February 1994.
60   B. Müller-Hill, 'The shadow of genetic injustice'. Reprinted with permission from *Nature*, **362**, 8 April 1993, pp. 491–492. © 1993 Macmillan Magazines Limited.
61   Reprinted from S. Jones, *Language of Genes*, 1993, by permission of HarperCollins Publishers Limited.
62   Reprinted from Clifton K. Meador, 'The last well person', in *The New England Journal of Medicine*, **330** (6) 1994, pp. 440–441. © 1994. Massachusetts Medical Society.

# General introduction

Since the first edition of this Reader was published in 1984, there has been a steady expansion of research and publication relevant to the subjects of health and disease. The field has become ever more diverse and has drawn an increasingly varied range of authors and commentators within its expanding boundaries. What was once the preserve of medical experts and academics in a few medically-oriented disciplines, has become a major subject for investigation and debate by a wide spectrum of natural and social scientists, statisticians, economists, demographers and epidemiologists, historians, poets and politicians, journalists, analysts of every conceivable policy and strategy, and laymen and laywomen whose claim to expertise lies in their personal experience.

The editors have selected the sixty-two articles in this Reader to represent the richness of the field broadly known as 'health studies'. There are contributions from most of the major academic disciplines engaged in active research into some aspect of health and disease, together with extracts from official reports and policy documents, letters, essays, fiction and interviews. Some contributions are deeply embedded in the concepts and viewpoints of a constrained sphere of interest; others bridge traditional disciplinary boundaries and attempt a synthesis of views, or reach into the future to speculate about the shape of things to come. Many difficult decisions had to be made on what to include and what to leave out. Roughly one third of the articles in this edition of the Reader were included in the first edition, though some of these have been re-edited and reduced in length; generally, these are 'classic' texts, which are difficult to find in print. Five articles have not been published previously.

The diversity of the material can be exemplified by considering the articles that, in some measure, cast light on health and disease by focusing on death. Mortality rates and their different distribution within societies, between nations and across time, figure prominently in articles as varied as Frederick Engels' account of industrial slums in nineteenth century Britain, and the analysis of famines by Jean Drèze and Amartya Sen. The Medical Services Study Group points to unhealthy lifestyles and disregard for medical advice as causes of premature death, in sharp contrast to J. N. Morris, Margaret Whitehead and Göran Dahlgren who identify poverty and social disadvantage as the main culprit. Jenny Morris challenges the willingness of able-bodied people to assume that a severe physical disability is reason enough for someone to want to die, while Sally Vincent explores the moral minefield that stands between active and passive euthanasia. The often-neglected but commonplace experiences of elderly people caring for a dying spouse are revealed by Ann Bowling and Ann Cartwright's study, and David Field investigates the thoughts and feelings of nurses striving to cope with terminally-ill patients. J. D. Bernal banishes death altogether in his vision of a future in which 'the flesh' is reduced to a disembodied and immortal brain.

There is a growing recognition that the investigation of any aspect of health and disease can benefit not only from a multi-disciplinary approach, but one that also values the subjective and illuminative as well as the objective and quantifiable. The borderland between these formerly separate perspectives has become fruitful territory for exploration, a development that is well represented by several articles in this Reader. For example, the sociologist Mildred Blaxter addresses the question 'What is health?' by analysing the vocabulary and ideas expressed by 900 people in a nation-wide survey. Each respondent's experience provides both a unique insight into an individual's personal world and an entry in a data-matrix from which generalizable conclusions can be extracted.

The articles and other readings differ greatly in style, content, focus and intent; they were originally written with very different audiences in mind, for a wide range of publications including academic journals, government departments and newspapers. Given this diversity and the broad reach of the selection, the editors have imposed a degree of order by grouping the contributions under seven headings: Part 1 – Concepts of health, disease and healing; Part 2 – Experiencing health and disease; Part 3 – Influences on health and disease; Part 4 – The role of medicine; Part 5 – The social context of health care; Part 6 – Health work; and Part 7 – Prospects and speculations. Each part of the book has a short introduction prepared by the editors, which aims to draw the reader's attention to common themes and sharp discontinuities.

Within each part of the book the emphasis has been on choosing material that adequately represents the range of disciplines, perspectives and styles of writing. To this end, we have edited the majority of articles to reduce their length from the original texts, thereby enabling us to include a larger selection; in some cases, the editors had the assistance of authors or trustees in carrying out this task. Where substantial and significant parts of a text have been omitted, this has been acknowledged in the note at the end of the article, which also contains a brief description of the author(s) and a full reference to the original source in which the unabridged material was published.

This Reader has been assembled as part of an Open University second-level course for undergraduate study and professional development, entitled *Health and Disease* (course code U205). This course explores in depth the possibilities of a multi-disciplinary approach to a whole range of health and disease topics. It consists of this Reader, eight specially-prepared distance-teaching textbooks (published by Open University Press and listed on the back cover of this book), and audiovisual materials. This Reader is indispensable for students taking the course, but it has also been designed to stand alone as a coherent and self-contained collection, accessible to a wide readership, which includes health workers and social workers of all kinds, students of the many disciplines represented here, and the general public.

# Part 1
# Concepts of health, disease and healing

## INTRODUCTION

Most societies maintain some myth of a Golden Age which, while usually set in the past, may be considered to be attainable in the future if the appropriate policies and practices are adopted. René Dubos, a microbiologist, who wrote 'Mirage of health', the first article in this part of the book, argues that the concept of health as arising from a harmony with nature is an attractive but essentially false illusion. It is opposed by a different conception of health, represented in Greek mythology by the god Asclepius, which identifies causes of ill health in precisely located malfunctions of the body. Dubos' preferred synthesis rests on the interaction between the two conceptions of health.

In 'The history of pernicious anaemia from 1822 to the present day', the painstaking isolation, through logical deduction and experimentation, of the precise cause of a particular disease is then described by Irvine Loudon, a retired general practitioner and medical historian. This represents the Asclepian tradition in thinking about health, geared towards establishing the localized pathologies upon which precisely targeted cures may then act. Upon such thinking are based many of the 'success stories' of modern medical science. It is common to contrast this reductionist vision of the body with the apparently 'unscientific' views of lay persons. Lay beliefs are explored in 'Feed a cold, starve a fever' by Cecil Helman, an anthropologist and general practitioner, who identifies the idea that ill health is due to an imbalance between the person and forces of nature. Thus, lay beliefs are placed by Helman firmly within the camp that Dubos earlier identified as that of the Greek goddess Hygeia, who embodied the precept *mens sana in corpore sano* (a healthy mind in a healthy body), and attracted the perception that health arose when people lived wisely.

The issue of moral responsibility for illness figures strongly in the lay beliefs described by Helman, and also in the accounts reported by the sociologist Mildred Blaxter in the next article, 'What is health?' Blaxter's research shows more variety in lay beliefs than does Helman's. Some are quite close to the medical, Asclepian view of health consisting of the absence of disease; others take it to incorporate much broader notions of the 'healthy life', which again contain moral and characterological connotations. The idea that disease confers a particular quality of character upon a person is also explored by Susan Sontag, in an extract from her book *Illness as Metaphor*, in which she writes about romanticized images of tuberculosis sufferers. The medieval theory of illness as caused by an imbalance of blood, bile or some other 'humour' was associated with a view that did not distinguish mind from body. This is referred to by Sontag, where she discusses the 'melancholy' character attributed to TB sufferers.

A belief in 'holistic medicine' is shared by advocates of alternative therapies in modern times. Ursula Sharma, a sociologist, stresses this in 'Using alternative therapies', her account of people's reasons for consulting alternative practitioners. She argues that, dissatisfied with the directive approach of orthodox doctors and fearful of the harmful effects of some medical therapies, people seek alternatives in the more democratic relationship offered by acupuncturists, chiropractors, homoeopaths, herbalists and the like. Her own view, that such alternatives address central problems in modern medicine, is clearly stated.

However, David Armstrong, who is a doctor and medical sociologist, takes a much more critical view of the claims of holistic practitioners in 'The problem of the whole-person in holistic medicine'. In this respect, he returns us to themes evident in Dubos' article, presenting a sceptical account of the Golden Age myth with which Sharma is struggling. Holism, with its idealized construction of what it is to be 'natural' is in Armstrong's eyes an ideological view designed to promote the claims of its practitioners. However, he cautions us against being too critical of alternative medicine, arguing, for example, against the view that such practices are a subtle form of surveillance and social control. He argues that it is, rather, a creative activity, offering new ways of thinking about ourselves and our health.

The idea that medicine can act as a means of social control is illustrated by the account given by two psychiatrists, Roland Littlewood and Maurice Lipsedge, of encounters between 'Ethnic minorities and the psychiatrist'. The doctor is graphically presented as ally to the policeman in maintaining a definition of 'disturbed' behaviour as deviant and in need of sedation and restraint. This is accompanied by explanations for the illness that may differ markedly from that given in the culture of the patient. Attempts to 'democratize' the relationship by abandonment of symbols of medical authority, such as the white coat, may simply be read as confusing by a patient untrained in the meaning that such actions are intended to have. Nor do they change the essential imbalance of power that exists between the two parties.

Imbalance of power is evident, too, in the historian Mary James' account of the medical view of hysteria in Paris during the nineteenth century. In 'Hysteria and demonic possession', she describes the work of the pioneering physician Charcot in seeking a medical understanding of a phenomenon previously explained by religious ideas about demon possession. James suggests that display of the 'symptoms' of hysteria might have been encouraged by a subtle process of suggestion by male doctors to their relatively powerless female patients.

This part of the book ends with an ambitious attempt by Sarah Nettleton, a sociologist, to apply to the case of dentistry the view that medical knowledge is a social construction, rather than an objective description of external reality. In the case of mental illness, or a general philosophical orientation towards a view such as 'holism', it is perhaps easy to pick out instances where the observer has distorted reality (which itself feels hard to 'pin down') to suit their own preconceptions or cultural beliefs. We are taught, however, to see some events – such as tooth decay – as having an objective physical existence, and we may resist efforts to depict it as having a variable meaning. Toothache appears to have a singular and most pressing meaning to the sufferer, and tooth brushing appears to be an incontrovertibly sensible, rational and inevitable response to conditions in mouths. See if you feel differently about brushing your teeth when you have read Nettleton's article, 'Protecting a vulnerable margin: towards an analysis of how the mouth came to be separated from the body'.

The relationship between medical, lay and alternative concepts of health, disease and healing is intricate and problematic. Different people may be pursuing different interests in advocating a certain perspective. The articles in Part 1 show that this is not just a matter of disagreement about how best to promote health or deal with ill health, as if these concepts had some fixed, objective meaning. The very objects of study – health, disease and healing – are contested concepts.

# 1
# Mirage of health

## RENÉ DUBOS

### The Gardens of Eden

The illusion that perfect health and happiness are within man's possibilities has flourished in many different forms throughout history. Primitive religions and folklores are wont to place in the remote past this idyllic state of paradise on earth. In the Old Testament the Patriarchs are said to have lived hundreds of years, while their descendants can hardly aspire to more than threescore and ten. The ancient Greeks believed in the existence of happy races, vigorous and virtuous, in inaccessible parts of the earth. According to their legends, the Hyperboreans and the Scythians in the north, the Ethiopians in the south, lived exempt from toil and warfare, from disease and old age, in everlasting bliss like the dwellers in the Isles of the Blest at the edge of the Western Sea.

### The return to Nature

Like primitive peoples, men in civilized societies commonly believe in the possibility of an ideal state of health and happiness. But, instead of expressing this belief through legends and folklore, they are apt to rationalize it in the form of philosophical theories and to assert that a healthy mind in a healthy body can be achieved only by harmonizing life with the ways of nature. The latter part of the eighteenth century proved particularly receptive – in theory at least – to the gospel that all human problems could be solved by returning to the ways of nature. Jean Jacques Rousseau asserted that man in his original state was good, healthy, and happy and that all his troubles came from the fact that civilization had spoiled him physically and corrupted him mentally. 'Hygiene,' Rousseau claimed, 'is less a science than a virtue.' Sickness being the result of straying away from the natural environment, the blessed original state of health and happiness could be recaptured only through abiding by the simple order and purity of nature – or, as Voltaire said in maliciously paraphrasing Rousseau, through learning again to walk on all fours.

Since very ancient times the theory that most of the ills of mankind arise from failure to follow the laws of nature has been endlessly reformulated in every possible form and mood, in technical and poetical language, in ponderous treatises and witty epigrams. In particular, the Taoist philosophy which has so profoundly influenced Chinese life and art is pervaded by reverence for nature. Lao-tzu, the Jean Jacques Rousseau of ancient China, was followed by many translators and imitators. Chuang-tzu wrote of the time when 'the ancient men lived in a world of primitive simplicity .... That was the time when the *yin* and the *yang* worked harmoniously, and the spirits of men and beasts did not interfere with the life of the people, when the four seasons were in order and all creation was unharmed, and the people did not die young.'

Modern man has done many odd things to display his faith in the fundamental goodness of nature. Following in the steps of Rousseau, one hundred million Central Europeans went botanizing in the hope of discovering among lowly flowers both the soul of the universe and natural remedies for chest troubles. More prosaic twentieth-century man tries to re-establish contact with this forgotten biological past in count-less country clubs, hunting or ski lodges and beach bungalows, through clambakes in the moonlight and barbecue parties in suburban gardens and picnic groves. Whatever his inhibitions and tastes, Western man believes in the natural holiness of seminudism and raw vegetable juice, because these have become for him symbols of unadulterated nature.

## The concept of Nature

It is probable that a few people now and then in limited periods of history have enjoyed relative peace in a fairly constant physical and social environment. But the state of equilibrium never lasts long and its characteristics are at best elusive, because the word 'nature' does not designate a definable and constant entity. With reference to life there is not one *nature*; there are only associations of states and circumstances, varying from place to place and from time to time.

Living things can survive and function effectively only if they adapt themselves to the peculiarities of each individual situation. For some sulphur bacteria, nature is a Mexican spring with extremely acid water at very high temperature; for the reindeer moss, it is a rock surface in the frozen atmosphere of the arctic. The word 'nature' also means very different things to different men. Man, by manipulating the external world, renders 'natural' for his individual taste many kinds of environments which display an astonishingly wide range of moods.

Harmonious equilibrium with nature is an abstract concept with a Platonic beauty but lacking the flesh and blood of life. It fails, in particular, to convey the creative emergent quality of human existence. [For man] the seasons and the soil, the plants and the beasts, the permanent dwellers and the distant visitors with which he came into contact during his long journey, all the factors of his total environment, differed from one place to another, from one period to another, and their temporary associa-tion constituted the 'nature' to which he had to adapt in each situation and at each moment.

## The doctrine of specific etiology

Until late in the nineteenth century disease had been regarded as resulting from a lack of harmony between the sick person and his environment. Louis Pasteur, Robert Koch, and their followers took a far simpler and more direct view of the problem. They showed by laboratory experiments that disease could be produced at will by the mere artifice of introducing a single specific factor – a virulent microorganism – into a healthy animal.

From the field of infection the doctrine of specific etiology spread rapidly to other areas of medicine; a large variety of well-defined disease states could be produced experimentally by creating in the body specific biochemical or physiological lesions. Microbial agents, disturbances in essential metabolic processes, deficiencies in growth factors or in hormones, and physiological stresses are now regarded as specific causes of disease. The ancient concept of disharmony between the sick person and his environment seems very primitive and obscure indeed when compared with the precise terminology and explanations of modern medical science.

Unquestionably the doctrine of specific etiology has been the most constructive force in medical research for almost a century and the theoretical and practical achievements to which it has led constitute the bulk of modern medicine. Yet few are the cases in which it has provided a complete account of the causation of disease. Despite frantic efforts, the causes of cancer, of arteriosclerosis, of mental disorders, and of the great medical problems of our times remain undiscovered. It is generally assumed that these failures are due to technical difficulties and that the cause of all diseases can and will be found in due time by bringing the big guns of science to bear on the problems. In reality, however, search for *the* cause may be a hopeless pursuit because most disease states are the indirect outcome of a constellation of circumstances rather than the direct result of single determinant factors.

It is true that in a few cases – far less common than usually believed – the search for *the* cause has led to effective measures of control. But it does not follow that these measures provide information as to the nature of the trouble that they correct. While drenching with water may help in putting out a blaze, few are the cases in which fire has its origin in a lack of water. Effective therapies do not constitute evidence for the doctrine of specific etiology.

## Darwin and Bernard

By equating disease with the effect of a precise cause – microbial invader, biochemical lesion, or mental stress – the doctrine of specific etiology had appeared to negate the philosophical view of health as equilibrium and to render obsolete the traditional art of medicine. Oddly enough, however, the vague and abstract concepts symbolized by the Hippocratic doctrine of harmony are now re-entering the scientific arena. Hippocratic medicine has acquired a more profound significance from the implications of the discoveries that Darwin and Claude Bernard were making around 1850 – even before Pasteur and Koch had made their contributions to the etiology of disease. Darwinism implies that the individual and species which survive and multiply selectively are those best adapted to the external environment. Claude Bernard supplemented the doctrine of evolutionary adaptation by his visionary guess that fitness depends upon a constant interplay between the internal and the external environment of the individual. He emphasized that at all levels of biological organization, in plants as well as in animals, survival and fitness are conditioned by the ability of the organism to resist the impact of the outside world and maintain constant within narrow limits the physicochemical characteristics of its internal environment. In other words, life depends not only upon the reactions through which the individual manages to grow and to reproduce itself but also upon the operation of the control mechanisms which permit the maintenance of individuality. The dual concept of fitness to the external environment and fixity of the internal environment is the modern expression of the Hippocratic dictum that health is universal sympathy.

## The gods of health

The word 'hygiene' now conjures up smells of chlorine and phenol, pasteurized foodstuffs and beverages in cellophane wrappers, a way of life in which the search for pleasurable sensations must yield to practices that are assumed to be sanitary. Its etymology, however, bears no relation to this pedestrian concept. Hygiene is the modern ersatz for the cult of Hygeia, the lovely goddess who once watched over the health of Athens. She was the guardian of health and symbolized the belief that men could remain well if they lived according to reason.

Throughout the classical world Hygeia continued to symbolize the virtues of a sane life in a pleasant environment, the ideal of *mens sana in corpore sano*. Hygeia was not an earthbound goddess of ancient origin. Her name derives from an abstract word meaning health. For the Greeks she was a concept rather than a historical person remembered from the myths of their past. She was not a compelling Jeanne d'Arc but only an allegorical goddess Liberty and she never truly touched the hearts of the people. From the fifth century BC on, her cult progressively gave way to that of the healing god, Asclepius.

To ward off disease or recover health, men as a rule find it easier to depend on healers than to attempt the more difficult task of living wisely. Asclepius, the first physician according to Greek legend, achieved fame not by teaching wisdom but by mastering the use of the knife and the knowledge of the curative virtues of plants. In contrast to Hygeia, the name Asclepius is of very ancient origin. Apparently Asclepius lived as a physician around the twelfth century BC. He was already known as a hero during Homeric times and was created a god in Epidaurus around the fifth or sixth century BC. His popularity spread far and wide, even beyond the boundaries of Greece. Soon Hygeia was relegated to the role of a member of his retinue, usually as his daughter, sometimes as his sister or wife, but always subservient to him. In most of the ancient iconography from the third century on, as well as in all subsequent representation, Asclepius appears as a handsome, self-assured young god, accompanied by two maidens: on his right Hygeia and on his left Panakeia. Unlike Hygeia, her sister, Panakeia became omnipotent as a healing goddess through knowledge of drugs either from plants or from the earth. Her cult is alive today in the universal search for a panacea.

The myths of Hygeia and Asclepius symbolize the never-ending oscillation between two different points of view in medicine. For the worshippers of Hygeia, health is the natural order of things, a positive attribute to which men are entitled if they govern their lives wisely. According to them, the most important function of medicine is to discover and teach the natural laws which will ensure to man a healthy mind in a healthy body. More skeptical or wiser in the ways of the world, the followers of Asclepius believe that the chief role of the physician is to treat disease, to restore health by correcting any imperfection caused by the accidents of birth or of life.

## Hippocratic wisdom

Hippocratic writings occupy a place in medicine corresponding to that of the Bible in the literature and ethics of Western peoples. Just as everyone quotes from the Bible, it is the universal practice to look to Hippocrates for statements that give the sanction of authority and of time to almost any kind of medical views, profound or banal. For twenty-five centuries Hippocrates has personified in the Western world the rational outlook of the philosopher, the objective attitude of the scientist, the practical approach of Asclepius, and the human traditions of Hygeia.

It is implicit in the Hippocratic teachings that both health and disease are under the control of natural laws and reflect the influence exerted by the environment and the way of life. Accordingly, health depends upon a state of equilibrium among the various internal factors which govern the operations of the body and the mind; this equilibrium in turn is reached only when man lives in harmony with his external environment. [Hippocrates'] writings are pervaded with the concept that the life of the patient as a whole is implicated in the disease process and that the cause is to be found in a concatenation of circumstances rather than in the simple direct effect of some external agency.

## The modern public health movement

Rudolf Virchow deserves special mention at this point because of his immense prestige as experimenter, scientist, and writer in several medical and other biological fields. During his student days, Virchow had been influenced by the political philosophy of the German Social Democratic Party. At the age of twenty-six in 1847, he was appointed member of a commission organized by the Prussian government to study the epidemic which was then raging in the industrial districts of Upper Silesia. In a minority report Virchow traced the origin of the epidemic to unfavourable meteorological conditions. Heavy rains had ruined the year's crops and this had resulted in famine. Furthermore, the winter following had been extremely severe, forcing the poor people to huddle together in their homes, cold and hungry. It was then that typhus had broken out, first spreading rapidly through the poor population and eventually reaching the wealthier classes. His experience in Silesia led Virchow to start in 1848 the new journal, *Medizinische Reform*. In it he professed, as did his French predecessors inspired by the philosophers of the Enlightenment, that poverty was the breeder of disease and that it was the responsibility of physicians to support social reforms that would reconstruct society according to a pattern favourable to the health of man. Thus, according to Virchow, the treatment of individual cases is only a small aspect of medicine. More important is the control of crowd diseases which demand social and, if need be, political action. In this light medicine is a social science.

Despite its vigorous intellectual and social basis, the early nineteenth-century health movement in France and Germany was rather ineffective in the way of practical reforms. The goals of the French and German philosophers and physicians were to a large extent political and therefore difficult to reach except by revolutionary action. Furthermore, their doctrines were presented to the public in somewhat abstract terms. In England, by contrast, the leadership was taken by practical men who succeeded in finding a formula that appealed to elementary emotions and was meaningful to everyone. To a group of public-minded citizens guided by the physician Southwood Smith and the engineer Edwin Chadwick it appeared that, since disease always accompanied want, dirt, and pollution, health could be restored only by bringing back to the multitudes pure air, pure water, pure food, and pleasant surroundings.

This simple concept was synthesized in the movement 'The Health of Towns Association', the prototype of the present-day voluntary health associations throughout the world. Its aim was to 'substitute health for disease, cleanliness for filth, order for disorder . . . prevention for palliation . . . enlightened self-interest for ignorant selfishness and bring home to the poorest . . . in purity and abundance, the simple blessings which ignorance and negligence have long combined to limit or to spoil: *Air, Water, Light.*'

Faith in the healing power of pure air, with much contempt for the germ theory of disease, was also the basis of Florence Nightingale's reforms of hospital sanitation during the Crimean War. 'There are no specific diseases,' she wrote. 'There are specific disease conditions.'

The conquest of epidemic diseases was in large part the result of the campaign for pure food, pure water, and pure air based not on a scientific doctrine but on philosophical faith. It was through the humanitarian movements dedicated to the eradication of the social evils of the Industrial Revolution, and the attempt to recapture the goodness of life in harmony with the ways of nature, that Western man succeeded in controlling some of the disease problems generated by the undisciplined ruthlessness of industrialization in its early phase.

## Defining health

Health and disease cannot be defined merely in terms of anatomical, physiological, or mental attributes. Their real measure is the ability of the individual to function in a manner acceptable to himself and to the group of which he is part.

For several centuries the Western world has pretended to find a unifying concept of health in the Greek ideal of a proper balance between body and mind. But in reality this ideal is more and more difficult to convert into practice. Poets, philosophers, and creative scientists are rarely found among Olympic laureates. It is not easy to discover a formula of health broad enough to fit Voltaire and Jack Dempsey, to encompass the requirements of a stevedore, a New York City bus driver, and a contemplative monk.

Among other living things, it is man's dignity to value certain ideals above comfort, and even above life. This human trait makes of medicine a philosophy that goes beyond exact medical sciences, because it must encompass not only man as a living machine but also the collective aspirations of mankind. A perfect policy of public health could be conceived for colonies of social ants or bees whose habits have become stabilized by instincts. Likewise it would be possible to devise for a herd of cows an ideal system of husbandry with the proper combination of stables and pastures. But, unless men become robots, no formula can ever give them permanently the health and happiness symbolized by the contented cow, nor can their societies achieve a structure that will last for millennia. As long as mankind is made up of independent individuals with free will, there cannot be any social status quo. Men will develop new urges, and these will give rise to new problems, which will require ever new solutions. Human life implies adventure, and there is no adventure without struggles and dangers.

René Dubos, microbiologist and experimental pathologist, was formerly Professor at the Rockefeller University of New York City. These extracts are taken from his book *Mirage of Health*, published by Harper Colophan, New York (1979).

# 2
# The history of pernicious anaemia from 1822 to the present day

## IRVINE LOUDON

First of all the history of pernicious anaemia is discussed as an interesting story in its own right, starting with the earliest clinical reports which led to the recognition of the disease, and ending with recent views on its nature.

The story is then presented as a characteristic example of the way that advances in the theory and practice of medicine occur and are influenced, sometimes adversely, by currently fashionable ideas on the causation of disease.

It has always been obvious that if you were severely wounded, or lost blood for any other reason, you could become weak or ill or even die, and blood is essential for life. But the idea that the blood could be deficient, not from excessive bleeding, but from a disease of the blood *sui generis*, was essentially a concept of the early nineteenth century when the term anaemia first came into general use. Once anaemia was recognised as common it was found that most cases responded well to an adequate diet and medicine. Iron, which had been used as a tonic or stimulant for a long time, was soon recognised as the treatment of choice for anaemia.

In 1849, Thomas Addison (1793–1860), a physician at Guy's Hospital in London, published a brief account of a form of anaemia which was unusual. He called it 'A remarkable form of anaemia which, although incidentally noticed by various writers [Dr Combe in Edinburgh had described a case in 1822] has not attracted . . . the attention it really deserves.' This form of anaemia occurred, he wrote, in males aged twenty to sixty '. . . commencing insidiously and proceeding very slowly'; and it was invariably fatal. No treatment, not even iron, was of the slightest benefit.

As interest in pernicious anaemia grew through the late nineteenth and early twentieth century, cases were commonly seen in the wards of the hospitals because they were selected as examples of a particularly interesting disease. Within the community, however, pernicious anaemia, because it was fairly uncommon and affected people mostly towards the end of their lives, was not in quantitative terms a serious health problem.

At first, Addison's brief report attracted little attention until a Swiss doctor, Biermer, described some cases in 1872 of the same kind of anaemia and named it 'progressive pernicious anaemia'. After that, it became known as Addisonian pernicious anaemia, or, more briefly, pernicious anaemia.

Anaemia is by definition a deficiency in the number of red blood cells in the circulation, or a deficiency in haemoglobin (the oxygen-carrying pigment in the red cells), or both. Blood is formed in the bone marrow, and the red cells, after evolving through several stages to full maturity, are released into the circulation. After an average period of 120 days the obsolete red cells are destroyed. In health, production and destruction continue at the same rate, ensuring that the number of red cells in the circulation remains constant.

In order to understand the history and nature of pernicious anaemia, a simple analogy is helpful. The analogy is that of a car factory in a country where it is the only one, and no cars are imported. The factory (the bone-marrow) manufactures the cars (the red cells) which appear on the roads (the blood vessels) until they become worn out and are scrapped. Now, suppose there is a sudden deficiency in a vital piece of equipment used in the final stage of manufacture. At first, finished cars held in stock can be used up, but when that stock is exhausted the number of cars on the road begins to fall. Meanwhile the factory continues to produce cars that are nearly, but not quite, fit to be sold. A few of these incomplete cars slip past the inspectors and appear on the road, but soon break down. In the factory itself unfinished cars accumulate until, because they are crammed to capacity, some of the unfinished cars are broken up and stored as scrap iron. Meanwhile, the number of cars on the road falls gradually but relentlessly.

Advances in medicine in the 1850s, particularly the ability to estimate the number of red cells in the blood and measure the amount of the pigment haemoglobin, led to discoveries about pernicious anaemia similar to those in the imaginary car factory. Thus, in 1875 and 1876, Pepper in the USA and Cohnheim in Germany demonstrated that in cases of pernicious anaemia the number of red cells in the circulation was greatly diminished but the bone marrow was hyperplastic (= over active), overloaded with iron and packed with immature, abnormal precursors of the red cells. Moreover, the blood contained some abnormal red cells, corresponding to the unfinished cars that slipped past the inspectors.

Clearly, the bone marrow was responding to the anaemia by trying to manufacture red cells, but it lacked the ability to produce the finished product. It is interesting that in the first description of pernicious anaemia by Combe in 1822, he suggested the fault might lie in the digestive processes. However, proof of this did not come until the end of the nineteenth century. Then it was shown, first of all, that the stomachs of patients dying of pernicious anaemia were often atrophic (= wasted or worn out). This was followed by the finding that hydrochloric acid, present in normal gastric juices in abundance, was absent in cases of pernicious anaemia. The obvious conclusion, that pernicious anaemia was due to lack of hydrochloric acid, was soon shown to be untrue. Feeding hydrochloric acid by mouth did not cure it. Then it was suggested that the function of the acid in the stomach was to provide an antiseptic barrier, and that patients with pernicious anaemia were suffering from 'toxins' produced by swallowed bacteria, which poisoned the bone marrow. This theory can be found in textbooks published between 1910 and 1925.

Bacteriology was, at this time, a relatively new exciting branch of medical science.

The temptation to attribute all diseases whose nature was obscure to bacterial sepsis or bacterial toxins was very strong. Thus it was widely believed that people could harbour toxin-producing bacteria in their tonsils, sinuses or teeth, even though these were, to all appearances, perfectly healthy; and that they could swallow these 'toxins' and become ill as a consequence. This was the theory of *focal sepsis*, and pernicious anaemia was for a time thought to be just such a disease. The unfortunate result was that a number of patients had healthy tonsils and teeth removed in obedience to a false theory. There were critics of this view of pernicious anaemia, but in general, the probability that a bone-marrow poisoned by toxins would appear hypoplastic (= under-active) rather than hyperplastic (= over-active) was ignored.

The next and most important stage of the story contains an element of luck, or at least trial and error. Whipple and his associates in the USA in 1920 carried out experiments that consisted of feeding various diets to dogs already made anaemic by bleeding them. They found that liver was the most effective food for stimulating new blood formation. This encouraged two other Americans, Minot and Murphy, in 1926 to try various diets, including liver in large quantities, on patients suffering from various kinds of anaemia. They found that cases of pernicious anaemia responded to liver in large quantities and some other foods (although not so well) including meat. These foods, it seemed, contained an anti-pernicious factor, but how this factor worked remained unknown. Whipple, Minot and Murphy were awarded a Nobel Prize for their work, and by 1928 an extract of liver which could be safely injected had been made and was soon brought into general use. Pernicious anaemia was, at last, treatable.

Treatment rapidly became available to all sections of the community and the hospital patients slowly dying of pernicious anaemia disappeared from the wards. As so often happens, when a really effective method of curing or preventing a medical disorder (but obviously not a surgical one) is discovered, it is nearly always a simple method that can be, and is, administered by general practitioners. Today, cases of pernicious anaemia are rarely seen in hospital wards, but every general practitioner has a number of cases for whose maintenance treatment he and his nursing staff are responsible.

Returning to the 1920s, the most imaginative and important advance was made by Castle in 1929. He postulated that blood formation required some dietary factor, found in high concentration in liver, which he called the *extrinsic* factor. However, the absorption of that factor was dependent on the secretion by the stomach of another factor, the *intrinsic* factor. Pernicious anaemia, Castle suggested, was a disorder of the stomach, and patients with pernicious anaemia had lost the ability to secrete not only hydrochloric acid (which was irrelevant to blood formation) but also the essential intrinsic factor. This proved to be correct. The most hopeful line of research was seen to be to try and isolate the extrinsic factor. This was done by 1948, when it was shown to be a vitamin and was named vitamin $B_{12}$. The nature of intrinsic factor is less important practically as it cannot be isolated and used in treatment, but the function of intrinsic factor is this. It 'escorts' the extrinsic factor (vitamin $B_{12}$) across the barrier of the wall of the gut, ensuring that all the $B_{12}$ ingested in the diet is absorbed into the blood stream. In the absence of intrinsic factor (i.e. in pernicious anaemia) only a small percentage of ingested $B_{12}$ can be absorbed by a process of slow diffusion across the gut wall. Thus by eating a diet with huge quantities of $B_{12}$, the patient with pernicious anaemia may just be able to absorb enough to stop the anaemia from getting any worse, but he has to continue to do so, day after day.

What is the function of this vitamin B$_{12}$? Vitamin B$_{12}$ is not so much an essential constituent of red cells; it is more a component required for certain chemical processes involved in the manufacture of normal red cells. The equivalent in the analogy of the car factory would be that the cars remained unfinished because a certain machine-tool was lacking and that tool was essential for finishing the manufacture of the car. To continue the analogy, there were plenty of the machine-tools available outside the factory gates, but the process of getting them through the factory gates and to the work bench had broken down. In this analogy the factory gates represent the stomach. *Pernicious anaemia is essentially a disease of the stomach made manifest through its effects on the blood.*

What does this mean in terms of medical practice today? Pernicious anaemia is rare below the age of 35; most cases occur at age 60 or over. It is found in 1 in every 250 people aged 60 in the United Kingdom, but there are large regional variations. Thus, it is more than three times as common in Scotland as it is in the South-east of England. It is much less common in the population as a whole than the ordinary iron deficiency anaemia by a ratio of about 9 to 1. It can occur in both sexes, not, as Addison thought, in males only. The usual history is that a patient is seen who is tired, often breathless and very pale; usually the pallor is described as of a lemon-yellow tint, but Addison's original description of the 'colour of bad wax' is much better. Pernicious anaemia is suspected, and a sample of blood is taken for examination. The blood shows a marked reduction in the number of red cells and the presence of some abnormal red cells (the unfinished cars which escaped on to the roads). The amount of vitamin B$_{12}$ in the blood can be estimated, and in pernicious anaemia this is abnormally low. There are now known to be a number of diseases similar to pernicious anaemia, which are called as a group the megaloblastic anaemias. To be absolutely certain the patient really is suffering from Addisonian pernicious anaemia, the gastric contents can be examined and the absence of hydrochloric acid confirmed, and a specimen of bone-marrow can be examined for the characteristic appearance found in pernicious anaemia. Because treatment has to be life-long, and the characteristic signs disappear once treatment has begun, the tests must be completed first. Once the diagnosis is certain, vitamin B$_{12}$ is given by injection and, once the blood has returned to normal, continued permanently. The injections are given regularly every three months, or more often if blood tests show it to be necessary. The commencement of treatment is the equivalent of removing the obstruction to the admission of machine-tools at the factory gates. In the analogy, the obvious result would be the sudden appearance on the roads of a large number of new, finished cars. Brand new cars would, for a while, form a much larger percentage of the total than usual. So it is with pernicious anaemia. The administration of vitamin B$_{12}$ leads to a sudden rise in the number of new red cells. These are slightly different from ordinary red cells and are called reticulocytes. There are always some reticulocytes in the blood, just as there are always some new cars on the roads, but the rise in the percentage of reticulocytes when vitamin B$_{12}$ is injected (the 'reticulocyte response') is further confirmation of the diagnosis of pernicious anaemia. Not only the blood, but also the bone marrow, rapidly return to normal. Usually the illness has come on so slowly and for such a long time that the patient has almost forgotten what it feels like to be well. For this reason, the treatment of pernicious anaemia can be one of the most striking and dramatic of all medical treatments as the patient is rapidly transformed back to health.

The history of pernicious anaemia is an unusually rich example of the nature of biomedical advances, and of the historical periods in which they have taken place. It began as a clinical observation in the first half of the nineteenth century by astute physicians who recognised there was a 'new' form of anaemia different from the majority of cases. All advances at this time came from bed-side observation and post-mortem studies. The next stage occurred in the era of laboratory investigations, in the second half of the nineteenth century, when blood counts became available. This allowed the various kinds of anaemia to be identified and classified with a new certainty. Progress to this stage had followed a logical path but had provided no treatment for a fatal disease.

The next stage depended on the use of biochemical tests in the investigation of disease and also illustrated the importance of chance observations. It was the analysis of gastric juices that led to the unexpected discovery of 'achlorhydria' (= absence of hydrochloric acid) as an invariable feature of pernicious anaemia. This in turn led to three developments of a kind so common in medical research:

1. First it indicated, correctly, that the cause of pernicious anaemia lay in the stomach.
2. Second, it suggested (incorrectly) that pernicious anaemia could be cured by administering hydrochloric acid; in other words, that the acid was the missing factor.
3. When that failed, it led to the unfortunate theory of bacterial toxins as the cause, and the subjection of many patients to the unnecessary removal of tonsils and teeth. Persistence of this kind of error was due to the popularity of a general theory of focal sepsis, then in vogue.

The next stage depended in the beginning on animal experiments, for it was Whipple's work on experimental anaemia that led to the discovery that liver contained the anti-pernicious anaemia factor.

Often, medical research is seen as the slow but steady progression through a logical series of steps. More often, it is actually a series of sudden jumps, some false (such as the focal sepsis theory), but others of outstanding importance. Often the sudden jumps seem obvious in retrospect, but Castle's theory of an extrinsic *and* an intrinsic factor was an example of a brilliant imaginative leap, and he confirmed the hypothesis by showing that ground beef (also a rich source of vitamin $B_{12}$) partially digested in the stomach of a 'normal' man induced a remission when fed to a patient with pernicious anaemia. The experiment may not sound attractive, but it was conclusive. Something in the gastric juice of healthy people was essential for the complete absorption of anti-pernicious factor. After this, the story was essentially one of logical but painstaking biochemical research to isolate the extrinsic factor: vitamin $B_{12}$.

It is easy to present the history of pernicious anaemia as one of the 'triumphs of biomedical research'. But one of the fashionable criticisms of modern medicine is that all too often it treats only the symptoms of a disease and fails to discover the root cause. This could be said of pernicious anaemia. The cause of the atrophy of the stomach that results in the failure to secrete intrinsic factor and hydrochloric acid (and, incidentally, is associated with an increased incidence of cancer of the stomach) is unknown. It tends to run in families and is therefore said to be 'an inherited constitutional weakness'. But that is no explanation. Recent work suggests that pernicious anaemia is an example of the failure of 'self-recognition' by the immune systems of the body. This means that pernicious anaemia belongs to a group of diseases in which there is a great deal of current interest, the auto-immune diseases. It is a group that contains, for example, certain forms of arthritis. The body contains an immune system whose function is to protect the body against the invasion by any foreign substances, such as bacteria or toxins. To perform this function, the immune system has to be able to distinguish between normal body tissues, or 'self', and foreign material, or 'not self'. If the recognition process breaks down, then the immune system can attack certain parts of the body. It is a kind of civil war waged by the immune system, or a situation such as an army shelling soldiers belonging to its own side. Why a part of the stomach should fail to be recognised as self and thus be singled out for attack in pernicious anaemia, rather than some other organ, is unknown. Indeed, the stomach is, sometimes, not the only target. There is another feature of pernicious anaemia not mentioned so far and which only appears in a minority of cases, and then, usually, only in the later stages. Occasionally, this other condition can occur even without any anaemia, but, when it does, it is always associated with the same disorder of the stomach and with absence of hydrochloric acid. This disorder, which consists of patchy damage to parts of the spinal cord, is called sub-acute combined degeneration of the cord; it results in numbness and weakness, both progressive, in the limbs. Existing damage cannot be reversed, but all progress of this disorder is prevented by injections of vitamin $B_{12}$. Thus it can be said that the cause of pernicious anaemia and of the spinal cord disease associated with it is unknown. It can even be argued that treatment with vitamin $B_{12}$, when the inability of the patient to absorb that substance is by-passed by injections, is an example of symptomatic treatment. Therefore, it can be argued that pernicious anaemia is a treatable disease, but not a curable one, and that the 'root cause' remains a mystery. Arguments of this kind, for all their philosophical interest, pale into trivial insignificance when set against the practical experience of a patient who, suffering from the disease, is restored to health by a few injections a year. Nevertheless, research into the nature of pernicious anaemia will, and should, continue – better methods of treatment, or even prevention, may well be discovered.

## References

Readers who wish to follow the history of pernicious anaemia from original sources will find the early description of a case by Combe in:

Combe, J. S. 'A history of a case of anaemia', *Transactions of the Medical-Chirurgical Society of Edinburgh*, 1, 194 (1822);

and Addison's first report in:

Addison, T. 'Anaemia – disease of the supra-renal capsules', *The London Medical Gazette*, 3rd series, 8, 517 (1849).

Minot and Murphy's work appeared in the *Journal of the American Medical Association*, 87, 470 (1926).

Castle's discovery was published in the *American Journal of Medical Sciences*, 178, 748 (1929).

Very good summaries of the history of pernicious anaemia with full references can be found in:

Haden, R. L. 'Pernicious anaemia from Addison to folic acid', *Blood*, 3, 22–31 (1948). The same issue of the journal, *Blood*, contains a reprint of Minot and Murphy's original paper.

Jacobs, A. 'Pernicious anaemia 1822–1929', *Archives of Internal Medicine*, 103, 329–333 (1959).

Major, R. *Classic Descriptions of Disease*, 2nd edn. Charles C. Thomas, Springfield and Baltimore (1939). Contains under one cover the papers of Addison, Combe, and Minot and Murphy.

Irvine Loudon, a retired general practitioner, was a Research Fellow at the Wellcome Unit for the History of Medicine, University of Oxford, when this article was written. It was first published in the first edition (1984) of this Reader.

# 3
# Feed a cold, starve a fever

**CECIL HELMAN**

The National Health Service, set up thirty-three years ago, was designed to bring the best of scientific medicine to the whole population. Much of the ill-health that had previously been borne, as one writer put it, in 'the imposed silence of poverty,' was now accessible to free health care. But what has been the impact of three decades of health education, television programmes about health, and easy access to doctors and hospitals, on traditional beliefs about illness? Whatever happened to folk remedies and old wives' tales?

A study I conducted on medical folklore in a north London suburb suggests that these folk beliefs about illness and health *can* survive the impact of scientific medicine, and in some cases may even be reinforced by this contact. This is important because in Britain the majority of ill-health – especially minor complaints – is dealt with outside the formal health care system.

In one recent study, Ruth Levitt estimated that about threequarters of abnormal symptoms are dealt with by patients themselves, their friends, family, or even the local pharmacist – without ever consulting a doctor. Self-medication is common (in some studies twice as common as the taking of prescribed medication), for a whole variety of conditions. Even after a doctor's prescription is issued, patients frequently use – or don't use – their drugs in ways that 'make sense' to them, rather than in ways the doctor intended. This 'non-compliance' has been estimated at 30 per cent, or more.

So how patients perceive ill-health and its treatment, both before and after seeing a doctor, depends on lay beliefs about what causes illness. There is an increasing amount of research into this; my own study tackled folk beliefs about some common, minor ailments – 'chills', 'colds' and 'fever'. As both an anthropologist and a GP I was trying to find out the concepts underlying the often-heard aphorism, 'Feed a cold, starve a fever.'

It arises from a folk model, or scheme of classification, of illness which is widely accepted by the patients; and it relates to those conditions of impaired well-being

| | HOT | COLD |
|---|---|---|
| | (1) *Ear, Nose, and Throat* <br> FEVER + NASAL CONGESTION OR DISCHARGE | (1) *Ear, Nose, and Throat* <br> COLD + NASAL CONGESTION OR DISCHARGE, WATERY EYES, 'SINUS' CONGESTION |
| | (2) *Chest* <br> FEVER + PRODUCTIVE COUGH | (2) *Chest* <br> COLD + NON-PRODUCTIVE COUGH |
| WET | (3) *Abdomen* <br> FEVER + DIARRHOEA AND ABDOMINAL DISCOMFORT | (3) *Abdomen* <br> COLD + LOOSE STOOLS AND SLIGHT ABDOMINAL DISCOMFORT |
| | (4) *Urinary System* <br> FEVER + URINARY FREQUENCY AND BURNING | (4) *Urinary System* <br> COLD + SLIGHT URINARY FREQUENCY BUT NO PAIN |
| | (5) *Skin* <br> FEVER + RASH + NASAL DISCHARGE OR COUGH | |
| DRY | FEVER + DRY SKIN, FLUSHED FACE, DRY THROAT, NON-PRODUCTIVE COUGH | COLD + SHIVERING, RIGOUR, MALAISE, VAGUE MUSCULAR ACHES |

**Figure 3.1**   The folk classification of common 'hot' and 'cold' symptoms.

which the patients perceive as disequilibrium, and regard as 'illness', and which concern perceived changes in body temperature – either 'hotter' than normal, or 'colder'. In general, these feelings of abnormal temperature change are purely subjective; they bear little or no relation to biomedical definitions of 'normal' body temperature as 98.4°F or 37°C, as measured orally on a thermometer. The conditions where the patient 'feels hot' are classified as *Fevers*, those where he 'feels cold' in his body are classified either as *Chills* or *Colds*. Both Fevers and Colds/Chills are states of being – both classified as abnormal – which, in the folk model have different causes, different effects, and thus require different treatments.

There are two important principles underlying this folk classification of 'illness-misfortune': (1) the relation of man with *nature*, i.e. with the natural environment, in Colds and Chills, and (2) the relation of man to man, which exists within human *society*, in Fevers.

To a large extent the area covered by the folk model – which I have set out schematically in Figure 3.1 – corresponds to that area of disorders which biomedicine classifies as Infectious Diseases: that is, acute or chronic inflammatory conditions where the causative agent is known to be either a virus or a bacterium. These disorders, which occur very commonly in general practice, include disorders known as: upper respiratory tract infections; influenza; coryza; bronchitis; pneumonia; sinusitis; urinary tract infections; gastroenteritis; childhood fevers (e.g. rubella); and several

|  | HOT | COLD |
|---|---|---|
|  | HOT | COLD |
| WET | WET | WET |
|  | HOT | COLD |
| DRY | DRY | DRY |

**Figure 3.2**

others. This classification overlaps, to some extent, the area covered by the folk model but as will be described there are significant differences. Illnesses associated with temperature change are common in all sections of the population, as are the often associated symptoms of cough or rhinitis. Cough is apparently the commonest symptom complained of in general practice,[1] and it is common even among those who do not consult the doctor: in Dunnell and Cartwright's study[2] 32 per cent of adults reported 'cough, catarrh, or phlegm' in a sample two-week period, while 18 per cent had suffered from 'cold, influenza, or rhinitis'. To describe the folk model it is necessary to adopt a diachronic approach: what follows is mainly the folk classification reported by older patients; those born during or since World War Two, while sharing the basic underlying classification, have introduced new elements, particularly with regard to the germ theory.

### Structural analysis of the folk system

In Figure 3.1 I have listed the common groups of symptoms which relate to, or are accompanied by, perceived changes in body temperature. There are four diagnostic categories in all (see Figure 3.2); the basic division is between 'Hot' and 'Cold' conditions, but in addition there is a further division into 'Wet' and 'Dry' conditions. 'Wet' conditions are those where the temperature change is accompanied by other symptoms, and with a seemingly abnormal amount of 'Fluid' being present – either still within the body, or else emerging from its orifices; this 'Fluid' includes sputum, phlegm, nasal and sinus discharge, vomitus, urine, and loose stools. The symptoms here include nasal congestion or discharge, sinus congestion, productive coughs, 'congested' chests, diarrhoea, and urinary frequency. 'Dry' conditions are those where the abnormal temperature change is the only, or the paramount symptom – such as a subjective feeling of being cold, shivering or rigours on one hand – and a feeling of being 'hot', perhaps with a dry throat, flushed skin, slight unproductive cough, and possibly delirium, on the other. Skin rashes usually occur on the 'Hot' side of the classification. Other subsidiary symptoms – including pain – may occur in one form or another on both sides of the temperature division.

Thus there are four basic compartments into which common symptoms relating to temperature change can be fitted (see Figure 3.3): 'Hot/Wet' (Fever plus Fluid), 'Hot/Dry' (Fever), 'Cold/Wet' (Cold plus Fluid), and 'Cold/Dry' (Cold). Obviously these compartments are not watertight; there is always some overlap between divisions. In addition, not all conditions associated with abnormal temperature changes have been included; only the commonest, as encountered in general practice.

|       | HOT             | COLD            |
|-------|-----------------|-----------------|
| WET   | FEVER + FLUID   | COLD + FLUID    |
| DRY   | FEVER           | COLD            |

**Figure 3.3**

'Colds' and 'fevers' relate to two bodily states both perceived as being abnormal. The first is where you feel 'colder', the other 'hotter', than usual. But, in fact, both are subjective feelings, unconnected to actual measurements on a thermometer. Both can occur in a 'dry' form (the abnormal temperature change alone), or in a 'wet' form (where temperature change is associated with excess fluid). 'Wet' symptoms would include nasal congestion, 'runny noses', 'congested chests', coughing up mucus, diarrhoea or urinary frequency.

In *chills* and *colds*, the abnormal temperature change is usually seen as a by-product of one's personal battle with the natural environment – particularly with areas of lowered temperature. In this view, damp or rain ('cold/wet' conditions), or cold winds or draughts ('cold/dry'), can penetrate the boundary of the skin, and cause similar conditions within the body.

A cold, rainy day causes one to feel 'cold', with a runny nose. Sitting in a cold wind ('a draught') causes a feeling of coldness, though often without the excess fluid.

Wind at body temperature is not dangerous, and is merely 'fresh air'. Night air, however, is often considered dangerous by older patients. And 'the children get sick if you leave the bedroom windows open at night.'

Some areas of skin are seen as more vulnerable than others to penetration by environmental cold – particularly the top of the head, the back of the neck, and the feet. I found that 'colds' occurred when these areas were inadvertently exposed to draughts or damp – for example: 'getting your feet wet', 'walking around with damp hair', 'going out into the rain, without a hat on', or 'stepping into a puddle'. Elderly men, in particular, reported an increased vulnerability to 'head colds' after a haircut – when the back and top of the head are unprotected by their normal covering of hair.

Temperature changes between hot and cold environments were considered dangerous, especially the intermediate zone between the two temperatures – for example, 'going into a cold room after a hot bath', 'walking on a cold floor when you have a fever'. Changes in season were also risky – autumn, for example, where the 'hot' summer is changing to 'cold' winter. It was explained to me that 'summer colds' are more common since cheap air flights returned people suddenly from 'hot' Spain or Italy to 'cold' Britain, with disastrous results.

Cold, once it has entered the body, can move around. From damp feet it can migrate to cause a 'stomach chill', or it can shift even further upwards to cause 'a head cold' or 'sinus cold'. In general, *chills* occur below the waist ('stomach chill', 'bladder chill', 'kidney chill'), and *colds* above it ('a head cold', 'a cold in the sinuses', 'a cold in the chest').

Unlike fevers, cold and chills are more one's own responsibility. They are the result of carelessness, or lack of foresight – if 'you don't dress properly', 'allow your head to get wet', 'wash your hair when you don't feel well'. Colds are caused, as one middle-aged patient explained seriously, 'by doing something abnormal'.

So folk remedies for colds emphasise the return to 'normal' temperature and equilibrium, by treating 'cold' with 'hot'. Hot drinks, hot food, rest in a warm bed, and generating your own bodily heat by 'tonics' or food ('feed a cold . . .') were frequently advised. Other remedies stress the return from the 'wet' state to the 'dry' one: drying up the excess fluid by a variety of traditional remedies (goose fat was commonly used at one time), or patent decongestants bought from a chemist.

By contrast, *fevers* are thought to be due to invisible entities known – interchangeably – as 'germs', 'bugs' or 'viruses'. Some of these terms may be borrowed from modern medicine, but they are used and conceptualised in an entirely different way.

For example, 'germs' are described as living, invisible and malevolent entities. They have no free existence in nature, it seems, but exist only in or among people. They are thought of as occurring in a cloud of tiny particles, or as a tiny invisible 'insect'. They travel through the air between people, entering the body of their victim by one of the orifices (usually the mouth, or the nose, but also the ears, urethra, and so on). They signal their presence by causing a 'fever'. The germs that cause stomach upsets are more 'insect-like' than others ('a tummy bug'), and apparently larger in size.

Germs have personalities. These reveal themselves, or are expressed in, the sorts of symptoms they cause. 'I've got that germ, doctor, you know – the one that gives you the dry cough and the watery eyes,' or 'the one that gives you diarrhoea, and makes you bring up.' The germs are amoral in their selection of victims, but they can only cause harm once they do attack. There are no 'good' germs: *all* germs are bad, and patients do not differentiate between 'germs', 'bugs' and 'viruses'.

Once a germ enters the body, and causes a fever, it can move or expand to attack several parts of the body simultaneously. 'It's gone to my lungs,' 'I can feel it in my stomach,' 'It's moved to my chest', or, as one patient with a peptic ulcer said, 'I got the flu, but then it flew to the ulcer and that blew up.'

Because germs, unlike colds (at least to older patients), originate in other *people*, rather than in the natural environment, germ infection implies some sort of social relationship of whatever duration. Infection is an inherent risk in all relationships, though neither party is to blame if one 'picks up a germ.'

## Cough up the muck

In that case, the victim is less blameworthy than in the case of a cold, and more able to mobilise sympathetic friends or relatives around him. One of the obligations of close relationships is to risk infection, if necessary, in looking after another person.

'Fevers' particularly attack the weak, the old, and the poor. This vulnerability of the poor is often explained away by their association with the dirt and disorder of poverty. 'Dirt' is seen as concentrated, or condensed, germs.

Like colds and chills, fevers can occur in the 'dry' ('feeling feverish', with a flushed skin, dry mouth) or 'wet' form (accompanied by excess catarrh, phlegm, urine). Folk remedies for fevers aim to return the victim from the 'hot' state to normal temperature; but also to move him (with the aid of *fluids* which 'flush out' or 'wash out' the germ) from the 'dry' state to the 'wet' state.

Fluids of one sort or another are used to 'wash out' the germ from the chest, so that a 'dry' cough can 'loosen', bringing with it the offending germ. A variety of fluids, like tea, hot water, and now patent cough mixtures, are used for 'getting it off your chest', 'coughing up the muck', 'getting it out of your system'.

Patients complain that a dry cough 'hasn't broken', or 'hasn't loosened', so that they can 'cough it off my chest'. 'I gargled with salt water to get the catarrh out,' one man said, 'and I always swallow a bit of it to loosen the cough.'

Fluids are also used as folk treatments for other hot/wet conditions, like diarrhoea, vomiting, or urinary frequency accompanied by a fever, to flush out the offending germ. Other folk remedies induce sweating, allowing you to 'sweat it out' of your system – in this case through the skin itself. Antibiotics are seen as powerful chemicals that kill germs *in situ*, with the body being the battlefield of this great clash. Both 'germs' and 'viruses' are seen as vulnerable to the effects of antibiotics.

Most people who use the words 'germs' or 'viruses' have never *seen* either of these entities. They have no perceptual evidence for their existence. So that they can be thought of more as hypotheses, or theories of causality. There is some similarity between these western ideas of 'germs', and the invisible, malign 'spirits' said to cause illness by people in non-western and non-industrialised societies.

There is a marked difference in lay views of colds and fevers between older patients, and those born since the second world war – who constitute the world's first 'antibiotic generation'. Younger patients are more likely to ascribe both fevers and colds to 'germs' or 'viruses'.

The Germ Theory is one example of a medical concept that has gradually influenced patients' ways of thinking about illness. 'Germs', as a cause of illness, have gradually spread to include many of the 'cold' conditions as well. Instead of 'a chill on the bladder', you have 'a germ in the water'; instead of 'a cold in the head', you have 'picked up a virus'.

One result of this is that the amount of personal responsibility for illness (as in old-fashioned 'colds') seems to have gradually declined. If more and more conditions are due to 'germs', then the victims are increasingly blameless, and more able to mobilise a caring community around themselves.

Illness seems to have become more *social* in its origin, effects and even treatment. Where you have 'germs' as a believed cause for illness, then you have a greater need of doctors and their remedies. There is also the slight sense of increased danger in social relationships – the threat of infection. Young mothers – more often than their own mothers would have – now ask, 'My child's got a cold; can she mix with other children?'

The metaphor of 'germs' as invisible forces 'out there' which cause suffering to the innocent, seems to have become a pervasive social metaphor. Pollution, radiation, and social changes 'of epidemic proportions', are all expressions of this.

The main meeting place between lay health beliefs and the medical profession, is usually the GP's surgery. In Britain, according to Ruth Levitt, the health service GP is the first point of contact for about 90 per cent of those who *do* seek medical help. In the surgery, both doctor and patient have to agree on what is wrong with the patient, and what should be done about it.

This involves a process of 'negotiation', whereby each party tries to influence the other about the outcome of the consultation, and the treatment to be given. One aspect of this is that, in order to get their patients' cooperation, GPs have to couch their diagnoses and treatment in concepts that *make sense* in terms of the patients' view of ill-health. This, in turn, may reinforce those same ideas.

A patient who presents a list of symptoms is often given a diagnosis couched in the everyday idiom of the folk model: 'You've picked up a germ,' 'You've got a flu bug,' 'It's a viral infection,' 'It's just a tummy bug – there's one going around,' 'You've got a germ in the water,' 'I'm afraid it's gone to your chest,' or 'Oh yes, is that the one where you've got a runny nose, watery eyes, and you lose your voice? I've seen a dozen already this week.'

More precise medical diagnoses are less commonly given, especially to uneducated patients. In many cases, these conditions are trivial, and self-limiting. They won't get worse; they will soon go away of their own accord; and no one else will catch them. A precise 'technical' diagnosis may be unnecessary, and in fact impossible. Not every cough and cold can be subjected to complex and expensive laboratory tests to identify the precise virus or bacteria causing it. The four-to-seven minute GP consultation time also makes more precise diagnoses impractical.

Many doctors do not, or cannot, differentiate between bacteria and viruses. So neither do patients. Bacteria *are* treatable by antibiotics but viruses are not. The distinction, however, has become blurred. Doctors reinforce this when they over-prescribe antibiotics generally – and particularly when they prescribe them for viral illnesses. This blurring strengthens the lay view that all 'germs' are bad; all are similar in nature; and all of them therefore susceptible to antibiotics. It also increases dependence on the doctor for prescribed treatment, even for minor complaints.

## Receptionist power

Doctors' receptionists, who do a great deal of health counselling over the surgery telephone, can also help the process of reinforcing folk beliefs. As one receptionist was heard to say to a patient with diarrhoea and vomiting: 'Yes, there is a tummy bug going around. Starve yourself and take only sips of water for 24 hours. Otherwise, the more you feed it [the bug], the more it'll enjoy itself and cause diarrhoea and sickness.'

Not everything which GPs do in order to meet their patients' need to 'make sense' of the treatment given can be 'scientifically' justified. For example, it's been estimated that *six million gallons* of cough mixtures are prescribed in Britain every year under the NHS. (This excludes the vast amount bought over the counter.) Yet most medical textbooks cast doubt on the scientific efficacy of these preparations. Part of this ocean of cough mixture must represent the subtle pressure of patients' expectations on GPs to prescribe – in a modern form – the *liquids* believed to 'wash out' or 'flush out' the infection from one's chest.

We need to know more about how people understand their sickness, how they deal with it, and how they interpret medical treatment they are given. Because self-treatment and 'non-compliance' are so common, we also need to know what happens to health and illness *outside* the NHS.

Free access to GPs, and health education on the media, does not seem to have altered some of the traditional folk beliefs about illness. Obviously, medical concepts like the Germ Theory of disease are widely known to the lay public. But they may be understood in entirely a different way, and often in terms of a much older folk view of illness.

# References

1. Morrell, D. C. 'Symptom interpretation in general practice', *J. Roy. Coll. Gen. Prac.*, **22**, 297–309 (1972).
2. Dunnell, K. and Cartwright, A. *Medicine takers, prescribers and hoarders*, Routledge and Kegan Paul, London, p. 11 (1972).

Cecil G. Helman has been both a general practitioner and a social anthropologist, who worked in the Department of Social Anthropology, University College London. This article is made up from one published in *New Society*, 222–224 (5 November 1981) and an extract from an article of the same title published in *Culture, Medicine and Psychiatry* **2**, 107–137 (1978).

# 4
# What is health?

**MILDRED BLAXTER**

What do people mean when they talk of 'health'? A dichotomy has traditionally been seen between the biomedical or scientific model of health and a looser, more holistic model. These are sometimes falsely regarded as 'medical' and 'non-medical' ways of looking at health. Crudely, medical knowledge is seen as based on universal, generalizable science, and lay knowledge as unscientific, based on folk knowledge or individual experience. The lay concepts discussed here are not, however, being presented as necessarily or essentially different from medical concepts. In western societies, an intermixing is inevitable: lay people have been taught to think, at least in part, in biomedical terms. Nor is modern medicine entirely wedded, in practice, to a narrowly-defined biomedical science: holistic concepts are also part of medical philosophy. Lay concepts are, of course, sometimes less informed or expert than those of medical professionals. In other ways, however – since health must in part be subjectively experienced – they may be better informed. As other studies have found, they are often complex, subtle, and sophisticated.

The concepts of health discussed here are derived from answers to two questions asked in a survey of 9,000 individuals carried out by an interdisciplinary team at the University of Cambridge Clinical School: (1) Think of someone you know who is very healthy. Who are you thinking of? How old are they? What makes you call them healthy? (2) At times people are healthier than at other times. What is it like when you are healthy? The replies – sometimes quite long and thoughtful – were written down verbatim.

The discussion and analysis in this article is based on a random 10 per cent sample of respondents, in which it was possible to examine in a more qualitative way the precise vocabulary used and the combinations of ideas which each individual expressed. First, those people who found themselves unable to offer any definition of health will be considered.

**'Negative' answers**

Almost 15 per cent of the respondents could not think of anyone who was 'very healthy', and over 10 per cent said in reply to the question about health for themselves, 'I just don't think about it', 'I can't answer that'. A proportion of this group, especially among the elderly, were expressing pessimism about their own health status 'I'm never healthy so I don't know', 'It's so long since I was healthy that I can't tell you what it's like'.

However, higher proportions, especially of men under 60, were expressing the idea that health is the norm, is just 'ordinary', and so is difficult to describe:

I don't think I know when I'm healthy, I only know if I'm ill (office worker, aged 28).

How do you describe it? I don't know. I think if you are healthy you don't think about it. You only think about ill health (wife of a tractor driver, aged 51).

This group of people tended to be among those who, in other parts of the survey, did not rate health very highly as a value. They were also likely, among the elderly, to see their own health as poor. Whether old or young, they were commonly people who expressed a lack of concern for 'healthy' behaviour.

**Health as not-ill**

The more explicit description of health as not being ill — as not suffering any symptoms, never having anything more serious than a cold, never seeing the doctor, having no aches and pains — has also sometimes been seen as a 'negative' concept, in opposition to the positive concept of fitness. It was a more popular definition of health in another person rather than oneself, offering an easy way of 'proving' that the person was healthy:

She's healthy because she never seems to suffer with her chest. She has an occasional cold but she's never been seriously ill (woman 70, with severe bronchitis herself, speaking of her daughter).

For oneself, more frequently than for others, 'not-ill' was expressed in terms of experienced symptoms, rather than recourse to medical services, though the nature of the symptoms naturally tended to vary with age:

Health is when you don't have a cold (man of 19).

You don't have to think about pain — to be free of aches and pains (woman of 78).

It has sometimes been suggested that a definition of health as 'not-ill' (or without disease) is characteristic of people in poorer circumstances, and to lack a positive view of health as fitness is a mark of general social deprivation (Blaxter and Paterson 1982). Though the latter may be true, there was little sign in this large sample of any social differentiation in the use of the concept 'not-ill': it seems possible that the previous finding may demonstrate one of the pitfalls of small-scale surveys. Because a 'negative' definition is found to be common among working-class respondents, it is assumed to be in some way associated with their social position. The 'not-ill' description of health was very markedly associated with the speaker's own state of health. At all ages, but particularly among the elderly, those who themselves were in poor health; or suffering from chronic conditions were less likely to define health in terms of illness.

The 'not-ill' description of health was found to be more frequently used by the better educated and those with higher incomes. It was also very markedly associated with the speaker's own state of health. At all ages, but particularly among the elderly, those who themselves were in poor health or suffering from chronic conditions were less likely to define health in terms of illness.

## Health as absence of disease/health despite disease

It is not always easy, in the respondent's replies, to distinguish illness – the experience of symptoms or malfunctioning – from a more clearly biomedical definition of disease. Disease was specifically mentioned rather rarely, whether for others or oneself, though phrases such as 'never had to go to hospital', 'don't have any really serious illnesses', 'never had any big illnesses', might be held to represent this concept. To have no (chronic or serious) disease is certainly one dimension of health, though not one commonly expressed by these respondents.

Certainly, however, there were expressions of a concept of health despite disease. Many people said of themselves 'I am very healthy although I do have diabetes', or 'I am very healthy apart from this arthritis' (crippled and housebound woman of 61). The concept of health as overcoming or coping with disease could be extended to include misfortune also:

Although he has TB he's been aware of his problems and has got over them. Though he was made redundant, since then he's done his own thing, just worked the way and when he wanted to. He didn't worry about being redundant, and he hasn't taken on too much in the size of house and garden. He enjoys life (man of 64 explaining why he calls a friend of the same age healthy).

## Health as a reserve

The idea of 'healthy though diseased' often had some affinity with the 'reserve of health' noted by Herzlich (1973). Someone is healthy because 'when he is ill he recovers very quickly', 'he has had an operation and got over it very well', or even because he takes risks and suffers no consequences: as one respondent said, 'he goes out on the drink but he never gets a hangover or a headache'. Occasionally, respondents expressed the idea of an inborn reserve of health:

He never goes to the doctors and only suffers from occasional colds. Both parents are still alive at 90 so he belongs to healthy stock (woman of 51 talking of her husband).

### Health as behaviour, health as 'the healthy life'

'The healthy person' (but rarely oneself) was rather frequently defined in terms of their 'virtuous' behaviour. He or she is a vegetarian, or a non-smoker and non-drinker, or goes jogging, or does exercises:

> I call her healthy because she goes jogging and she doesn't eat fried food. She walks a lot and she doesn't drink alcohol (woman of 50 about her neighbour).

For these respondents, health was identical with the healthy life: the non-smoker, non-drinker must be healthy, though no evidence about their health could be offered. These respondents were also more likely to be those who, throughout the rest of the interview, stressed the role of 'bad habits' in the causation of disease and the importance of self-responsibility. As one lady said:

> Why do I call her healthy? She leads a proper respectable life so she's never ill.

### Health as physical fitness

Among younger people, physical fitness was very prominent. When thinking of 'the healthy person', young men in particular stressed strength, athletic prowess, the ability to play sports: 'fit' was by far the most common word used in their descriptions of health by men under 40. The 'healthy other' was, for them, likely to be either a well-known athlete or sportsman, or a personal acquaintance who ran marathons, played squash, engaged in karate or judo, or 'trained every week'. Weight-lifting and body-building were very frequently mentioned as a source of, and a proof of, fitness. Older men also mentioned sportsmen, though less frequently. Young women, too, commonly expressed a concept of health (in others) that involved sports and physical fitness.

This is one reason why the sex of the 'person thought of as healthy' was predominantly male. Among those who offered any answer, whatever concept of health they were expressing, 80 per cent of males mentioned a man, and 57 per cent of females also mentioned a man. Few women athletes appeared as role models.

Women rarely mentioned sports or specific physical leisure pursuits. They did, however, frequently define physical fitness in terms of its outward appearance. They commonly mentioned being (or feeling) slim. To be fit was to have a clear complexion, bright eyes and shining hair:

> Being healthy is when my skin is good and my hair isn't greasy and I can do all the things I want to without feeling tired (woman of 30).

### Health as energy, vitality

The last quotation combines the notions of an appearance of fitness with a feeling of energy or vitality. 'Energy' was in fact the word most frequently used by all women and older men to describe health, and for younger men it came a close second to 'fitness'. Sometimes physical energy was clearly meant, and sometimes a psycho-social vitality which had little to do with physique: most often, the two were combined.

The words used to describe this were 'lively', 'alert', 'full of get up and go', 'full of life', 'not tired', 'not listless' As one young man said:

> Health is when I feel I can do anything. I jump out of bed in the morning, I wash my car in the cold without a thought. I feel like doing things. Nothing can stop you in your tracks (engineer of 28).

Many young men, like this one, mentioned getting up early, or not going to bed so early at night: 'it's easier to get out of bed', 'I feel like getting up in the morning', 'I don't spend all morning in bed', 'You can afford to sleep less at night'. Even as a description of the healthy 'other', not staying in bed appeared to mark really positive healthiness:

> He regularly wakes up early in the morning, gets up, doesn't watch a lot of TV (man of 21).

For older men, the same concept of energy and vitality was most often expressed as enthusiasm about work:

> I can give myself to work a hundred per cent. Work is a pleasure. Work's not a problem (Council engineering employee, aged 49).

> You feel ready to get on with anything that needs doing. You feel that you can tackle any physical work (man of 74).

Women, too, very commonly defined healthiness in terms of energy and enthusiasm for work. It was notable, however, that few of any age, whether or not they had a job outside the home, mentioned paid work. The symbol of energy for women was 'going right through the house', 'cleaning the house from top to bottom': 14 per cent of all women under 60 mentioned enthusiasm about housework. For elderly women, being *able* to do housework might be a mark of health, but for the younger, who took their everyday work for granted, *enjoyment* of housework indicated special energy. Certain less popular jobs were singled out:

> I clean·the windows and rush round like a mad thing. When I'm not healthy is when I want to sit in front of the box (single-handed mother, kitchen assistant, aged 29).

> When I'm healthy I feel like tackling the cooker and getting it clean (female teacher, aged 47).

### Health as a social relationship

A notable difference between men and women was that women were considerably more likely to define health in terms of relationships with other people.

> She goes around looking after friends and shopping for them. She's active, her mind's alive. She paints and she's a member of the theatre club and a lot of other groups (woman of 51 speaking of her mother of 77).

For younger women, health was commonly defined in terms of good relationships with family and children – 'having more patience with them', 'coping with the family', 'enjoying the family'. For the older, serving other people, being in a position to help other people, having sufficient energy to care for other people, were often cited as the marks of good health.

## Health as function

Both health as energy, and health as social relationships, are concepts which overlap with the idea of health as function – health defined by being able to do things, with less stress upon a description of feelings. This was more likely to be expressed by older people: for the young, of course, the ability to cope with the tasks of life might be taken for granted, and it is only later in life that health may be seen as a generally restricting factor.

For men below retirement age, and especially those who did manual work, health for oneself or for others could be defined as being able to do hard work. Many women who identified a man (usually their husband) as 'someone who is very healthy' also gave as their reason the physically demanding nature of his work, or the fact that he was able to work long hours. Although women were chosen as a 'healthy other' because of their general social, family and community activity, it was notable that neither sex often chose women because of their demanding work, whether within the house or outside it.

However, many elderly men and women were identified as 'someone I know who is very healthy' because they were able to work despite an advanced age:

> She's 81 and she gets her work done quicker than me, and she does the garden (woman of 63).

## Health as psycho-social well-being

The concept of health as psycho-social well-being is often close to or combined with the notions of health as energy, health as social relationships, or health as function, which have been discussed. In this analysis the category was reserved, however, for expressions of health as a purely mental state, instead of, or as well as, a physical condition. Often, these were embedded in a very holistic view of health:

> She's a person with a spiritual core. She's physically, mentally and spiritually at one (single woman, aged 45, living in a religious community).

For health in oneself, psycho-social health was stressed at all ages, and for those in the middle years was the most popular concept. It tended to be used rather more frequently by women than by men, and by those with more education rather than less. 'Health is a state of mind' or 'health is a mental thing more than physical' were common statements. 'Feel like living life to the full', 'on top of the world', 'full of the joys of spring', were phrases very commonly repeated.

> I've reached the stage now where I say isn't it lovely and good to be alive, seeing all the lovely leaves on the trees, it's wonderful to be alive and to be able to stand and stare! (farmer's widow, aged 74).

## Conclusions

Firstly, the way in which health is conceived of differs over the life course, in not unexpected ways. Younger men tend to speak of health in terms of physical strength and fitness, and commonly cite athletes as the 'healthy other'. Young women, though they also talk of fitness or its appearance, favour ideas of energy, vitality, and ability to cope. In middle age, concepts of health become more complex, with an emphasis upon total mental and physical well-being. Older people, particularly men, think in terms of function, or the ability to do things, though ideas of health as contentment, happiness, a state of mind – even in the presence of disease or disability – are also prominent.

Secondly, there are clear sex differences. At all ages women, in general, gave more expansive answers than men, and appeared to find the questions more interesting. Women of higher social class or higher educational qualifications, in particular, expressed many-dimensional concepts. Many women, but few men, included social relationships in their definition of health.

## References

Blaxter, M. and Paterson, E. *Mothers and Daughters: a Three-Generational Study of Health Attitudes and Behaviour*, Heinemann, London (1982).

Herzlich, C. *Health and illness: a social psychological analysis*, Academic Press, London (1973).

Mildred Blaxter is Honorary Professor of Medical Sociology, at the School of Social and Economic Studies, University of East Anglia. This article is a heavily edited extract from Chapter 3 of her book *Health and Lifestyles*, published by Tavistock-Routledge, London (1990).

# 5
# Illness as metaphor

## SUSAN SONTAG

It seems that having TB had already acquired the association of being romantic by the mid eighteenth century. In Act I, Scene I of Oliver Goldsmith's satire on life in the provinces, *She Stoops to Conquer* (1773), Mr Hardcastle is mildly remonstrating with Mrs Hardcastle about how much she spoils her loutish son by a former marriage, Tony Lumpkin:

> *Mrs H*: And I am to blame? The poor boy was always too sickly to do any good. A school would be his death. When he comes to be a little stronger, who knows what a year or two's Latin may do to him?
>
> *Mr H*: Latin for him! A cat and fiddle. No, No, the alehouse and the stable are the only schools he'll ever go to.
>
> *Mrs H*: Well, we must not snub the poor boy now, for I believe we shan't have him long among us. Any body that looks in his face may see he's consumptive.
>
> *Mr H*: Ay, if growing too fat be one of the symptoms.
>
> *Mrs H*: He coughs sometimes.
>
> *Mr H*: Yes, when his liquor goes the wrong way.
>
> *Mrs H*: I'm actually afraid of his lungs.
>
> *Mr H*: And truly so am I; for he sometimes whoops like a speaking trumpet – [TONY *hallooing, behind the Scenes*] – O there he goes – A very consumptive figure, truly.

This exchange suggests that the fantasy about TB was already a received idea, for Mrs Hardcastle is nothing but an anthology of clichés of the smart London world to which she aspires, and which was the audience of Goldsmith's play.[1] Goldsmith

---

1. Goldsmith, who was trained as a doctor and practiced medicine for a while, had other clichés about TB. In his essay 'On Education' (1759) Goldsmith wrote that a diet lightly salted, sugared, and seasoned 'corrects any consumptive habits, not unfrequently found amongst the children of city parents.' Consumption is viewed as a habit, a disposition (if not an affectation), a weakness that must be strengthened and to which city people are more disposed.

presumes that the TB myth is already widely disseminated – TB being, as it were, the anti-gout. For snobs and parvenus and social climbers, TB was one index of being genteel, delicate, sensitive. With the new mobility (social and geographical) made possible in the eighteenth century, worth and station are not given; they must be asserted. They were asserted through new notions about clothes ('fashion') and new attitudes toward illness. Both clothes (the outer garment of the body) and illness (a kind of interior décor of the body) became tropes for new attitudes toward the self.

Shelley wrote on July 27, 1820 to Keats, commiserating as one TB sufferer to another, that he has learned 'that you continue to wear a consumptive appearance.' This was no mere turn of phrase. Consumption was understood as a manner of appearing, and that appearance became a staple of nineteenth-century manners. It became rude to eat heartily. It was glamorous to look sickly. 'Chopin was tubercular at a time when good health was not chic,' Camille Saint-Saëns wrote in 1913. 'It was fashionable to be pale and drained. Princess Belgiojoso strolled along the boulevards . . . pale as death in person.' Saint-Saëns was right to connect an artist, Chopin, with the most celebrated *femme fatale* of the period, who did a great deal to popularize the tubercular look. The TB-influenced idea of the body was a new model for aristocratic looks – at a moment when aristocracy stops being a matter of power, and starts being mainly a matter of image. ('One can never be too rich. One can never be too thin,' the Duchess of Windsor once said.) Indeed, the romanticizing of TB is the first widespread example of that distinctively modern activity, promoting the self as an image. The tubercular look had to be considered attractive once it came to be considered a mark of distinction, of breeding. 'I cough continually!' Marie Bashkirtsev wrote in the once widely read *Journal*, which was published, after her death at twenty-four, in 1887. 'But for a wonder, far from making me look ugly, this gives me an air of languor that is very becoming.' What was once the fashion of aristocratic *femmes fatales* and aspiring young artists became, eventually, the province of fashion as such. Twentieth-century women's fashions (with their cult of thinness) are the last stronghold of the metaphors associated with the romanticizing of TB in the late eighteenth and early nineteenth centuries.

Many of the literary and erotic attitudes known as 'romantic agony' derive from tuberculosis and its transformation through metaphor. Agony became romantic in a stylized account of the disease's preliminary symptoms (for example, debility is transformed into languor) and the actual agony was simply suppressed. Wan, hollow-chested young women and pallid, rachitic young men vied with each other as candidates for this mostly (at that time) incurable, disabling, really awful disease. 'When I was young,' wrote Théophile Gautier, 'I could not have accepted as a lyrical poet anyone weighing more than ninety-nine pounds.' (Note that Gautier says lyrical poet, apparently resigned to the fact that novelists had to be made of coarser and bulkier stuff.) Gradually, the tubercular look, which symbolized an appealing vulnerability, a superior sensitivity, became more and more the ideal look for women – while great men of the mid and late nineteenth century grew fat, founded industrial empires, wrote hundreds of novels, made wars, and plundered continents.

One might reasonably suppose that this romanticization of TB was a merely literary transfiguration of the disease, and that in the era of its great depredations TB was probably thought to be disgusting – as cancer is now. Surely everyone in the nineteenth century knew about, for example, the stench in the breath of the consumptive person. (Describing their visit to the dying Murger, the Goncourts note 'the odor of rotting flesh in his bedroom.') Yet all the evidence indicates that the cult of TB was not simply an invention of romantic poets and opera librettists but a widespread attitude, and that the person dying (young) of TB really was perceived as a romantic personality. One must suppose that the reality of this terrible disease was no match for important new ideas, particularly about individuality. It is with TB that the idea of individual illness was articulated, along with the idea that people are made more conscious as they confront their deaths, and in the images that collected around the disease one can see emerging a modern idea of individuality that has taken in the twentieth century a more aggressive, if no less narcissistic, form. Sickness was a way of making people 'interesting' – which is how 'romantic' was originally defined. (Schlegel, in his essay 'On the Study of Greek Poetry' [1795], offers 'the interesting' as the ideal of modern – that is, romantic – poetry.) 'The ideal of perfect health,' Novalis wrote in a fragment from the period 1799–1800, 'is only scientifically interesting'; what is really interesting is sickness, 'which belongs to individualizing.' This idea – of how interesting the sick are – was given its boldest and most ambivalent formulation by Nietzsche in *The Will to Power* and other writings, and though Nietzsche rarely mentioned a specific illness, those famous judgments about individual weakness and cultural exhaustion or decadence incorporate and extend many of the clichés about TB.

The romantic treatment of death asserts that people were made singular, made more interesting, by their illness. 'I look pale,' said Byron, looking into the mirror. 'I should like to die of a consumption.' 'Why?' asked a friend, who was visiting Byron in Athens in October 1810. 'Because the ladies would all say, "Look at that poor Byron, how interesting he looks in dying."' Perhaps the main gift to sensibility made by the Romantics is not the aesthetics of cruelty and the beauty of the morbid (as Mario Praz suggested in his famous book), or even the demand for unlimited personal liberty, but the nihilistic and sentimental idea of 'the interesting.'

Sadness made one 'interesting.' It was a mark of refinement, of sensibility, to be sad. That is, to be powerless. In Stendhal's *Armance*, the anxious mother is reassured by the doctor that Octave is not, after all, suffering from tuberculosis but only from that 'dissatisfied and critical melancholy characteristic of young people of his generation and position.' Sadness and tuberculosis became synonymous. The Swiss writer Henri Amiel, himself tubercular, wrote in 1852 in his *Journal intime*:

> Sky draped in gray, pleated by subtle shading, mists trailing on the distant mountains; nature despairing, leaves falling on all sides like the lost illusions of youth under the tears of incurable grief . . . The fir tree, alone in its vigour, green, stoical in the midst of this universal tuberculosis.

But it takes a sensitive person to feel such sadness; or by implication, to contract tuberculosis. The myth of TB constitutes the next-to-last episode in the long career of the ancient idea of melancholy – which was the artist's disease, according to the theory of the four humors. The melancholy character – or the tubercular – was a superior one: sensitive, creative, a being apart. Keats and Shelley may have suffered atrociously from the disease. But Shelley consoled Keats that 'this consumption is a disease particularly fond of people who write such good verses as you have done . . .' So well established was the cliché which connected TB and creativity that at the end of the century one critic suggested that it was the progressive disappearance of TB which accounted for the current decline of literature and the arts.

But the myth of TB provided more than an account of creativity. It supplied an important model of Bohemian life, lived with or without the vocation of the artist. The TB sufferer was a dropout, a wanderer in endless search of the healthy place. Starting in the early nineteenth century, TB became a new reason for exile, for a life that was mainly travelling. (Neither travel nor isolation in a sanatorium was a form of treatment for TB before then.) There were special places thought to be good for tuberculars: in the early nineteenth century, Italy; then, islands in the Mediterranean, or the South Pacific; in the twentieth century, the mountains, the desert – all landscapes that had themselves been successively romanticized. Keats was advised by his doctors to move to Rome; Chopin tried the islands of the western Mediterranean; Robert Louis Stevenson chose a Pacific exile; D. H. Lawrence roamed over half the globe.[2] The Romantics invented invalidism as a pretext for leisure, and for dismissing bourgeois obligations in order to live only for one's art. It was a way of retiring from the world without having to take responsibility for the decision – the story of *The Magic Mountain*. After passing his exams and before taking up his job in a Hamburg ship-building firm, young Hans Castorp makes a three-week visit to his tubercular cousin in the sanatorium at Davos. Just before Hans 'goes down,' the doctor diagnoses a spot on his lungs. He stays on the mountain for the next seven years.

By validating so many possibly subversive longings and turning them into cultural pieties, the TB myth survived irrefutable human experience and accumulating medical knowledge for nearly two hundred years. Although there was a certain reaction against the Romantic cult of the disease in the second half of the last century, TB retained most of its romantic attribute – as the sign of a superior nature, as a becoming frailty – through the end of the century and well into ours. It is still the sensitive young artist's disease in O'Neill's *Long Day's Journey into Night*. Kafka's letters are a compendium of speculations about the meaning of tuberculosis, as is *The Magic Mountain*, published in 1924, the year Kafka died. Much of the irony of *The Magic Mountain* turns on Hans Castorp, the stolid burgher, getting TB, the artist's disease – for Mann's novel is a late, self-conscious commentary on the myth of TB. But the novel still reflects the myth: the burgher *is* indeed spiritually refined by his disease. To die of TB was still mysterious and (often) edifying and remained so until practically no-body in Western Europe and North America died of it any more. Although the incidence of the disease began to decline precipitously after 1900 because of improved hygiene, the mortality rate among those who contracted it remained high; the power of the myth was dispelled only when proper treatment was finally developed, with the discovery of streptomycin in 1944 and the introduction of isoniazid in 1952.

If it is still difficult to imagine how the reality of such a dreadful disease could be

---

2. By a curious irony,' Stevenson wrote, 'the places to which we are sent when health deserts us are often singularly beautiful . . . [and] I daresay the sick man is not very inconsolable when he receives sentence of banishment and is inclined to regard his ill-health as not the least fortunate accident of his life.' But the experience of such enforced banishment, as Stevenson went on to describe it, was something less agreeable. The tubercular cannot enjoy his good fortune: 'the world is disenchanted for him.'

  Katherine Mansfield wrote: 'I seem to spend half of my life arriving at strange hotels . . . The strange door shuts upon the stranger, and then I slip down in the sheets. Waiting for the shadows to come out of the corners and spin their slow, slow web over the Ugliest Wallpaper of All . . . The man in the room next to mine has the same complaint as I. When I wake in the night I hear him turning. And then he coughs. And after a silence I cough. And he coughs again. This goes on for a long time. Until I feel we are like two roosters calling each other at false dawns. From far-away hidden farms.

transformed so preposterously, it may help to consider our own era's comparable act of distortion, under the pressure of the need to express romantic attitudes about the self. The object of distortion is not, of course, cancer – a disease which nobody has managed to glamorize (although it fulfils some of the functions as a metaphor that TB did in the nineteenth century). In the twentieth century, the repellent, harrowing disease that is made the index of a superior sensitivity, the vehicle of 'spiritual' feelings and 'critical' discontent, is insanity.

The fancies associated with tuberculosis and insanity have many parallels. With both illnesses, there is confinement. Sufferers are sent to a 'sanatorium' (the common word for a clinic for tuberculars and the most common euphemism for an insane asylum). Once put away, the patient enters a duplicate world with special rules. Like TB, insanity is a kind of exile. The metaphor of the psychic voyage is an extension of the romantic idea of travel that was associated with tuberculosis. To be cured, the patient had to be taken out of his or her daily routine. It is not an accident that the most common metaphor for an extreme psychological experience viewed positively – whether produced by drugs or by becoming psychotic – is a trip.

In the twentieth century the cluster of metaphors and attitudes formerly attached to TB split up and are parcelled out to two diseases. Some features of TB go to insanity: the notion of the sufferer as a hectic, reckless creature of passionate extremes, someone too sensitive to bear the horrors of the vulgar, everyday world. Other features of TB go to cancer – the agonies that can't be romanticized. Not TB but insanity is the current vehicle of our secular myth of self-transcendence. The romantic view is that illness exacerbates consciousness. Once that illness was TB; now it is insanity that is thought to bring consciousness to a state of paroxysmic enlightenment. The romanticizing of madness reflects in the most vehement way the contemporary prestige of irrational or rude (spontaneous) behaviour (acting-out), of that very passionateness whose repression was once imagined to cause TB, and is now thought to cause cancer.

Susan Sontag is a leading American critic and essayist, who has also published novels and stories. The extract above is the whole of Chapter 4 of her book, *Illness as Metaphor*, which was originally published in 1978 by Penguin books.

# 6
# Using alternative therapies: marginal medicine and central concerns

## URSULA M. SHARMA

Who uses alternative medicine? A hypothesis which seems to have informed some research, either explicitly or implicitly, is the idea that users of alternative medicine are possibly marginal *people* as well as users of marginal *medicine*.

The study which I undertook in 1986 was not designed to compare users of alternative medicine with non-users, but to discover the routes by which patients came to use it. I interviewed thirty people in the Stoke-on-Trent area who had used at least one form of alternative medicine in the past twelve months. The sample was largely obtained by inviting readers of the local newspaper to volunteer their experiences of alternative medicine. We cannot draw any conclusions about the representativeness of such a self-selected sample in terms of demographic or socio-economic characteristics, but this was not the purpose of the research.

The interviews were structured to the extent that they covered some standard questions and elicited a corpus of comparable data, but as far as possible I encouraged respondents to deliver this information in the context of their own 'story' of how they had come to use alternative medicine. This left them free to include in their accounts much that I would not have elicited through standardized questions in a set order. For most of the respondents the 'story of how they had come to use alternative medicine' was a narrative with a point, even a moral, which they wished to convey. In many cases the interviewee was describing a process which was by no means complete.

Using alternative medicine is therefore part of a *process*. While some interviewees could pinpoint predisposing factors in their family background (e.g. usage of herbal medicine by parents, horrific experiences of orthodox medical treatment by a close relative) most took as their starting point their own experience of some chronic disorder and their own subsequent dissatisfaction with the treatment they received for this under the NHS. All had consulted their GP about this illness in the first place and several had seen specialists in connection with diagnosis or treatment. I did not encounter any who had used alternative medicine because they had been brought up to do so, because it was the norm in their ethnic/religious group or for other 'cultural' reasons, apart from one woman whose parents had been ardent adherents of naturopathy, though a larger sample might well identify cases of this kind of usage.

It is important to discuss users' sources of dissatisfaction with orthodox medicine at some length because many of them do not relate straightforwardly to conventional medicine's failure to 'cure' disease so much as to its failure to 'cure' disease on terms that are acceptable to the particular patient. Two individuals did report a conflictual relationship with their GP, but in most cases dissatisfaction was not focused on the perceived incompetence of individual doctors or consultants. The problems with orthodox medicine as offered under the NHS which interviewees mentioned could be grouped as follows.

*The claim that conventional medicine fails to get at the 'root cause' of chronic illness or fails to take a preventative approach, and can therefore only treat the symptoms.* For example, a young man suffering from chronic depression had been referred to a psychiatrist and had received anti-depressant drugs which had some temporary effect. But he felt that the basic cause of his state had not been discovered and that therefore he would continue to be liable to periods of depression, a prospect which he did not wish to accept. The experience of acupuncture described by friends who had used it suggested to him that this therapy might effect a long term change in his condition. When he had tried acupuncture it so fascinated him that he decided to train as an acupuncturist himself, and whilst his depression has not entirely ceased to be a problem, the periods of disability are shorter and less frequent.

This is not to say that patients always required a detailed diagnosis or a technical description of what the healer saw as the problem; patients varied very much as to the degree of interest they took in the actual rationale or theory of the forms of healing used. What was more often reported was relief that their dissatisfaction with symptomatic 'cures' had been acknowledged as legitimate and reasonable, and an appreciative sense that the healer was tackling the problem at a more fundamental level than conventional doctors had managed to do.

*The fear of drugs which might become habit forming, or the dislike of side effects of particular drugs.* Sometimes this took a rather diffuse concern about drugs that are too 'strong' – an imprecise fear of the body being interfered with too drastically. Sometimes there was general anxiety that prolonged or frequent use of drugs would interfere with the body's ability to react to drugs in acute situations, especially with regard to the use of antibiotics for childhood ailments. In other cases the dissatisfaction was based on a very specific experience. For instance, one interviewee's consultant had prescribed drugs for high blood pressure which, she said, made her feel exhausted and weak, 'like an old woman'. When she discovered a herbalist who could treat her she was relieved to be offered medicine which, she said, controlled her condition with no side effects whatsoever. The same interviewee expressed concern over the state of health of her sister who suffered from arthritis and who, she said, had been given ever stronger drugs to control the condition without any real improvement.

*Fear or dislike of forms of treatment which are seen as too radical or invasive.* A middle-aged woman who suffered from back pain had been offered surgery under the NHS without, however, any guarantee that her condition would be cured. Indeed, she had been told that there was a slight risk that it might become worse. A major operation which did not have any certain outcome seemed to her too drastic a step to take and the risk of a deterioration dismayed her as her work required her to move and lift inmates in an old people's home. She visited a chiropractor at the suggestion of a colleague of her husband and after a fairly lengthy (and at first painful) course of treatment reported an almost complete recovery.

*The perceived inability of conventional medicine to cope with the social and experiential aspects of illness.* There is now more awareness of the need for personal support in severe or terminal illness, yet even apparently trivial conditions like eczema pose a need for personal support when they are chronic (as patients' self-help groups recognize). The sufferer needs to feel that the healer (of whatever kind) appreciates and does not dismiss the forms of distress or inconvenience which the illness causes. Some interviewees emphasized a desire for practical advice in the day-to-day management of their illness (useful adjustments to diet, suggestions for patterns of rest and exercise, stress management techniques etc.). It is not by any means the case that all conventional doctors are unable to offer this personal interest and support, nor is it the case that all sufferers found alternative healers willing to provide it. Many healers, however, allow for much longer consultation times than do GPs, especially for a first consultation which may (especially in systems like homoeopathy) involve taking a very detailed case history. A time-consuming form of treatment may be acceptable to the sufferer if s/he feels it is producing some lasting effect.

*Dissatisfaction with the kind of relationship between doctor and patient which interviewees feel that conventional medicine requires or presupposes.* In many of the interviews, patients communicated a conscious appreciation of the more active role they felt able to play in the management of their illness or the general pursuit of health. Usually this feeling of being in control was described as a by-product of their experiences rather than as the goal they had been seeking in the first place. A woman who had suffered from asthma for many years described her encounters with conventional and numerous forms of alternative medicine by saying:

> I am not criticizing other people . . . but I think that very often they go to the doctor and they just accept what the doctor says. I would advise anybody to go to the doctor first, but now I would always use alternative medicine to get a second opinion and treatment if you are not satisfied.

Many took an explicitly consumerist approach; one young man who had recently begun to consult an iridologist and to use herbal medicine described his and his wife's attitude to conventional medicine thus:

> If we need to, then we do go to our GP – we are not totally blinkered. We aim to get the best out of both systems.

Yet some interviewees recognized that this active, critical and perhaps eclectic approach to health care might be incompatible with the model of the doctor–patient relationship in which the doctor has total responsibility for the treatment and the patient has only to trust and comply. Most interviewees had avoided telling their GPs about any alternative treatment they had received because they intended to continue to use the GP's services and did not wish to be seen to violate this model of the GP–patient relationship.

Most interviewees in the sample described the initial decision to use alternative medicine as prompted by a recommendation to a specific practitioner by a specific member of their network (see Table 6.1). Table 6.1, however, refers to the *first*

**Table 6.1** How respondents heard about the 'alternative' healer they used first

| Source of information | Number of respondents |
| --- | --- |
| **'Public' sources** | |
| Advertisements/Yellow Pages | 3 |
| GP's recommendation | 1 |
| Local association/organization | 1 |
| **'Private' sources** | |
| Friends/acquaintances/colleagues | 23 |
| Relatives | 2 |
| Total | 30 |

**Table 6.2** Number of types of alternative medicine used by respondents (either serially or simultaneously)

| Types of alternative medicine used | 1 | 2 | 3 | 4 | 4+ | |
| --- | --- | --- | --- | --- | --- | --- |
| Number of respondents | | 9 | 8 | 4 | 7 | 2 (total 30) |

experience of alternative medicine, and many patients had used more than one form of alternative medicine, either for the same disease at different times, or more usually, for different diseases. If we include sources of information used for all consultations (not just the first) we find more diverse sources of information, with cultural and political organizations playing a greater part (for example, the Soil Association, vegetarian cookery classes, feminist groups).

Most patients, however, seemed to have gained the confidence to approach a non-orthodox healer in the first place after hearing some kind of success story about that healer from a relative, friend or colleague, and only used information from more impersonal sources once a personal recommendation had yielded some kind of useful experience.

What is striking about the interviewees' stories is that initial usage of one form of alternative medicine is often followed by use of other forms, either serially or simultaneously, for the same or for different illnesses. Some patients had used as many as five types in as many years (see Table 6.2). In only one case was this due to continued failure to obtain any relief. A young man who had a skin condition affecting his scalp and had seen a consultant dermatologist, but without any significant improvement, announced to me his dogged intention of trying as many different forms of medicine in turn until he found one which had some effect. What seemed more common was that some degree of satisfaction (not necessarily total) with the particular form of alternative medicine first sampled led to a more experimental attitude and eventually to trials of other kinds of healing.

In many cases this change to a more eclectic approach to health care was one which affected the whole family. This could happen in several ways. In some cases the interviewee had recommended a form of treatment which s/he had used to other members of the family or had used it for children. In other cases the treatment

**Table 6.3**   Types of usage of alternative medicine

| | |
|---|---|
| Conflictual relationship with GP plus occasional or regular use of alternative medicine | 2 |
| 'Experimental' or eclectic use of alternative medicine | 12 |
| Stable and regular use of one form of alternative medicine | 9 |
| 'Restricted' use of one form of alternative medicine (for a single illness) | 7 |
| Total | 30 |

involved the family indirectly insofar as the patient had to observe some regime (usually dietary) which affected the family. A woman who used a particular kind of diet recommended by a herbalist in treating chronic arthritis said that whilst she could not insist that her family eat the diet prescribed for herself, it was convenient to plan meals so that her work was not unnecessarily duplicated. Her family had accepted these changes in family eating patterns, indeed had come to appreciate them. In other cases the regime presented more problems, but only one patient reported downright uncooperative or dismissive attitudes on the part of household members to their usage of alternative medicine. In a few cases patients reported that a spouse or children had regarded their usage of alternative medicine in the light of an eccentric aberration but had not put any obstacles in the way of the interviewee's sticking to the regime prescribed.

When looking at the effects of use of alternative medicine on family health care practices it is important to place these changes in a broader context. Some of the dietary changes and shifts in lifestyle reported by patients as stemming from the recommendations of alternative healers are changes which are being recommended by many other sources of medical authority or information (GPs, popular medicine journals, health promotion campaigns) and are by no means peculiar to alternative medicine 'sub-cultures'. Reduced consumption of animal fats, high fibre diets, regimes of exercise and use of relaxation techniques might be examples. Such changes should be seen as part of more general shifts in thinking about personal and family health care voiced particularly effectively, but not exclusively, by holistic healers.

More significantly, there is little evidence that users of alternative medicine cease entirely to use orthodox medicine, though they may use it less, or for different purposes, or more critically. A sceptical attitude to orthodox medicine did not lead to its abandonment. Usually patients used alternative medicine for specific illnesses or problems and GPs for others. Interviewees had not abandoned the NHS even though dissatisfied with it. In Table 6.3 I have tried to summarize some of the main patterns of usage which I found among the individuals I interviewed. Most interviewees could think of occasions during the past twelve months when they had consulted their GP for themselves or for other members of their family, and could envisage other times in the future.

One very widespread idea which seems to me to be a misconception is that users of alternative healing are naively attracted by the ideological claims of alternative medicine. Jonathan Miller suggested in a recent newspaper article[1] that

much alternative medicine on offer – acupuncture or homoeopathy, for example – appeals to soft primitivism

a concept which he defines as

a belief that there was a time when men were harmonious and happy – the myth of the Golden Age – and possessed with wisdoms we are foolish to ignore and idiotic to forget (Miller, 1989).

Possibly this is so: certainly such ideas are frequently expressed in a variety of quarters. But this would not in itself suffice to explain the increasing use of alternative medicine, which seems related to quite pragmatic objectives such as obtaining a cure for a specific illness or leading a more active and healthy life. Only a very few of the people I interviewed gave explicitly ideological reasons for their initial attraction to alternative medicine, though some, as I have indicated, have altered their way of looking at care of the body and mind as a result of their encounter. So ideological commitment might explain why some people *continue* to use alternative medicine having once used it successfully, insofar as they are convinced by what they learn about it from practitioners, but it would not account for the initial resort to unorthodox medicine itself.

Yet most patients using alternative medicine would seem to be (negatively) dissatisfied with the service offered by orthodox medicine, coming on the whole from its areas of notable failure, rather than (positively) attracted by any alternative world view the former may claim to offer. Two themes recur very frequently in the interviews, and receive widespread mention in the literature on the subject:

1. The demand that the patient's experience and understanding of his or her disease should be acknowledged and treated with respect. Not all interviewees spoke in terms of a more 'equal' relationship with the doctor or healer, but many wanted to be better informed so that they could exercise more control in the management of their illness. Where alternative practitioners took the trouble to explain the rationale of treatment to the patient this was appreciated, and often contrasted with the failure of orthodox doctors to take time to provide information about treatment, or to take account of the patients' experience of his/her illness.
2. The demand for what could loosely be called a more holistic approach on the part of doctors. Patients do not always use the term holism, and when they do, they do not always refer to exactly the same thing. However, a recurrent theme in the interviews was the desire that the personal context of illness should be taken into account. The treatment by drugs, which is all that many patients can obtain under the NHS, was often seen as too narrow even where it was 'effective' in terms of sheer relief of symptoms.

Use of alternative medicine is still a minority choice, but from what I have said here, it will be clear that it is not a marginal issue. Though some patients do change their expectations about what doctors or healers should do, or about how illness is caused, as a result of their encounters with alternative medicine, most cannot be said to belong to a separate cultural group; where they express unease over the way in which orthodox medicine delivers its services, they are generally voicing anxieties which they share with many who do not use alternative medicine. Users of alternative medicine are making certain kinds of consumer choice, albeit choices which may have radical consequences for the entire household's lifestyle and habits. As with other patients, their choices derive from the interaction between the nature of their illnesses (chronic, difficult for orthodox medicine to treat) and the nature of their lay referral networks (access to information about specific healers, cultural and political resources).

Alternative medicine therefore is 'marginal' medicine in the obvious sense that it is still used by a minority (albeit a substantial one), and in the political sense that it has limited recognition by the state. Its study has raised issues concerning changes in household health care practice, consumer eclecticism and sources of dissatisfaction with orthodox medicine which should be of central concern to the medical professionals and social scientists alike.

## Reference

1. Miller, J. 'Neither fish, fowl nor red herring', the *Independent*, 7 January (1989).

This article is an edited version of a longer text, which was originally published in 1990, under the same title, in *New Directions in the Sociology of Health*, edited by P. Abbott and G. Payne, Falmer Press. Ursula M. Sharma is a Senior Lecturer in the Department of Sociology and Anthropology at Keele University, whose principal research interest has been in gender and work in India.

# 7
# The problem of the whole-person in holistic medicine

## DAVID ARMSTRONG

Being so recent, holistic medicine has hardly had time to establish a coherent account of its historical origins, but nevertheless it cannot for long exist in a temporal vacuum. Indeed one of the first tasks of any new discipline is the construction of a history which will explain the inevitability of its arrival, justify its existence and promote its future.[1]

A 'tradition' is important because it helps sidestep the awkward question of 'why now?' Holistic medicine is so 'obvious' that if it were in fact to be only recent it would be difficult to explain how preceding times failed to grasp its inherent truth, particularly as the whole-person has had universal existence. The advent of holistic medicine must therefore be construed as simply one event in a long process of gradual enlightenment and progress. The evocation of tradition is no doubt of assistance in promoting and establishing the recent growth of holistic medicine. But the endorsement of a 'tradition' in holistic medicine carries with it a significant explanatory difficulty, namely the historical ascendency of reductionist medicine.

From within holistic medicine (hospital based) medicine is criticized as 'reductionist' because it attempts to reduce all illness to a single intra-corporal lesion and thereby, through appropriate investigative procedures and treatments, reduces the body – and the whole-person – to a collection of separate systems, organs, tissues and cells. But if holistic medicine is somehow rooted in tradition, how was it possible for pathological medicine, the apparent antithesis of holistic medicine, to gain ascendency? What might be called the liberationist explanation within holistic medicine attempts to tackle this problem of historical discontinuity.

The liberationist explanation holds that there was a period of holistic medicine in the past but this tradition was repressed with the ascendency of reductionist medicine. Recently however that period of subjugation has been lifted by the rediscovery of traditional holistic practices. In effect the historical triumph of reductionist medicine is claimed to be an aberration and modern holistic medicine presented as a means of liberation from error. Yet this leaves unresolved how holistic medicine has only now begun to throw off the repression of reductionist medicine and, perhaps more importantly, it fails to explain how reductionist medicine triumphed in the first place over a medicine which was the natural and traditional attendant of the whole-person.

## The social control thesis

Critics from without, however, have advanced an analysis which challenges the liberationist claims of holistic medicine. In summary they would argue that far from holistic medicine escaping from the confines of reductionist medicine it has simply reinforced those elements of the dominant paradigm of which it has been so critical: if pathological medicine negated parts of the whole-person by its reductionist stance, holistic medicine has negated all of the whole-person by its totalizing perspective.

That there might be an unconscious danger in allowing medicine an extended position in social control was first pointed out by Zola in the early 1970s.[2] Though not attacking holistic medicine by name he pointed to the increasing intervention of doctors into all sorts of different facets of people's lives. A reductionist medicine which only monitored a component of the body had limited control functions over people's bodies, but a medicine which took a broader interest in the whole-person and offered advice and support on diet, exercise, stress, anxiety, etc., carried with it the incipient danger that the social control functions of medicine were getting out of hand and invading areas of people's lives to their ultimate detriment. While the stated claim of holistic medicine might be the enhancement of personal autonomy, its actual practical effect was to undermine it.

Zola's explanation for this increasing medicalization of everyday life was an expansionist medical profession matched by increasing reliance on experts to help run people's lives. This argument was taken further by Illich.[3] The problem, he argued, was much more extensive than Zola had imagined and, moreover, its causes were less innocent and the remedy therefore more radical. Illich – ironically in view of the similar focus of holistic medicine – placed the freedom and autonomy of the whole-person at the heart of his model of health, but anything, including the 'helping' professions, which encroached upon this autonomy was detrimental to personal well-being.

Marxists have argued that the modern industrial state has had to develop complex systems of medical control.[4] Thus a homeless patient has a problem in their environment, not in the politics which denies them homes; a depressed patient is drugged or counselled so that they can cope with their moods rather than being encouraged to challenge the system which made them depressed; and so on. From this point of view holistic medicine might claim to be radical but it is only radical chic; its proponents might be well-meaning but they are the unwitting advance guard of medical hegemony or the lackeys of a capitalist system; their wider concerns with the whole-person simply means that the whole-person must be brought into visibility and into control.

## Political anatomy

The argument that medicine is inherently an agency of social control and that holistic medicine is simply another manifestation of this function certainly offers a more coherent explanation for the rise of holistic medicine than holistic medicine itself offers. The difficulty with the social control argument however is that it tends to assume a conspiratorial or malevolent medicine; and yet the avowed and no doubt sincere intentions and practice of most advocates of holistic medicines is to provide a humanist medicine which truly serves the interests of the whole person. In this way the intentions, actions and probably effects of most of those within holistic medicine seem completely opposed to the charges of repression.

Thus far it would appear a simple choice between believing or disbelieving the purported goals of holistic medicine. But there is a third explanation for the rise of holistic medicine which manages both to accept the sincerity and goals of holistic medicine and to incorporate some of the key features of the social control argument. This third position is not a compromise one but a radical solution to the historical puzzle of holistic medicine: it starts with the rejection of the core assumption of both holistic and social control arguments that the whole person is a 'universal' being. Instead it argues that the patient is an 'invention' or construction.

Both holistic and social control perspectives tend to assume a golden age of medicine in the past, sometimes specified – perhaps Hippocratic medicine or pre-capitalism – more often left vague. No evidence is offered to support the existence of a golden age beyond a faith that it must have existed. It is important to note the historical context of these claims: they are certainly made about the past but only from the perspective of the last two decades. Does whole-person medicine therefore belong to the past or is it backward projection of the present? And if the whole-person has no immutable identity then he or she can neither be liberated nor repressed, in effect they can only be 'constructed'.

Pathological medicine first emerged at the end of the 18th century when disease became located to specific anatomical structures and hence illness could yield to a reductionist analysis. Pathological medicine treated the patient's body as a machine, as an object. This fundamentally new approach is one of the principal points of attack for holistic medicine which decries this new corporal positivism, this strategy which objectified 'real' people. But alternatively, the objectification of the individual can be seen as the first step in the actual creation of the individual whole person. The constructivist position is that reality does not exist independently of perception, thus the new medicine created its own reality and pathological medicine far from being repressive and negative was creative and positive.

The end of the 18th century and beginning of the 19th, which saw the birth of this new medicine, was a watershed period in Western history. The 'objectified' individual appeared for the first time in medicine but also in the school, the prison, the workshop and the barracks.[5] New techniques for examining individuals were devised; dossiers and case histories for the first time recorded the actions and states of ordinary individuals; the novel, which documented the lives of ordinary people, made its appearance; and the word 'individualism' entered the language.[6]

What existed before pathological medicine is difficult to know. It was a different world; there are no criteria by which it can be judged a golden age or not. What is more certain is that it was only since this period over the last two centuries that the 'whole-person' has had some form of rudimentary existence. It was not therefore a new 'dark ages', rather it was a period during which the reality of the body as an analysable object was slowly constituted, a period in which a new 'political anatomy' was forged and when the human sciences made their first appearance.[5] Before the advent of reductionist medicine bodies were not explored: doctors did not physically examine their patients, post-mortems were not conducted and case histories were not written because the body itself contained no secrets, no truth to be revealed. The ascendency of reductionist medicine therefore established the body as the material core of a new individuality and ushered in a new realm of humanist concerns.

In 1935 Brackenbury published a book on whole-person medicine.[7] To be sure the patient as viewed by Brackenbury was less than complete, being a rather passive object, but it was in the first few decades of the 20th century that a new analysis of the nature of the patient and illness was commenced. As before, when at the end of the 18th century a certain analysis constructed a particular object, so too the identity of the patient began to be transformed by a new medicine which sought to explore the social and conceptual spaces surrounding the individualized body.[8]

From the beginning of the 20th century medicine began to focus on 'social' diseases which were in some way linked to the social contact of one body with another and as it did so the old public health gave way to a new discipline of social medicine. The body became seen as inhabiting a social as well as physical space; in consequence it became a social as well as physical phenomenon. For example, in the 19th century psychiatric disease had been virtually restricted to insanity and its precursors; in the 20th century medicine 'discovered' the neuroses. When the mind had been restricted to a faculty of rationality, madness was its only disease. When, on the other hand, the mind was seen as the interface between body and outside world then it became the faculty of 'coping' and the neuroses could be invented to identify failure and difficulty with the management of affect.[9]

Since the 1950s these elements of an extended patient identity have been reinforced and extended. Certainly reductionist medicine continues to fabricate a discrete and analysable body but the mind and social context of that body have been interrogated to construct a psycho-social identity for patienthood. How was it possible for the placebo effect only to be extensively recognized from the 1950s? How was it possible that the 'problem' of doctor–patient relationship could only be identified during the 1950s and 1960s? How was it that the importance of 'the patient's view' had to wait until the 1970s?[10] That the psychological adjustment of the dying patient could only be recognized from the 1960s?[11] And so on. In the last three decades medicine has investigated a series of new phenomena and problems which have as their common goal and assumption the existence of the patient as a subjective 'whole-person': the actual practice of medicine has presupposed and reinforced the independent existence of a particular patient identity. The whole-person is therefore a construction of this new perspective in medicine, as is its supposed 'universal' status.

## References

1. Kuhn, T. S. *The Structure of Scientific Revolutions*, Chicago (1962).
2. Zola, I. K. 'Medicine as an institution of social control', *Sociological Review*, 20, 487–504 (1972).
3. Illich, I. *Medical Nemesis*, Caldar Boyars (1974).
4. Ehrenreich, J. (ed.) *The Cultural Crisis of Modern Medicine*, Monthly Review Press (1978).
5. Foucault, M. *Discipline and Punish; the Birth of the Prison*, Tavistock (1977).
6. Lukes, S. *Individualism*, Blackwell (1973).
7. Brackenbury, H. B. *Patient and Doctor*, Hodder & Stoughton (1935).

8. Armstrong, D. *Political Anatomy of the Body: Medical Knowledge in Britain in the 20th Century*, Cambridge University Press (1983).
9. Armstrong, D. 'Madness and coping', *Sociology of Health and Illness*, 2, 293–316 (1980).
10. Armstrong, D. 'The patient's view', *Social Science and Medicine*, 18, 737–744 (1984).
11. Arney, W. R. and Bergen, B. *Medicine and the Management of Living*, Chicago University Press (1982).

David Armstrong is a Senior Lecturer at Guy's Hospital Medical School. This article is an edited version of the original which appeared in *Holistic Medicine*, 1, 27–36 (1986).

# 8

# Ethnic minorities and the psychiatrist

## ROLAND LITTLEWOOD AND MAURICE LIPSEDGE

The meeting between psychiatrist and patient does of course involve two people who have their own particular expectations. If the situation is familiar to them, they will probably make an effort to live up to the other person's expectations.[1]

The psychiatrist is likely to regard psychiatric illness as he does physical illness. He also has less clear expectations of how the patient is likely to behave and what, in different societies, the limits of normality and abnormality are. In addition to his background and training, the psychiatrist's attitude to the minority patient will be formed by his own personal problems, conscious or unconscious racist assumptions and the particular setting in which the two meet. He is, amongst other things, an employee of the state and responsible to it for maintenance of its beliefs and disposal of its funds.

Patients too have their expectations: to be sick in our society offers us freedom from many social obligations and from responsibility for the illness, but it presumes a desire to get well and a motivation to ask for medical help.[2] The extent to which a patient sees himself as ill and in need of treatment varies with his culture. What may be endured in India requires therapy in New York. What is insane behaviour in Barbados may not be in Jamaica. Acceptance of the role of a mental patient depends on our beliefs about the nature of mental illness and whether any stigma is associated with it. Psychiatrists are rare in developing countries and admission to a mental hospital is an uncommon – perhaps unheard of – event. There is one psychiatrist in Britain for every twenty thousand people compared with one for over a million in India and one for four million in Nigeria. The immigrant family may be hesitant about agreeing with a doctor who tells them that their relative is mentally ill. They may not even see the problem as a medical one: the patient may come from a rural community in which all Western medicine is regarded with distrust. Many societies carry out similar religious healing ceremonies for both physical and emotional distress and do not make our customary separation between the two.

The immigrant patient may well see the psychiatrist as a doctor rather than specifically as a psychiatrist. Not burdened with our folk-lore about psychiatrists (and endless cartoons of bearded doctors sitting next to patients on couches), he looks for themes familiar to him from his experiences with other doctors and hospitals: the ward with its rows of beds and quiet discipline, the uniformed nurses and white-coated doctors; authority, certainty, a minimum of questioning and immediate treatment. Ironically these are the very aspects of medicine which psychiatrists are discarding, in the belief that they may actually perpetuate psychological difficulties.[3] As psychiatry has sought to relinquish the magical symbols of medicine, many of these have been confusingly adopted by other professions: porters, clerks and domestic staff may now wear the clinical white coat.[1]

A common mode of arrival of immigrant patients at a hospital is to be brought in by police, often at night.[4] Does the psychiatrist see himself as an ally of the police or the patient, or perhaps of both? Is his overriding reaction to dispose of the problem as soon as possible and get back to bed?

To observe another person is always to some extent to diminish their individuality – especially in a hospital interview. For the patient the stress of the interview is increased when the doctor starts by talking privately with the police who are waiting on the ward, taking them aside, reading the admitting form and glancing periodically at the patient. If he then dismisses the police, greets the patient, shakes his hand and talks to him as if he is about to explain this embarrassing situation, the doctor will soon find himself in a difficult position. The patient sees a friend and confides his denunciation of the police to him while the doctor listens patiently. The psychiatrist is then startled by a request from the patient to return home. He feels irritated – the patient has taken advantage of his kindness. With the police gone, the nurses will be reluctant to help him to restrain a person he may now believe to be in urgent need of medical attention; their looks suggest he has made a fool of himself and wasted their time; he cannot persuade the increasingly anxious patient even to continue to talk to him. The patient begins to realize that the doctor has not really been sympathizing with him and that he has other plans. The doctor changes: his tone becomes hectoring and tense, and he provides increasingly unpleasant arguments for the patient to stay.

In the end the patient is sedated with the help of the nurses or dishonestly promised that he will be allowed home in the morning. In either case, he feels betrayed – he is not going to be so trusting again. Since his attempt at understanding the patient produced an unsatisfactory result, the psychiatrist also decides not to waste time talking next time. No more messing about – in future he will sedate the patient straight away. He rationalizes this by saying that it is not fair to the patient to deceive him and that it is easier anyway to talk the next morning, when he will be able to listen to a comfortably sedated patient with their respective roles clearly defined and his own anxieties diminished.

The immigrant brought to a psychiatric ward by the police will regard the whole business with suspicion, if not panic. He is puzzled by the doctor's insistence that he is there to *help*. The doctor's behaviour does not bear this out. If the patient is in the hospital because of behaviour associated with unusual religious experiences, he may wonder whether the doctor thinks these are 'genuine experiences'. If the doctor says they are, he is placating the patient, who realizes he is lying – why otherwise would he keep the patient in hospital? If the doctor ventures a medical explanation of the phenomenon the patient knows he has no chance of a fair hearing – the doctor will continue to try to persuade him to accept his own interpretation.

However sympathetic he may be initially to a patient who is anxious to spread the news of his divine mission, the psychiatrist will soon change. He must observe the patient and 'take a history' in accordance with the expectations of medical practice and the watching nursing staff. He tentatively suggests the patient is ill. If the patient disagrees, wakes the other patients or throws things about the ward, the doctor writes down 'no insight' and moves, reassured, into his more rewarding decision-making role.

Whatever interest doctor and patient may take in each other, the confrontation is limited by time. The interview is limited to a few key questions. The doctor wants to know whether the voices talk among themselves or talk directly to the patient. Such a question seems irrelevant to the patient. He is initially concerned with whether they are going to harm him. Why is the black patient feeling so suspicious? Maybe the police and the hospital are behaving in this extraordinary manner because they have a grudge against him. How widespread is this conspiracy? How much will it be wise to say to the doctor? The psychiatrist is meanwhile looking for such 'first-rank symptoms of schizophrenia' as whether the patient experiences his thoughts being controlled by external influences. If these are found, the patient's own explanation of his situation can again be dismissed. He is now firmly told he is sick and must have some medicine; patient and doctor have achieved their definitive roles.

The patient is told he must stay in hospital, he is asked to strip and the doctor examines him physically. The psychiatrist may be unsympathetic and harsh and he may make the wrong diagnosis, but by tradition he must on no account miss any physical illness. Further reduced to an object, the patient lies there as the doctor applies various instruments and listens and peers. The doctor gives instructions and leaves; the patient tells the nurses his age, address and occupation and accepts sedation for the night. The black patient may be reassured by the fact that the nurses, who are frequently black themselves, accept without question the medical definition of his experience. Often he is not.

Until both doctor and patient can agree on common grounds, there is unlikely to be a basis for friendship or even an acceptance of help. At present this tension is resolved only when the patient accepts the doctor's view of the situation and entirely rejects his own. Over the next few days responsibility is gradually withdrawn from the patient: for his liberty, his clothes and his beliefs.[3,5,6] His most popular move will have been to present a typical symptom to the doctor, resulting in swift and standard procedures to deal with his condition and a lessening in uncertainty for the staff. His further progress depends on the rapidity with which he accepts the new concepts and opportunities open to him.

An immigrant patient who has had many admissions to mental hospitals will have been given repeated explanations that he is not entirely responsible for his actions. The doctor should not then be surprised to find that the patient will not take any further responsibility for his problems and that he now passively expects the doctor to find him a job and accommodation and to solve his various domestic difficulties. The psychiatrist is confirmed in his belief that one of the effects of mental illness is a long-term loss of initiative and motivation. Unless he offers the unlikely option of psychotherapy, the psychiatrist now steps back and explains that medicine is not the solution to all problems but only those accepted by the patient as divine intervention, spirit possession or sorcery. Psychiatry thus deals with that part of the immigrant's experience associated with his original society but not with those related to problems in Britain – discrimination, housing and unemployment. It de-Caribbeanizes and de-authenticates him. While depriving the patient of much of his tradition, it does not seem to offer much in return. [. . .]

If we take class and age differences into account, are there any differences in treatment offered to blacks and whites in Britain? No one has yet looked at this methodically. Although less likely than the British-born to see a GP for psychiatric reasons, West Indian men are more likely to be admitted to psychiatric hospitals.[7] Psychotic black patients are twice as likely as British-born and white immigrants to be in hospital detained involuntarily, 'sectioned' under the Mental Health Act.[8,9] Four out of ten of them in one study were involuntary patients at some point in their admission.[4] Asian-born patients in Britain are also more likely to be involuntary patients in psychiatric hospitals and less likely to refer themselves.[10] A study of the use of psychiatric facilities in a London hospital over a three-week period suggested that immigrant patients, both black and white, are particularly likely to refer themselves to hospital as emergencies but they are less likely than the British-born to attend appointments booked for them.[11] Black patients are more likely than white patients to see a black member of the psychiatric team and to see a junior rather than a senior doctor. When differences in diagnosis are allowed for, they are still more likely to receive the powerful phenothiazine drugs and to receive electro-convulsive therapy. A large proportion of Jewish patients receive convulsive treatment; this is, however, related to a greater incidence of depression among Jews.

Racialism in psychiatric treatment may occur in many forms. Overt discrimination in Britain is rare, perhaps because of the considerable number of psychiatrists and psychiatric nurses who are themselves members of ethnic minorities. Members of minorities are less likely to get the more 'attractive' type of psychiatric care such as individual or group therapy because they are regarded as not meeting the 'ideal' criteria for psychotherapy (including the type of problem or middle-class mode of describing their feelings) which are traditionally associated with the best response to this type of therapy in Europe. What is particularly lacking is the commitment of psychotherapists to work with ethnic minorities.

Between a white doctor and a black patient the colour difference may be either exaggerated or it may be ignored. Exaggeration is likely to lead to stereotypes of 'West Indian psychosis' and neglect of individual emotional difficulties unrelated to discrimination. A sympathetic doctor may see his patients as so scarred by racialism as inevitably to be a passive victim with no secure identity and little self-respect; he may then bend over backwards to support him, to avoid any guilt the patient brings out in *him*. Underestimating the difference in culture by the white psychiatrist leads to an avoidance of the problems of discrimination and to a lack of sensitivity in understanding non-medical approaches to emotional difficulties.

The meeting of a white patient with a black psychiatrist produces *a status contradiction* for the doctor. Patients and relatives have to reconcile their rather different attitudes to immigrants and to doctors. In our experience they are often patronizing, feel they are getting second-class treatment and complain to a white psychiatrist that a black doctor cannot understand them or even has too many problems of his own to be helpful.

Status contradiction also occurs with black patient and black psychiatrist. The mutual awareness that both are immigrants is usually concealed beneath class and professional differences. The patient regards the doctor as really 'white', while the psychiatrist, often from quite a different society from the patient, agrees with his white colleagues that psychotherapy with a working-class patient (not of course a *black* patient) is rather unrewarding. The patient suspects that an English doctor might have helped him more. Neither recognize themselves in the other.

Racism is neither a science nor a disease but a set of political beliefs which legitimates certain social and economic conditions. It is pointless to ask which is primary – prejudice, or exploitation. They developed historically together, each validating the other.

## References

1. Goffman, E. *The Presentation of Self in Everyday Life*, Allen Lane, London (1959).
2. Parsons, T. *The Social System*, Routledge and Kegan Paul, London (1952).
3. Wing, J. K. and Brown, G. W. *Institutionalism and Schizophrenia*, Cambridge University Press (1970).
4. Lipsedge, M. and Littlewood, R. 'Compulsory hospitalisation and minority status' 11th Biennial Conference of the Caribbean Federation for Mental Health, Gosier, Guadeloupe (1977).
5. Goffman, E. *Asylums*, Penguin, Harmondsworth (1968).
6. Scheff, T. J. *Being Mentally Ill*, Aldine, Chicago (1966).
7. Cochrane, R. 'Mental illness in immigrants to England and Wales. An analysis of mental hospital admissions', *Social Psychiatry*, **12**, 23–35 (1977).
8. Lipsedge, M. and Littlewood, R. 'Transcultural psychiatry'. In *Recent Advances in Psychiatry*, 3rd edn, Churchill Livingstone, London (1959).
9. Rwegellera, G. G. C. 'Mental illness in Africans and West Indians of African origin living in London', M.Phil. thesis, University of London (1970).
10. Pinto, R. T. 'A study of psychiatric illness amongst Asians in the Camberwell area', M.Phil. dissertation, London University (1970).
11. Littlewood, R. and Cross, S. 'Ethnic minorities and psychiatric services', *Sociology of Health and Illness*, **2**, 194–201 (1980).

At the time of writing Roland Littlewood was a psychiatrist and a Research Fellow at the Institute of Social Anthropology at Oxford University. Maurice Lipsedge was a Consultant in Psychological Medicine at Guy's Hospital, London. This is an edited extract of pages 25–28 and 65–66 from their book *Aliens and Alienists, Ethnic Minorities and Psychiatry*, published by Penguin (1982). This was published in a revised edition in 1989 by Routledge (Unwin Hyman).

# 9
# Hysteria and demonic possession

## MARY JAMES

## Introduction

Jean-Martin Charcot (1825–1893) was a figure of major importance in French medicine at the end of the nineteenth century. In 1856, when he first took a post at the vast and ancient Salpêtrière hospital in Paris, doctors and students alike were reluctant to work there. Charcot, however, was quick to recognize the enormous potential this institution held for medical research. Its population of some 5,000 old and ailing women suffered from a great variety of chronic illnesses, especially diseases of the nervous system, which had yet to be classified and diagnosed.

In 1862, as head of one of the hospital's largest sections, Charcot embarked upon the enormous task of methodically examining every one of his patients, completing his clinical notes, where possible, by correlating symptoms with lesions at postmortem. Charcot's special talent in this field was to produce most fruitful results. By the late 1860s virtually all the most chronic neurological diseases on his wards had been systematized. By the time of his death, in 1893, he had constructed the basic framework of modern neuropathology and the Salpêtrière had been transformed into one of the world's leading teaching hospitals.

Although Charcot studied a number of different diseases, by 1872 hysteria had become his main area of interest, especially in its convulsive form which he termed *la grande hystérie* (major hysteria). The Paris Medical Faculty, at that time, considered hysteria to be unsatisfactorily defined as a disease because of its highly variable manifestations for which no cause could be found. Charcot, however, was confident that the method responsible for his neurological achievements could be extended to explain hysteria as a disorder of the nervous system. By prolonged clinical observation the seemingly formless attacks of *la grande hystérie* were schematized into four distinct stages occurring with various degrees of intensity according to the patient.

The aims of this article are twofold. The first is to explore Charcot's concept of *la grande hystérie* by looking closely at his description of the four stage classical attack.

It will then be possible to examine how this diagnosis was used at the Salpêtrière to reinterpret certain historical accounts of supernatural phenomena as instances of hysterical pathology.

Implicit in Charcot's project of reinterpretation was the rejection of religious and metaphysical explanations of phenomena. His view that only systematic observation and experiment were capable of yielding genuine knowledge was informed by the positivist tradition of scientific explanation. The belief that one can only have knowledge of observable phenomena and the law-like relations between them was well established in Charcot's day. It exerted a profound influence on many branches of intellectual activity and was crucial to his understanding of hysteria.

Given this, Charcot needed to demonstrate the law-governed regularity of hysteria before this condition could be satisfactorily explained. This meant that Charcot needed evidence that *la grande hystérie* was not limited to any specific time or place. As proof that it existed in former times Charcot used various historical paintings and written accounts of saints in ecstasy and the demonic possessed. By making meticulous, point by point comparisons with his *grandes hystériques* (major hysterics) he was able to highlight significant similarities that lent support to his claim. This process of identifying historical instances of hysteria was known as *retrospective diagnosis*.

In order to examine more closely how this was done at the Salpêtrière and to bring to light the conceptual and methodological difficulties that it entailed, the second part of this paper focuses on the case history of one of his *grandes hystériques*, Geneviève, known by the doctors at the Salpêtrière as 'La Succube' (that is a female demon supposed to have sexual intercourse with sleeping men). Her photographically illustrated case history was published in 1877–78 in the *Iconographie Photographique de la Salpêtrière*.[1]

This case is interesting for a number of reasons. Most importantly it illustrates how, at the Salpêtrière, clinical and religious interpretations became intertwined. It also offers a rich source for insights into the relationship between hysterical symptoms and socio-cultural context in which they occur.

*La Grande Hystérie*

When, in 1870, Charcot first turned his attention explicitly towards hysteria, considerable controversy surrounded its diagnosis. Convulsive hysteria, on account of its resemblance to epileptic fits, was known as hystero-epilepsy and many doctors believed it to be a combination of the two disorders. Charcot, however, held that where epileptic fits seemed to occur simultaneously with the symptoms of convulsive hysteria the condition was in fact only very severe hysteria. Although Charcot decided to retain the term hystero-epilepsy, he preferred the designations *la grande hystérie* or hysteria major, as they were less likely to arouse confusion.

Influenced by Pierre Briquet's study of hysteria in 1859, Charcot showed that *la grande attaque hystérique* (attack of major hysteria) in its most perfect form could be reduced to a very simple formula. In the complete attack four distinct phases succeeded one another with mechanical regularity. However, the concept of a *pure type* of hysteria was an abstract one to which patients, in reality, only very rarely conformed. Nevertheless Charcot believed that any inconvenience that arose from this was compensated by its potential for imposing order on the chaos of seemingly random hysterical manifestations.

According to the degree of intensity of any one of the stages of the *grande attaque*, different varieties were identified. At the Salpêtrière each aspect of patients' hysterical attacks was observed, documented, photographed and sketched in minute detail. The multiplicity of observations recorded were interpreted in the framework of the four stage model.

The classical *grande attaque* began with a warning *prodrome* or *aura*, usually of only a few minutes duration. This was generally marked by excessive sensitivity around the ovaries with the sensation of a ball rising from the abdomen to the throat, causing a feeling of suffocation. Other characteristic signs were palpitations of the heart, beating at the temples and whistling in the ears, often accompanied by mental excitation and sometimes by hallucinations.

The attack proper commenced with the stage designated *épileptoid* because of its similarity to an epileptic fit. Involuntary muscular contractions contorted the patient's face and body. Typically the eyeballs convulsed upwards, respiration was snorelike and foam appeared at the mouth. This stage was estimated to continue for about four minutes in all.

Next came the stage termed *grandes mouvements* (great movements) on account of the immense struggling purposelessness that it entailed. Beginning after a moment of calm, it was said to be motivated by an exaggerated expenditure of muscular force, enabling the patient to perform feats of staggering strength and agility. The bizarre postures and contortions of this period were known as *attitudes illogiques* (illogical postures), in which no overall rhythm or order could be identified. It was described as a fit of rage in which the subject, howling like a wild beast, tore or broke anything within reach, and attacked anyone who tried to approach.

The third stage to occur was the *période des attitudes passionnelles* (period of postures denoting strong emotion). In this phase the patient experienced hallucinations, the content of which was expressively acted out in mime. A certain sentiment, either cheerful (*gaie*), or sad (*triste*) was said always to predominate and sometimes patients switched from one to the other in succession. Romantic or religious joy were usually the subject of *hallucinations gaies*, whilst fires, wars, revolutions and murders were most often the basis of the *tableaux tristes* (mimes portraying sadness). Sometimes expressive poses were adopted in which the patient appeared as a living statue. Charcot said that this phase was generally short and might not occur at all.

The attack drew to a close with the fourth or terminal period. The patient came back to self-awareness, but only in part, often being prey to deliria and to symptoms very similar to those of the initial aura. The four-part attack generally lasted for around a quarter of an hour, but it could recur to constitute a series sometimes of two hundred or more attacks.

### Retrospective diagnosis and the *attaque démoniaque*

Meticulous clinical observation at the Salpêtrière revealed the *attaque démoniaque* (demonic attack) to be a frequently occurring variation of the classical *grande attaque hystérique* that has just been described. It consisted in the predominance of the second stage of *grandes mouvements*. Charcot drew a close parallel between the bizarre contortions and violent outbursts of this period and the behaviour which had historically been understood as demonic possession. For instance, in both cases the superhuman muscular strength and agility of seemingly frail women often astounded spectators.

To establish this point historical literature on demonic possession was sometimes quoted at length in the case histories of hystero-epileptics. Works such as *La Piété Affligée*, published in 1700 by the exorcist involved in occurrences of possession at a convent in Louviers, and *L'Histoire des Diables de Loudun*, an eyewitness account by a protestant minister of possession in a convent in Loudun, published in 1693, were used to confirm the similarity between the *attaque démoniaque* and all the major characteristics of demonic possession.

Works of art were also subjected to medical scrutiny. For instance, a sketch of a person possessed by devils, by the Flemish painter Rubens (1577–1640), was used to illustrate the case of the *grande-hystérique*, Celina.[2] Analogies were drawn between the sketch and photographs of her in the throes of a 'demonic' attack.

Retrospective diagnosis served a dual purpose. The fact that the classical symptoms of hysteria, as enumerated by Charcot, had already been fully described hundreds of years before was taken as proof that *la grande hystérie* was objectively real and could not be the result of suggestion (this is a covert or inadvertent influence) proceeding from any current medical theory. It also meant that supernatural accounts of demonic possession could be replaced by reference to natural causes alone, thereby extending the boundaries of scientific knowledge. This approach to diagnosis was, however, problematic in several respects, not least because Charcot's focus of attention on superstitious beliefs brought them to the fore, making the Salpêtrière itself into a kind of 'theatre of possession'.[3,4] Once the concept of the *attaque démoniaque* had been set in place not only were doctors more likely to identify and emphasize those characteristics which could be subsumed within this category, but patients, in turn, became more inclined to supply them with good cause. At the Salpêtrière the results of a complex process of suggestion, autosuggestion and expectation were subtle and far-reaching.


## Geneviève – *La Succube*


The demonic connotations of hysteria are especially interesting and intricate in the case of Geneviève. The second part of her case history, entitled *Succube*, was compiled in 1878 by Charcot's colleague and former student D. M Bourneville (1840–1909). He stated that less than two centuries ago she would have been thought of as possessed by a demon.[5] This identity was attributed to her, not on account of her hysterical crises, which did not conform to the *attaque démoniaque*, but because of her generally bizarre and unruly behaviour and the strange hallucinations she experienced. The seventeenth century accounts of demonic possession at the convents in Loudun and Louviers were referred to throughout to illustrate the point. For Bourneville, Geneviève was 'living proof' that the nuns had been hysterics.

Geneviève's case history records that she was first taken into hospital in 1851, when she was eight years old. She could not, however, remember why. Throughout the rest of her childhood and adolescence many periods were spent as a hospital patient. Although she received no formal schooling, nursing nuns taught her to read religious texts. When not in hospital she lived with a foster family and worked on their farm.

At the age of fourteen, she was courted by a young man named Camille. Eighteen months later she was devastated when he died of brain fever. Her foster family tried to prevent her from attending his funeral, but she escaped and attempted to throw herself in the grave. This experience left her depressed and angry and she often refused to speak. The following year, when her foster mother died, her condition deteriorated and she was taken back into hospital at Poitiers.

Six months later, in better health, she took work as a chamber-maid in the town. Soon her employer began to make sexual advances and although she tried to defend herself her feelings towards him were ambivalent. It was in this frame of mind that she suffered her first convulsive attack. She was taken back to the hospital and for the next five or six months had attacks every day.

By the time Geneviève became one of Charcot's patients, in March 1872, she was twenty nine years old and had already spent a considerable amount of time at the Salpêtrière. She first went there in 1864 as a psychiatric patient, and then, as her condition improved, stayed on as a nursing assistant. In 1865 she was taken to the section for epileptics, but after being granted permission to go into town with a nurse, had escaped and run to the house of a lover she had met in Paris.

Over the next fifteen months she moved from one hospital to another, her status oscillating between patient and nursing assistant. However in July 1866, after violently assaulting the *chef du service* (chief of staff) at La Pitié hospital in Paris, she was sent back to the section for the insane at the Salpêtrière. Later that year she was transferred to an asylum at Toulouse, but, having gained the confidence of the nursing nuns, she soon absconded. For the next three months, dressed in hospital uniform and clogs, she made her way back to Paris on foot, sleeping rough and begging for alms. Upon her return she went to join her lover and in August 1867 gave birth to a daughter at the Salpêtrière.

Bourneville's account of Geneviève's history clearly depicts her as rebellious and recalcitrant both to medical control and diagnosis. As a patient of Charcot's she often tried to run away by climbing on the roof and jumping over the fence, sometimes accompanied by the 'demonic' Celina. Behaviour of this kind was used to draw comparisons with the nuns of Loudun whose exploits in the acrobatic field included shinning up trees and climbing onto the convent roof.

However, what is perhaps most significant about the demonic interpretation of Geneviève's hysteria is that she was born in Loudun and grew up in that area. Throughout her childhood and adolescence she was in close contact with nursing nuns who, because of her boisterous and headstrong character, frequently beat and punished her. Whilst supplying these details, Bourneville did not acknowledge that they may have influenced her 'demonic' behaviour.

The demonic possession at the Ursuline convent is perhaps Loudun's only claim to fame, and stories of the nuns' bizarre and often lewd behaviour were well known. Until 1861, when Geneviève first came to Paris, she had been immersed in this milieu of possession. Whilst Bourneville recognised the influence of convent life upon her marked religiosity (for instance she spent much time kneeling in prayer in front of a large crucifix which she kept constantly by her), it was supposed that her unruly outbursts shed light on the strange conduct of the possessed nuns of the seventeenth century rather than vice versa.

The numerous comparisons drawn between Geneviève and the demonic possessed were intended to show not just that the nuns were hysterics, but that Geneviève's hysteria was objectively real. Most notably, Geneviève's hallucinations, in which she received nocturnal visits of a sexual nature from a Dr X, were said to have an historical counterpart. The possessed nuns had claimed that they had been necromantically seduced by Urbain Grandier, Loudun's handsome, young parish priest. He was, consequently, tried and burned at the stake as a sorcerer in 1634.

Geneviève's extravagant antics before and after attacks were also likened to those of demoniacs. In particular, her insensitivity to cold and pain and her tendency to take off all her clothes and cavort about naked in all weathers, were said to resemble in every detail descriptions of the Ursuline Mother Superior, Madame de Belfiel, one of Grandier's accusers.

Ostensibly it was on account of these resemblances to *les possédées* (the possessed) that Geneviève was referred to as 'La Succube'. This terminology is interesting in two respects. Not only does it make medical and historical discourse interchangeable, but it subtly distorts the issue at hand. Geneviève believed Dr X visited her in her hospital bed in order to have sexual intercourse. However by naming *her* La Succube she is misleadingly represented as the female demon which folk lore characterizes as having sexual intercourse with sleeping men.

This inversion of meaning not only attributes to her a demonic identity that is inappropriate under the circumstances, it also suggests that she is sexually culpable. This implication is amplified by the connotation of prostitution that the term carries from the Latin *succuba* (i.e. prostitute). Thus this label had moral as well as medical significance, stereotyping the sexually unconventional Geneviève as a whore. (The idea that an actual seduction by Dr X might have occurred did not enter the question and is now beyond the reach of time.)

## Conclusion

Charcot's method of retrospective diagnosis, whilst it brought many interesting comparisons to light, was nevertheless seriously flawed in its deployment of the evidence. Historical depictions of demoniacs, on the one hand, were taken as evidence of the authenticity of certain hysterical phenomena witnessed by Charcot and his colleagues. On the other hand contemporary manifestations of 'demonic' behaviour were 'living proof' that the demoniacs of former times were actually hysterics. This strategy entails the uncomfortable consequence of explanatory reciprocity, that is to say the 'objective' evidence supporting either claim was itself defined in terms of the condition it was intended to guarantee.

At the Salpêtrière, two systems of representation, the clinical and the religious, were constantly intermingling and contaminating one another. The medical discourse drew heavily on the religious superstitions it was trying to dispel, often becoming entangled and confused in the process. The unintended result was the accentuation of the very demonic connotations that the positivist approach aimed to counteract. Ironically the demonic phenomena exhibited at the Salpêtrière arose from and were closely related to Charcot's main clinical objective, namely to provide a scientific explanation for hysteria as an objectively real, law-governed phenomenon, on the basis of clinical observation.

## Notes and references

1. Bourneville, D. M. and Regnard, P. *Iconographie Photographique de la Salpêtrière*, Vol. 1, Observation IV (1876–7), Vol. 2, Observation IV (1878). Progrès Médical, Delahaye and Lecrosnier, Paris.
2. Plate XI in Volume 1 of Bourneville and Regnard (1877).
3. Page 501 in Carroy-Thirard, J. 'Possession, extase, hystérie au XIXe siècle'. *Psychanalyse à l'université*, 5 (19), pp. 499–515 (1980).
4. Chapter 5 in James, M. *The Therapeutic Practices of Jean-Martin Charcot (1825–1893) in their Historical and Social Context*. Ph.D. thesis, University of Essex (1989).
5. Page 202 in Volume 2, Part II of Bourneville and Regnard (1878).

*Further sources for this article*
Charcot, J.-M. *Lectures on Diseases of the Nervous System*, Vols 72, 90, 128. Translated and edited by George Sigerson, New Sydenham Society, London (1877–89).
Charcot, J.-M. and Richer, P. *Les Démoniaques dans l'Art*, Delahaye and Lecrosnier, Paris (1887).
Didi-Huberman, G. 'Charcot, l'histoire et l'art', postface to J.-M. Charcot and P. Richer, *Les Démoniaques dans l'Art* (1887), Macula, Paris, 1984.

This article was first published by the Open University in 1994 as a supplementary article to *Medical Knowledge: Doubt and Certainty*, for students studying the second-level course *U205 Health and Disease*. Mary James wrote her doctoral thesis on the work of the French doctor, Jean-Martin Charcot, who described various specific aspects of hysterical manifestations in his writings with the French terms used in this article (since no corresponding English terms exist in most cases, a rough translation only has been given in brackets). Mary James currently lectures in the Department of History at the University of Essex.

# 10

# Protecting a vulnerable margin: towards an analysis of how the mouth came to be separated from the body

## SARAH NETTLETON

### Introduction

In 1841 George Waite published the document *An Appeal to Parliament; the Medical Profession and the Public on the present state of Dental Surgery*, in which he argued that the legislature should recognize dental surgery as a legitimate branch of medicine. Eighteen years later the London School of Dental Surgery was established, followed by the first Dental Act in 1878 which created a dental register and the founding of the British Dental Association in 1880 to uphold this Act.[1] Finally, in 1921 the Dentists Act abolished unregistered practice and dentistry became a recognizable organized occupation with state support.[2]

These developments represented the appearance of a new knowledge: a knowledge of the mouth containing the teeth. That the mouth should come to be the focus of a new profession with a distinct body of knowledge presents a sociological puzzle. Identified as an object of knowledge in the mid-nineteenth century, it became by the end of that century and throughout the twentieth century the focus of a whole new system of beliefs and associated practices.

Conventional historical accounts have assumed that people in the population increasingly experienced dental disease during and towards the end of the nineteenth century.[3,4] This has been associated with an increase in sugar consumption.[5,6] Those suffering pain sought the services of the local barber-surgeon. With time these surgeons became increasingly aware of their skills, and so grouped together to make demands that their expertise be recognized. Political pressure groups were established, for example the College of Dentists in England and the Odontological Society. In 1921 their demands were finally met and dentistry established as a profession.[7]

[In these accounts] no consideration has been given to the object of dental knowledge. The appearance of the dental profession, it has been assumed, took place only in response to diseased mouths. This paper however, argues that to assume the mouth as a discrete entity, which suffered from increasing amounts of dental disease, does not permit an adequate analysis of the appearance of dentistry.

## A discourse on public health

In the nineteenth century, the numbers of the poor and the sick who were seen to be suffering from communicable diseases, for example cholera, were growing.[8] Indeed the whole population was at risk from epidemics. The sources of disease were seen to lie in the natural environment; in the water, soil, air and food. Increasingly however throughout the twentieth century the public health movement influenced by 'discoveries of bacteriology' has shifted from the environment to the individual.[9]

Disease by the turn of the century was seen to arise from

... people and their points of contact. It was people who carried health from the natural world into the social body and transmitted it within.[10]

Writing in his Annual Report of 1910 the Chief Medical Officer wrote:

... the fact emerges that the centre of gravity of our public health system is passing in some degree from the environment to the individual and from problems of outward sanitation to the problems of personal hygiene.[11]

With reorientation of public health from the environment as the source of danger and the individual being perceived as the victim, to the person as the transmitter of disease, the surveillance of all bodies came to be of utmost importance. The points of contact between people came to be crucial in the control of bodies. A regulation of the mouth however did not so much involve the repression of the population but rather produced a new knowledge of it.

Certainly when we look to the medical texts of the end of the nineteenth, and beginning of the twentieth centuries we can see the evidence of 'points of contact' that came to be significant. It was argued that a healthy body was only possible with a healthy mouth, for example a school medical officer reported:

... with such dreadful oral conditions and constant absorption of septic materials the chances of a healthy childhood are small in most infants.

The Medical Officers Association reported on the care of children's teeth and in 1910 wrote that:

... it is a peculiarity of dental disorders that they bring innumerable evils in their train, not least of which is lowering the body's vitality and thus opening wide a door for other diseases to enter.[12]

Further, Wallis, an active figure in the development of the dental service, was anxious to point out in 1908:

... it has been proved by actual practice that the health of children has been markedly raised through dental treatment, and dental treatment aids in the prevention of disease and in the war against tuberculosis.[13]

Wheatly (1912) suggested that prevention of dental disease would do 'more for the improvement of the health of the people than the extermination of any other disease, even TB'.[14] It was suggested [in 1929] that

> ... if your children are to enjoy the blessing of a firm and intelligent countenance, see to it that their mouths have unremitting, careful attention.[15]

In 1920, in *Practical Preventive Medicine*, Boyd described the significance of the 'portals through which infective agents enter the body':

> The principal body orifices play an important part 'particularly' the orifices of entrance, rather than those of exit ... the mouth and the nose are the portals of entrance of the greatest importance from the standpoint of the number of infective agents which are introduced through them.[16]

The mouth was conceived of as the boundary between the internal body and the external sources of pollution. Specified or unseen matter, which crossed the boundary of the mouth was indeed 'matter out of place'. The mouth then was to be rigorously protected from the pollutants that lay 'out there'. Hyatt wrote in 1929 that:

> We are zealously taught and trained from our earliest years to guard against and repel visible foes external to our bodies. How much more important it is to exercise the utmost vigilance to see that the more insidious foes ... do not gain access to the marvellous and delicate organs that compose the hidden mechanism of the human body. By far the greatest number of germ infections that assail us gain their entrance by the mouth. Air breathed in through the nose is comparatively innocuous, physicians state, because the hairs in the nose serve as traps for bacteria, and by far the largest proportion of those that try to get in are ejected with succeeding exhalation.[15]

The use of common drinking cups and utensils was discouraged [by Boyd in 1920] and it was important to avoid the mouths of persons who 'laugh and talk loudly in an explosive manner'.[16]

## A discipline of the mouth

Once the mouth was established as a socially significant object, it was deemed necessary to find the 'truth' about it; to analyse, describe and to understand it. The focus towards the mouth took place in a wider process in which attention was being directed towards individual bodies and populations. The individual, it has been suggested [by Foucault 1985], was part of the machinery of power, a power that creates the body, isolates it, explores it, breaks it down and rearranges it.[17] A knowledge of the body therefore required a mechanism of discipline; that is, a machinery of power that was part of the production of knowledge. Discipline was the 'political anatomy of detail', that is to say the body became known and understood as a series of useable parts which could be manipulated, trained, corrected and controlled. The outcome was to be a cumulation of increasingly detailed observations which simultaneously and inescapably produced knowledge of individuals.

Foucault has argued that this mechanism of discipline required and developed three conditions for its implementation.[17] First it was cellular, in that it referred to the space into which individuals were located, they were isolated into individual units. For example in the school [of 1910]:

> basins should be provided with water taps over them and unbreakable cups, a toothbrush for *every* child with its own number, racks where they may be placed with names and numbers on. The 'toothbrush drill' will then be a reality instead of a farce and this wholesome recreation will save much money in the future.[12]

A second condition of discipline concerned the control of activity, exemplified by the timetable. Behaviours were allocated to strict temporal regimes: teeth were brushed in the morning and before bed. Harvey (1928) wrote a text on the *Care of the Mouth and Teeth* in which he detailed for various age groups the precise times when these children should eat and the nature of their food.[18]

A third dimension of discipline was 'the correct use of the body, which makes possible the correct use of time' (Foucault 1985); for example, the correct way to brush teeth was described to the finest detail. An extract from a lengthier description [written in 1921] of a method of brushing reads:

> With the bristles of the brush pointing upward and the end of the thumb on the back of the handle, brush the roof of the mouth and the inside gums and surfaces of the teeth with a fast in-out-stroke, reaching back on the gums as far as you can go. Go back and forth across the roof of the mouth with this in-and-out stroke at least four times. Hold the handle of the toothbrush in your fist with the thumb lying across the back of the handle and brush the gums and teeth with an in-out-stroke, using chiefly the tuft end or the toe of the brush. Reach back in the mouth on the gums below the last tooth on both sides and brush with a fast, light in-and-out stroke.[19]

People were trained and supervised to control their own mouths, individuals were recruited to the 'army' to fight the 'ravages of decay',[20] children had to practise their 'toothbrush drill', for example:

> The drill proper is given when the children are seated, while the assistants pass up and down the aisles helping the children to hold the brushes correctly. There are four positions for holding the brush and two movements in each drill. The children brush to a count in a stereotyped form, it being intended to teach merely the correct form of brushing, and not meant for the actual cleaning of teeth . . . the children repeat the drill standing, and brushes are wrapped in waxed paper to be taken home.[19]

This is what Foucault referred to as the art of 'composing forces in order to obtain an efficient machine' that is 'the individual body becomes an element, that may be placed, moved and articulated on others.'[17] There was no space for idiosyncrasies, each individual was part of a greater whole; a 'body segment in a whole ensemble over which it is articulated . . . the body is constituted as a part of a multisegmentary machine'.[17]

By drawing on Foucault's concept of the disciplinary regime we can better appreciate how the mouth came to be policed. It was policed not by the dominator controlling the dominated but through the operation of examining (the dental check up) measuring and comparing (dental epidemiological records) and normalizing the mouth. The toothbrush drill was an example of the micro-mechanisms of power that since the late eighteenth century have played an increasing part in the management of people's lives through direct action on their bodies.

The regular dental examination is perhaps one of the more readily tangible illustrations of the disciplinary regime. Foucault wrote of the examination that 'in this slender technique are to be found a whole domain of knowledge, a whole type of power.'[17] Each mouth was to be subjected to systematic examination, a neglected mouth would inevitably result in disease. Cunningham (1905) said the case for bringing the doctor and dentist into the school for regular inspections was unanswerable.[21] The regular dental examination placed the patient in a situation of perpetual observation and facilitated a knowledge of the population. Knowledge was extracted from the patient by the dentist and documented, recorded, classified and compared. A record of each individual's teeth was kept in the dental case notes. Each tooth, and each tooth surface (palatal, buccal, mesial, distal, occlusial and lingual) was recorded and arranged for epidemiological data. The examination, wrote Foucault, of all the mechanisms of power is highly ritualized because:

> In it are combined the ceremony of power and the form of experiment, the deployment of force and the establishment of truth. At the heart of the procedures of discipline it manifests the subjection of those who are perceived as objects and the objectification of those who are subjected.[17]

The examination of the individual which provided a knowledge of the population was part of a technique of knowledge; the epidemiological survey. In this way it established over individuals a visibility through which mouths were measured, compared and distributed. Epidemiology acted as a process of 'normalization', every mouth could be placed in relation to every other, no mouth could escape categorization.

The mouth had emerged as a discrete object at the same time as the invention of the child as an object of medical attention. The mouth was but one of other areas of the body that was to be used, manipulated and subjected to surveillance. As Armstrong (1983) noted:

> At the same time as the body of every child was subjected to educational surveillance through the introduction of compulsory education the child entered medical discourse as a discrete object with attendant pathologies.

The Chief Medical Officer's Annual Report of 1915 announced that, in 1914, 130 of the 317 education authorities had established dental clinics for the examination of school children's teeth.[22] The dentist could be added to the list of 'experts' who generated a knowledge of increasingly diversified categories associated with the child's body and mind.[23]

## Conclusion

Dentists did not emerge simply as an outcome of an increasing demand for the relief of toothache. The increasingly skilled dentist did not merely draw the tooth from the suffering patient, but rather a population of bodies produced a dental knowledge as they were caught up in the machinery of dentistry. The mouth became an object of surveillance, a subject of the mechanisms of discipline which were inherent in the twentieth century public health movement. It was then that dentistry could become established as an accepted profession, the largest specialized sub-branch of medicine peering intently into the mouths of the population. It was then that knowledge of the mouth and teeth could be accumulated in texts and journals and transmitted in specialized schools. It was only at this moment that oral and dental hygiene could become embedded in the routinized and everyday practices of the whole population.

## References

1. Bennett, N. G. 'The BDA: its origins, progress and advance', *British Dental Journal*, 51(11), 565–587 (1930).
2. Richards, N. D. 'Dentistry in England in the 1940s: the first movements towards professionalisation', *Medical History*, 12, 137–152 (1968).
3. Gelbier, S. and Randall, S. 'Charles Edward Wallis & the rise of London's school service', *Medical History*, 20, 395–404 (1982).
4. Norman, H. D. 'Public health dentistry before 1948', *Dental Public Health: An Introduction to Community Dentistry*, John Wright & Sons, Bristol (1981).
5. Quick, A., Sheiham, H. and Sheiham, A. *Sweet Nothings*, Vol. 3, Health Education Council, London (1981).
6. Hardwick, J. L. 'The incidence and distribution of caries throughout the ages in relation to the Englishman's diet', *British Dental Journal*, 108, 11–12 (1960).
7. Freidson, E. *The Profession of Medicine*, Dodd Mead, New York (1970).
8. The occurrence of disease was recorded in reports throughout the country. The most often quoted is Chadwick's *Report on the Enquiry into Sanitary Conditions of the Labouring Population in Great Britain* (1850). The General Health Board produced many reports, for example the *Report on the Epidemic of Cholera of 1848–1849* (1850).
9. Starr, P. *The Social Transformation of American Medicine*, see pp. 189–194, Basic Books, New York (1982).
10. Armstrong, D. *The Political Anatomy of the Body*, Cambridge University Press, Cambridge (1983).
11. Newman, G. *Annual Report of the Chief Medical Officer of the Board of Education for 1908*, London (1910).
12. Denson Redley, R. *The Care of Teeth During School Life*, Medical Officers Association, Churchill, London (1910).
13. Wallis, E. *The Care of Teeth in Public Elementary Schools with Special Reference to what is done in Germany*, Medical Officers Association, London (1908).
14. Wheatly, J. 'Dental caries as a field of preventive medicine', *Public Health*, 25, 406–414 (1912).
15. Hyatt, T. P. *Hygiene of the Mouth and Teeth*, Brooklyn Dental Publishing Co., New York (1929).
16. Boyd, M. F. *Practical Preventive Medicine*, W. B. Saunders & Co., London (1920).
17. Foucault, M. *Discipline and Punish: The Birth of the Prison*, Penguin Books, London (1985).
18. Harvey, J. *Care of the Mouth and Teeth*, Burkhard, London (1928).
19. Turner, C. L. *Hygiene, Dental and General*, Kimpton, London (1921).
20. Militaristic words and phrases like these are used frequently throughout the dental literature.
21. Cunningham, G. 'The teeth and physical deterioration', *British Dental Journal*, 26(17), 817–825 (1905).
22. Chief Medical Officer Board of Education *Annual Report*, London Cd. 8055 (1915).
23. Foucault (1985) notes that 'judges of normality are present everywhere. We are in a society of the teacher-judge, the doctor-judge, the educator-judge, the social worker-judge; it is on them that the universal reign of the normative is based.' To this list we could add the dentist-judge.

This article is a heavily edited version of a much longer text, which was originally published in 1988, under the same title, in the journal *Sociology of Health and Illness*, volume 10 (No. 2), pages 156–169. At the time of writing, Sarah Nettleton was a researcher at King's College School of Medicine and Dentistry in London, and is now a Lecturer in Social Policy and Social Work at the University of York. This article was further developed in her book, *Power, Pain and Dentistry*, published in 1992 by Open University Press.

# Part 2
# Experiencing health and disease

## INTRODUCTION

In the second part of the book, we turn aside from attempts to define what constitutes health, disease and healing, and focus on the individual's experience of these states. Yet even here, the theme developed in Part 1 continues to surface: some of the accounts that follow demonstrate that the experience of being well or ill, of living with a physical impairment or a latent infection, of giving birth or failing to conceive, carries with it a mixed bag of prejudices and beliefs about the nature of the condition which can have a profound effect on personal experience, over and above coping with its physical manifestations. The collection of articles ranges widely across the spectrum of experience of health and disease; they include accounts of giving or receiving care within the family and of encounters with health and social care professionals. Some were written by academic researchers, others by writers whose work falls outside the academic sphere; what they have in common is an acute sensitivity to the felt experience of their subjects.

The first article sets the scene for those that follow. In 'The insanity of place', the American sociologist Erving Goffman contrasts the experience of physical illness with that of mental breakdown, viewing both from the standpoint of the patient's family. As long as the sick person is recognizably 'themselves', as is usually the case with a physical ailment, he or she can maintain their habitual place within the family culture and indicate in countless ways that they appreciate the services rendered necessary by their illness. But the whole structure of the family is threatened when one member becomes mentally disturbed: no matter how the family tries to maintain life as they knew it, their efforts are undermined, the patient tears down his or her familiar identity and 'the family is turned inside out'.

In the nine articles that follow Goffman's, there are many examples of the difficulties faced by families – as well as by individuals – when an illness, or a state that is confused with illness, cannot be 'contained' within recognizable boundaries of social relationships. Most obvious among them is the account by Julia Burton-Jones of Tom and Dot, a couple she interviewed during research into the experience of people who are caring for a seriously ill relative at home. Dot has Alzheimer's disease and during the long slow decline into complete dependency, Tom struggles to keep her looking 'normal' to the outside world. The unremitting physical labour of looking after Dot would be so much more bearable, he feels, if only she could still recognize him.

'The social impact of childhood asthma' by the sociologists Andrew Nocon and Tim Booth, catalogues the multiple sources of anxiety for parents of an asthmatic child. Not only do they experience the worry of their child's episodic illness and the disruption to family plans and attendance at work, but they must keep vigilant in the face of a world full of potential triggers for an attack – smoke from birthday cake candles, horsehairs on a sister's clothes, dust in the bedroom carpet. And yet, in these accounts, the child itself seems scarcely aware of the attention lavished on an illness which seems no more than an occasional inconvenience in its otherwise active life. This mirrors the experience of David Oldman, described in the next article 'Coping with migraine'. Oldman is a lifelong sufferer from migraine who learned early on how to cope with his attacks and relate to them simply as episodes of incapacity in his healthy life. His co-author, Sally Macintyre, had a different experience; she was encouraged by her medical attendants to seek explanations for her migraines within herself, in disordered biological or mental states. Where Oldman took responsibility for *managing* his migraines, Macintyre struggled to take responsibility for *having* hers. In this respect, she resembled a few of the parents of asthmatic children in Nocon and Booth's study, who agonized about whether they had somehow caused their child's asthma.

Variations in coping styles, from active control to agonizing over the condition, are central to David Kelleher's article, 'Coming to terms with diabetes'. His research illustrates the extent to which the same biological disorder – inadequate regulation of glucose in the body – can be experienced in many different ways, depending on whether the diabetic feels that he or she is in control of, or is controlled by, their deficient insulin. In some individuals, the responsibility for managing the diabetes is devolved to their doctors, who are believed to 'know best'; this is a recurrent theme in this Reader and one that we will revisit shortly. Diabetes is not a condition that evokes revulsion or fear of contagion among non-diabetics, in sharp contrast to the subject of the next article, 'Living with HIV and AIDS', by Neil Small. Like Kelleher, Small is a sociologist, sensitive to the need to address the 'meaning' placed on an illness – or the threat of an illness – by those affected. He argues that HIV infection should be clearly distinguished from AIDS. Like AIDS itself, HIV is equated with guilt and death, an assumption that contaminates the experience of being HIV-positive and in good health. The attribution of guilt for becoming infected contributes to the isolation that many HIV-positive people feel. Society separates into 'us and them', a common reaction to life-threatening, disabling or disfiguring conditions.

This is reflected in the experience of people whose normal life includes coping with a severe physical impairment, like Jenny Morris, the author of 'Pride against prejudice: "Lives not worth living"'. Morris chronicles a number of high-profile cases in which a person with multiple physical impairments wished to die, but lacked the physical means or ability to commit suicide. Their desire for death was interpreted by the media and the courts as the understandable reaction of a sane person to an intolerable life; Morris argues that their suicidal depression should instead be attributed to the social rejection which denies them the high level of support necessary to deliver a tolerable quality of life. The severity of their physical impairments challenged the ability of able-bodied people to recognize them as 'like us', individuals with a life worth living. This is an extreme example of society shutting the door on those of its members whose experience of health and disease is considered to fall outside 'the norm'. One of the most pervasive beliefs in western culture is that it is normal for adults to become parents; it follows that those who cannot conceive a child are treated as outsiders and a few become desperate seekers after medical help. In 'The stigma of infertility', Naomi Pfeffer continues the exploration of cultural attitudes that profoundly affect the experience of health and disease. People who are infertile are characterized as though suffering from a sickness; in reality they are generally healthy and their invisible physical impairment is only revealed if they attempt to procreate. Pfeffer considers the vested interest of doctors in promoting infertility as an intrinsically desperate state that requires medical intervention, rather than one that produces manageable episodes of despair. Her research is part of a feminist sociology of medicine, to which Ann Oakley has also made a major contribution (her article 'Doctor knows best' appears in Part 6 of this Reader).

Jocelyn Cornwell also explores the relationship between patient and professional in 'Hard-earned lives: experiences of doctors and health services', but she does so through the personal accounts of a small group of women belonging to an extended family in London's East End. Their experiences of health care enabled Cornwell to distinguish a pattern and a hierarchy. The hospital doctors who treated these women for what they considered to be 'real' illnesses, were accorded respect and compliance no matter how late, how apparently uninterested, uncaring or uninformative the doctors were. GPs were held in less awe, but were still judged to be experts; however, their pronouncements could occasionally be taken with a pinch of salt or questioned out of earshot. No such privileged status attached to midwives and health visitors, whose expertise was considered to be at best simple common sense and did not achieve even that standard some of the time. Pregnancy and labour were not experienced as illnesses by these women, and they rejected attempts by their birth attendants to claim superior medical knowledge about these processes. Midwives and health visitors were seen as similar to social workers – all species far below doctors in the hierarchy of health care.

The experiences recounted in the last article are those of Mrs Williams, a woman of eighty-seven who has no great respect for social workers either. In an interview with Tony Parker, she robustly describes her independent but isolated life in a council flat as blindness closes in and her children and the vicar stop visiting. She isn't ill and she doesn't need much help, but she wishes the council would stop sending round 'Some bloody do-gooding cow' to see if she will accept meals-on-wheels or a card to display in her window to call for help. When she uses the card, no-one notices it for three days. Her experience of growing old in contemporary Britain strikes a chord with other articles in Part 2; coping alone, or behind the closed doors of the family, seems to be woven into British culture.

# 11
# The insanity of place

**ERVING GOFFMAN**

In the last twenty years we have learned that the management of mental illness under medical auspices has been an uncertain blessing. The best treatment that money has been able to buy, prolonged individual psychotherapy, has not proven very efficacious. The treatment most patients have received – hospitalization – has proven to be questionable indeed. Patients recover more often than not, at least temporarily, but this seems in spite of the mental hospital, not because of it. Upon examination, many of these establishments have proven to be hopeless storage dumps trimmed in psychiatric paper.

Given the life still enforced in most mental hospitals and the stigma still placed on mental illness, the philosophy of community containment seems the only desirable one. Nonetheless, it is worth looking at some implications of this approach for the patient's various 'others', that is, persons he identifies as playing a significant role in his life. To do this we must examine the meaning of the patient's symptoms for his others. If we do this we will learn not only what containment implies, we will learn about mental disorder.

The interesting thing about medical symptoms is how utterly nice, how utterly plucky the patient can be in managing them. There may be physical acts of an ordinary kind he cannot perform; there may be various parts of the body he must keep bandaged and hidden from view; he may have to stay home from work for a spell or even spend time in a hospital bed. But for each of these deviations from normal social appearance and functioning, the patient will be able to furnish a compensating mode of address. He gives accounts, belittles his discomfort, and presents an apologetic air, as if to say that in spite of appearance he is, deep in his social soul, someone to be counted on to know his place, someone who appreciates what he ought to be as a normal person and who is this person in spirit, regardless of what has happened to his flesh. He is someone who does not will to be demanding and useless. Tuberculosis patients, formerly isolated in sanitaria, sent home progress notes that were fumigated but cheerful. Brave little troops of colostomites and ileostomites make their brief appearances disguised as nice clean people, while stoically concealing the hours of hellish toilet work required for each appearance in public as a normal person. We even have our Beckett player buried up to his head in an iron lung, unable to blow his own nose, who yet somehow expresses by means of his eyebrows that a full-fledged person is present who knows how to behave and would certainly behave that way were he physically able.

And more than an air is involved. Howsoever demanding the sick person's illness is, almost always there will be some consideration his keepers will *not* have to give. There will be some physical cooperation that can be counted on; there will be some task he can do to help out, often one that would not fall to his lot were he well. And this helpfulness can be *absolutely* counted on, just as though he were no less a responsible participant than anyone else. In the context, these little bits of substantive helpfulness take on a large symbolic function.

Now obviously, physically sick persons do not always keep a stiff upper lip (not even to mention appreciable ethnic differences in the management of the sick role); hypochondriasis is common, and control of others through illness is not uncommon. But even in these cases I think close examination would find that the culprit tends to acknowledge proper sick-role etiquette. This may not only be a front, a gloss, a way of styling behaviour. But it says: 'Whatever my medical condition demands, the enduring me is to be dissociated from these needs, for I am someone who would make only modest reasonable claims and take a modest and standard role in the affairs of the group were I able.'

The family's treatment of the patient nicely supports this definition of the situation, as does the employer's. In effect they say that special licence can temporarily be accorded the sick person because, were he able to do anything about it, he would not make such demands. Since the patient's spirit and will and intentions are those of a loyal and seemly member, his old place should be kept waiting for him, for he will fill it well, as if nothing untoward has happened, as soon as his outer behaviour can again be dictated by, and be an expression of, the inner man. His increased demands are saved from expressing what they might because it is plain that he has 'good' reasons for making them, that is, reasons that nullify what these claims would otherwise be taken to mean. I do not say that the members of the family will be happy about their destiny. In the case of incurable disorders that are messy or severely incapacitating, the compensatory work required by the well members may cost them the life chances their peers enjoy, blunt their personal careers, paint their lives with tragedy, and turn all their feelings to bitterness. But the fact that all of this hardship can be contained shows how clearly the way has been marked for the unfortunate family, a way that obliges them to close ranks and somehow make do as long as the illness lasts.

Now turn to symptoms of mental disorder as a form of social deviation. In our society, what is the nature of the social offence to which the frame of reference 'mental illness' is likely to be applied?

The offence is often one to which formal means of social control do not apply. The offender appears to make little effort to conceal his offence or ritually neutralize it. Mental symptoms are not, by and large, *incidentally* a social infraction. By and large they are specifically and pointedly offensive. As far as the patient's others are concerned, the troublesome acts do not merely happen to coincide partly with what is socially offensive, as is true of medical symptoms; rather these troublesome acts are perceived, at least initially, to be intrinsically a matter of wilful social deviation.

It is important now to emphasize that a social deviation can hardly be reckoned apart from the relationships and organizational memberships of the offender and offended, since there is hardly a social act that in itself is not appropriate or at least excusable in some social context. The delusions of a private can be the rights of a general; the obscene invitations of a man to a strange girl can be the spicy endearments of a husband to his wife; the wariness of a paranoid is the warranted practice of thousands of undercover agents.

Mental symptoms, then, are neither something in themselves nor whatever is so labelled; mental symptoms are acts by an individual which openly proclaim to others that he must have assumptions about himself which the relevant bit of social organization can neither allow him nor do much about.

It follows that if the patient persists in his symptomatic behavior, then he must create organizational havoc in the minds of members. This havoc indicates that medical symptoms and mental symptoms are radically different in their social consequences and in their character. It is this havoc that the philosophy of containment must deal with. It is this havoc that psychiatrists have dismally failed to examine and that sociologists ignore when they treat mental illness merely as a labelling process. It is this havoc that we must explore.

Mental hospitals can manage such diffusions and distortions of identity without too much difficulty. In these establishments much of the person's usual involvement in the undertakings of others and much of his ordinary capacity to make contact with the world are cut off. There is little he can set in motion. A patient who thinks he is a potentate does not worry attendants about their being his minions. That he is in dominion over them is never given any credence. They merely watch him and laugh, as if watching impromptu theatre. Similarly, when a mental hospital patient treats his wife as if she were a suspect stranger, she can deal with this impossible situation merely by adjusting downward the frequency and length of her visits. So, too, the office therapist can withstand the splotches of love and hate that the patient brings to a session, being supported in this disinvolvement by the wonderfully convenient doctrine that direct intercession for the patient, or talk that lasts more than fifty minutes, can only undermine the therapeutic relationship. In all of these cases, distance allows a coming to terms; the patient may express impossible assumptions about himself, but the hospital, the family, or the therapist need not become involved in them.

Matters are quite different, however, when the patient is outside the walls of the hospital or office – outside, where his others commit their persons into his keeping, where his actions make authorized claims and are not symptoms or skits or something disheartening that can be walked away from. Outside the barricades, dramatically wrong self-identification is not necessary in order to produce trouble. Every form of social organization in which the patient participates has its special set of offences perceivable as mental illness that can create organizational havoc.

The maintenance of the internal and external functioning of the family is so central that when family members think of the essential character, the perduring personality of any one of their numbers, it is usually his habitual pattern of support for family-organized activity and family relationships, his style of acceptance of his place in the family, that they have in mind. Any marked change in his pattern of support will tend to be perceived as a marked change in his character. The deepest nature of an individual is only skin-deep, the deepness of his others' skin.

In the case of withdrawals – depressions and regressions – it is chiefly the internal functioning of the family that suffers. The burden of enthusiasm and domestic work must now be carried by fewer numbers. Note that by artfully curtailing its social life, the family can conceal these disorders from the public at large and sustain conventional external functioning. Quiet alcoholism can similarly be contained, provided that economic resources are not jeopardized.

It is the manic disorders and the active phases of a paranoid kind that produce the real trouble. It is these patterns that constitute the insanity of place.

The beginnings are unclear and varied. In some cases something causes the prepatient – whether husband, wife, or child – to feel that the life his others have been allowing him is not sufficient, not right, and no longer tenable. He makes conventional demands for relief and change which are not granted, perhaps not even attended. Then, instead of falling back to the *status quo ante*, he begins his manic activity. As suggested, there are no doubt other etiologies and other precipitating sequences. But all end at the same point – the manic activity the family comes to be concerned with. We shall begin with this, although it is a late point from some perspectives.

The manic begins by promoting himself in the family hierarchy. He finds he no longer has the time to do his accustomed share of family chores. He increasingly orders other members around, displays anger and impatience, makes promises he feels he can break, encroaches on the equipment and space allocated to other members, only fitfully displays affection and respect, and finds he cannot bother adhering to the family schedule for meals, for going to bed and rising. He also becomes hypercritical and derogatory of family members. He moves backward to grandiose statements of the high rank and quality of his forebears, and forward to an exalted view of what he proposes soon to accomplish. He begins to sprinkle his speech with unassimilated technical vocabularies. He talks loudly and constantly, arrogating to himself the place at the centre of things this role assumes. The great events and personages of the day uncharacteristically evoke from him a considered and definitive opinion. He seizes on magazine articles, movies, and TV shows as containing important wisdom that everyone ought to hear about in detail right now.

In addition to these disturbances of rank, there are those related to the minor obligations which symbolize membership and relatedness. He alone ceases to exercise the easy care that keeps household equipment safe and keeps members safe from it. He alone becomes capricious in performing the little courtesy-favours that all grown members offer one another if only because of the minute cost of these services to the giver compared to their appreciable value to the recipient. And he voices groundless beliefs, sometimes in response to hallucinations, which imply to his kin that he has ceased to regulate his thought by the standards that form the common ground of all those to whom they are closely related.

The constant effort of the family to argue the patient out of his foolish notions, to disprove his allegations, to make him take a reasonable view – an argumentation so despaired of by some therapists – can similarly be understood as the family's needs and the family's effort to bring the patient back into appropriate relationship to them. They cannot let him have his wrong beliefs because they cannot let him go. Further, if he reverses his behaviour and becomes more collected, they must try to get him to admit that he has been ill, else his present saneness will raise doubts about the family's warrant for the way they have been treating him, doubts about their motivation and *their* relationship to him. For these reasons, admission of insanity has to be sought. And what is sought is an extraordinary thing indeed. If ritual work is a means of retaining a constancy of image in the face of deviations in behaviour, then a self-admission that one is mentally ill is the biggest piece of ritual work of all, for this stance to one's conduct discounts the greatest deviations. A week of mayhem in a family can be set aside and readied to be forgotten the moment the offender admits he has been ill. Small wonder, then, that the patient will be put under great pressure to agree to the diagnosis, and that he may give in, even though this can mean that he must permanently lower the conception he has of his own character and must never again be adamant in presenting his views.

The issue here is not that the family finds that home life is made unpleasant by the sick person. Perhaps most home life is unpleasant. The issue is that meaningful existence is threatened.

Let me repeat: the self is the code that makes sense out of almost all the individual's activities and provides a basis for organizing them. This self is what can be read about the individual by interpreting the place he takes in an organization of social activity, as confirmed by his expressive behaviour. The individual's failure to encode through deeds and expressive cues a *workable* definition of himself, one which closely enmeshed others can accord him through the regard they show his person, is to block and trip up and threaten them in almost every movement that they make. The selves that had been the reciprocals of his are undermined. And that which should not have been able to change – the character of a loved one lived with – appears to be changing fundamentally and for the worse before their eyes. In ceasing to know the sick person, they cease to be sure of themselves. In ceasing to be sure of him and themselves, they can even cease to be sure of their way of knowing. A deep bewilderment results. [Consider] now some further aspects of the family's response.

One issue concerns the structure of attention. Put simply, the patient becomes someone who has to be watched. Each time he holds a sharp or heavy object, each time he answers the phone, each time he nears the window, each time he holds a cup of coffee above a rug, each time he is present when someone comes to the door or drops in, each time he handles the car keys, each time he begins to fill a sink or tub, each time he lights a match – on each of these occasions the family will have to be ready to jump.

Three points are to be made concerning the family's watchfulness. First, households tend to be informally organized, in the sense that each member is allowed considerable leeway in scheduling his own tasks and diverting himself in his own directions. He will have his own matters, then, to which he feels a need to attend. The necessity, instead, of his having to stand watch over the patient blocks rightful and pleasurable calls upon time and generates a surprising amount of fatigue, impatience, and hostility. Second, the watching will have to be dissimulated and disguised lest the patient suspect he is under constant surveillance, and this covering requires extra involvement and attention. Third, in order to increase their efficiency and maintain their morale, the watchers are likely to engage in collaboration, which perforce must be collusive.

The family must respond not only to what the patient is doing to its internal life, but also to the spectacle he seems to be making of himself in the community. At first the family will be greatly concerned that one of its emissaries is letting down the side. The family therefore tries to cover up and intercede so as to keep up his front and theirs. This strengthens the collusive alignment in the family against the patient.

As the dispute within the family continues and grows concerning the selves in whose terms activity ought to be organized, the family begins to turn outward, first to the patient's kinsmen, then to friends, to professionals, to employers. The family's purpose is not merely to obtain help in the secretive management of the patient, but also to get much needed affirmation of its view of events. There is a reversal of the family information rule. Acquaintances or other potential sources of aid who had once been personally distant from the family will now be drawn into the centre of things as part of a new solidarity of those who are helping to manage the patient, just as some of those who were once close may now be dropped because apparently they do not confirm the family's definition of the situation.

Finally, the family finds that in order to prevent others from giving weight to the initiatory activity of the patient, relatively distant persons must be let in on the family secret. There may even be necessity for recourse to the courts to block extravagances by conservator proceedings, to undo unsuitable marriages by annulments, and the like. The family will frankly allow indications that it can no longer handle its own problems, for the family cat must be belled. By that time the family members will have learned to live exposed. There will be less pride and less self-respect. They will be engaged in establishing that one of their members is mentally ill, and in whatever degree they succeed in this, they will be exposing themselves to the current conception that they constitute the kind of family which produces mental illness.

The family's conspiracy is benign, but this conspiracy breeds what others do. The patient finds himself in a world that has only the appearance of innocence, in which small signs can be found – and therefore sought out and wrongly imputed – showing that things are anything but what they seem. At home, when his glance suddenly shifts in a conversation, he may find naked evidence of collusive teamwork against him – teamwork unlike the kind which evaporates when a butt is let in on a good-natured joke that is being played at his expense. He rightly comes to feel that statements made to him are spoken so as to be monitored by the others present, ensuring that they will keep up with the managing of him, and that statements made to others in his presence are designed and delivered for his overhearing. He will find this communication arrangement very unsettling and come to feel that he is purposely being kept out of touch with what is happening.

In addition, the patient is likely to detect that he is being watched. He will sense that he is being treated as a child who can't be trusted around the house, but in this case one who cannot be trusted to be frankly shown that he is not trusted. If he lights a match or takes up a knife, he may find as he turns from these tasks that others present seem to have been watching him and now are trying to cover up their watchfulness.

In response to the response he is creating, the patient, too, will come to feel that life in the family has become deranged. He is likely to try to muster up some support for his own view of what his close ones are up to. And he is likely to have some success.

The result is two collusive factions, each enveloping the other in uncertainties, each drawing on a new and changing set of secret members. The household ceases to be a place where there is the easy fulfilment of a thousand mutually anticipated proper acts. It ceases to be a solid front organized by a stable set of persons against the world, entrenched and buffered by a stable set of friends and servers. The household becomes a no-man's land where changing factions are obliged to negotiate daily, their weapons being collusive communication and their armour selective inattention to the machinations of the other side – an inattention difficult to achieve, since each faction must devote itself to reading the other's furtive signs. The home, where wounds were meant to be licked, becomes precisely where they are inflicted. Boundaries are broken. The family is turned inside out.

## Acknowledgement

I am much indebted to Edwin Lemert and Sheldon Messinger and to Helen and Stewart Parry for help in writing this paper.

Erving Goffman, late Professor of Sociology at the University of Pennsylvania, was author of *Asylums, Stigma* and *The Presentation of Self in Everyday Life*. This article consists of edited extracts from an article that originally appeared in *Psychiatry: Journal for the Study of Interpersonal Processes*, XXXII, No. 4 (November 1969).

# 12

# Tangled feelings: an account of Alzheimer's disease

## JULIA BURTON-JONES

Tom and Dot were childhood sweethearts. They first met each other in their early teens and became boyfriend and girlfriend a couple of years later. They married in 1950 when Tom was 23 and Dot 22. Tom is proud to say that Dot was the only girlfriend he ever had.

In the first 34 years of their marriage, Dot and Tom enjoyed the best of health. Then, out of the blue, in 1984, Dot began to do strange things. The change that came about is marked in Tom's memory by an occasion when his wife attempted to boil eggs in a dry pan. Then he noticed that her concept of time was affected. She would prepare Tom's tea at odd hours. She was only 57 and Tom could not face the possibility that Dot's mind might be sick. He tried to ignore her strange behaviour and memory lapses but knew in his heart of hearts that something was badly wrong. This period of growing awareness of his wife's illness remains in Tom's mind as the worst time of all. He knew only too well that an older brother and sister of Dot's had suffered from Alzheimer's disease, but was horrified by the suggestion that his cherished wife might be going the same way.

Tom felt very alone in his suffering. To the outside world, there did not seem to be too much wrong with Dot. She looked a picture of health and even managed to continue working part-time. She retired in 1984 from the electronics company where she had been a valued member of staff, but continued for several years working as a cleaner for the city university under the supervision of her sisters-in-law.

Sadly, Tom felt his GP failed him. Had the doctor acted more responsibly, Tom sees now, his experience of caring could have been so different. Dot herself refused to accept anything was wrong with her and the GP said there was nothing he could do without Dot's consent. It seemed as though no one, neither relatives, nor professionals, understood the heartache Tom was experiencing. Isolated and driven to distraction coping with a sick wife, Tom reached rock bottom. He even considered committing suicide and taking Dot with him. Around about this time, Dot sprained an ankle out cleaning. Tom was overjoyed when she agreed to visit the doctor for help, anticipating that at last her more fundamental problem would be identified and help would swiftly follow. 'You look very well for your age! I hope I look as well as you do,' was the doctor's remark. Although it was not their own GP, Tom had hoped some mention of the concerns he had expressed earlier about Dot's health would appear in her notes. No reference to them was made, however, and once more Tom was left feeling that no one in the world grasped the reality of the situation he faced.

It was not until 1989, five years into Tom's ordeal, that he was eventually put in touch with an effective support system. A neighbour, whose husband was a stroke victim, mentioned Tom's plight to her social worker. The social worker visited Tom and, realising the enormity of his problem, contacted his [new] GP, his former GP having died. Help came swiftly from that point onwards. In September 1989, shortly after finishing her cleaning job, Dot was diagnosed as having Alzheimer's disease.

Tom has made it his business to acquire knowledge about Alzheimer's disease. He belongs to the Alzheimer's Disease Society, has read books and attended conferences on the illness, and talked to professionals in the field. The result is that he now knows what to expect in the future and can see how Dot has passed through many of the phases Alzheimer's patients endure. Initially it was Dot's memory that was lost. She would also suspect people of stealing things from her. She was like a squirrel, Tom says, too. She would wrap things up and hide them away in obscure places so that, in some cases, Tom would not find them again for several years. She would turn on the gas oven without igniting it.

In 1987, Tom began to see signs of the next stage of the illness, what he calls the 'wanderlust'. Dot began to disappear and would be found wandering miles from her home. This phase reached a climax in 1989 and was the most trying of all the problems. If Tom was not constantly vigilant, Dot would be out of the house in an instant. Throughout this phase, two further symptoms began to emerge. The first was one of continence. Dot became doubly incontinent, a factor which altered the form of care she needed from Tom dramatically. Also, she gradually lost the ability to speak so that she is now able to say nothing.

Up until this time, Tom was able to continue working full-time. He worked as a clerk of works for a housing association in the neighbouring city. Tom loves his work. He has strong views about it, believing the need for good housing to be the most important human need of all. Tom struggled on as long as he could, returning at 5.30 pm each day to face a gruelling evening of changing and cleaning Dot, preparing supper and somehow fitting in the time for washing, ironing and housework. Eventually it became too much for him and he began in 1990 to work part-time (from 8.30 until lunch-time each day). Dot spends the mornings during the week in a local authority home where she has her breakfast and lunch.

Tom now feels fortunate to have access to a range of support services. It was through Dot's hospital assessment in 1989 that Tom became aware of the help he could receive. He speaks highly of the consultant psycho-geriatrician at the local hospital who has given Tom two weeks' respite care for Dot when he has become over-tired. The consultant has also helped Tom fight for Mobility Allowance, a benefit denied him several times, but granted eventually by a tribunal in January 1991. Through the hospital Tom has received the advice of a community psychiatric nurse who has helped Tom receive continence pads that are far more effective than the ones previously supplied by the district nurses.

He still has moments of frustration caused by the inertia or incompetence of professional people. An occupational therapist agreed, when she assessed Tom and Dot's home, that they needed special rails and a shower in the bathroom. Tom had too many savings to qualify for a shower, but the rails were promised. While they waited to have hand rails fitted, however, Dot had a nasty fall in the bath and broke her nose. It was a traumatic experience for Tom, dressing her as she bled profusely, and rushing her to the hospital. In his exasperation, Tom went out the very same day and bought, out of his own resources, the items required to make the bathroom secure and, that evening, fitted them himself.

It was after Dot's diagnosis that Tom's relatives came to the dawning realisation that he was struggling at home. His brother lives in the next street and now calls in to see Tom every evening for half an hour and shops with him for a couple of hours on Saturdays. His wife cooks Tom's main, lunch-time meal of the day and takes it round when Tom gets in from work and at the weekends. This is a great help, as it means Tom only has to cook a snack in the evenings.

Tom can see that Dot has now moved into the next stage of Alzheimer's disease. Far from wandering constantly, she is now unable to stand on her own. He has to lift her from her chair and push her up the stairs to the bathroom when she needs changing. Once in the bath, he has to exert considerable strength in pulling her out. The incontinence is now a part of life. The day before I visited was the worst of all. Dot needed changing three times. Tom admitted to feeling so exasperated with Dot that he almost hit her. Of course, he felt very remorseful, but in that heated moment there was a real risk of him lashing out at Dot.

Because Dot is now unstable on her feet, she falls frequently, injuring herself quite badly. She strangely feels no pain, though, so does not complain, even on occasions, such as one several months ago, when she fell backwards and fractured her skull. The constant trips to casualty are very stressful for Tom, who is in a state of exhaustion anyway. He gets up at around 2.30 am every night to take Dot to the toilet or to change her. He then gets up at 6.15 am, cleans and dresses her, taking her to the toilet. At 8.00 am he leaves Dot at the old people's home and sets off for work. At 1.00 pm he collects Dot. He puts her on the commode (which is downstairs), and, if necessary, changes her. At 6.30 pm he then changes her pad and clothes again. Dot's incontinence generates mountains of washing and ironing. As Tom said, she needs treble the amount of clothes others have, as she wears three outfits a day. This costs Tom a lot of money as well as effort. Dot can no longer feed herself, so that Tom has to feed her.

By far the hardest thing about caring for a wife with Alzheimer's disease, says Tom, is the loneliness. He says he would much rather Dot's illness were a physical one. At least then he could still talk to her. At weekends, he can spend hours exchanging no words with anyone. He is so grateful for his brother's regular visits. Another friend who comes round faithfully for a chat on Saturdays is someone with whom Tom started a judo club back in 1950. Other friends, though, do not come anymore. The couple have no children and Dot's own living relatives have never shown any concern, let alone visited.

There are opportunities for Tom to spend time away from home, when Dot is in respite care, but he does not have the heart to go away on holiday and leave her, or even to have a night out at the pub. Tom is grateful for all the help he receives, only wishing he had known early on what he knows now. However helpful the people who visit are, though, he recognises that he is the one left with Dot, providing the care, when they leave.

Despite the many trials and the absence of rewards, Tom dreads the time when his wife's condition is so severe he can no longer look after her at home. He can hardly bear to think of Dot as she was, but says she was a devoted wife. He glows with pride as he remembers how spotless she kept the house, while working full-time, how she did all the cooking and baked her own bread. She was a very attractive woman, he boasts, and wore only the best clothes. He spent some time looking at old photos of her recently, but the memory was so painful he had to put them away again.

Tom's care of Dot is devoted. He respects her dignity totally, making sure she is always clean and continuing to buy for her the expensive clothes in which she always took pride. He knows only too well how horrified Dot would have been if she could have seen the state she is in now. He recognises his efforts are futile, in one sense, in that one day soon Dot will die, but the only defence he has is to avoid facing up to that reality. At moments when he is likely to start thinking too deeply about the tragedy of the situation, Tom finds something to do to take his mind off it. His small consolation is in knowing that Dot still just about recognises and feels at home with him. He is determined to keep her in the home they have shared now for almost 40 years for as long as possible. But he admits that life will be tough next year when he retires and spends all his time at home.

The future does not look rosy. Tom knows Dot will soon reach the stage when she spends most of her time sleeping. Then will come the phase when she stops eating. For now, he lives a day at a time, striving to give the ultimate care to a woman to whom he feels he owes a debt of gratitude and who will never be able to repay him.

This edited case-study is one of several in Julia Burton-Jones' book *Caring for the Carers*, published in 1992 by the Scripture Union, 130 City Road, London EC1V 2NJ. The book focuses on the experiences of people caring for a chronically ill or disabled family member at home and is based on interviews carried out by the author while she was a Researcher for the Jubilee Centre in Cambridge, and as part of the training programme, 'Action for Family Carers', organized by the Scripture Union Training Unit.

# 13
# The social impact of childhood asthma

## ANDREW NOCON AND TIM BOOTH

Asthma affects large numbers of people of all ages. One child in ten suffers from some form of asthma before the age of ten. In most cases, the asthma disappears before the child reaches adulthood but, for about one adult in twenty, it will reappear later in life.

A good deal of research has been, and continues to be, carried out on the causation and control of asthma. Less is known about the way that asthma affects sufferers' everyday lives. Nevertheless, asthma is responsible for time lost from school and from work, it can restrict sufferers' social lives and the lives of the people they live with, and it can affect sufferers' personal well-being and family relationships.

The focus of this report is on the social impact of asthma on sufferers and their families. It describes [part of] a research study carried out with asthma sufferers in Sheffield. [Interviews were conducted with the parents of 32 children, all but one of whom was under 10 years old, who had all been admitted to a Sheffield hospital in the previous year as a result of their asthma.]

### Restrictions on general activities

While some respondents experienced difficulties at all times, others only had problems when their asthma was bad. For the children, walking uphill caused the greatest degree of difficulty, affecting 28 per cent of the children most of the time. Some types of sport caused some difficulty most of the time for six of the 14 school-age children, while a further two had difficulties when their asthma was worse: most of these children experienced some difficulty with running. In another case, a child was unable to do any horse-riding because of an allergy to horses. A total of nine (64 per cent) of the school-age children thus experienced some degree of difficulty with some sport because of their asthma. However, as will be seen below, none of the children were in fact prevented by their asthma from taking part in sports activities at school. Outside school, some children were not always able to keep up with their friends, and one boy in the cubs had to do some physical activities in stages rather than all at once. Another child sometimes developed asthma if she went on a jumping castle.

Smoke in the atmosphere could trigger asthma attacks in some children and therefore made it difficult (or indeed impossible) for them to visit some relatives or friends of the family or to use some public transport (though the latter restriction was now less frequent as no smoking areas were generally available). One four-year-old boy had to keep well away from bonfires (and had to stay in on bonfire night); he also had to avoid fireworks and the smoke from birthday cake candles. Four children had to avoid places where animals might trigger their asthma, one could not go to parks with flowers or into hothouses where there was dense greenery; another could not paddle or play in cold water. A two-year-old child with severe and easily triggered asthma was unable to attend a playgroup (because excitement set off her asthma), play outside in spring or autumn (when the weather could turn cold), and her parents had to ensure they brought her back home early in the evening if they went out (as she was otherwise liable to become tired and wheezy); her parents also adopted precautionary measures such as keeping her away from bonfires.

## Household arrangements

[A] number of respondents [had] made practical changes around the home because of asthma. The most common change was the replacement of bedclothes, usually of feather pillows and duvets with synthetic ones. The parents of two children said that they adopted a generally more health-conscious approach to food because of their child's asthma; [the parents] of 22 per cent of the children avoided particular foods because they provoked allergic response.

Some respondents noted that, while they had been advised to make some changes in their living arrangements, they had not done so. Two respondents, for instance, had been advised to remove bedroom carpets in order to reduce the potential sources of asthma triggers but they had decided against this: the mother of a four-year-old girl said that she did not want the bedroom to seem 'clinical'. Another mother said she had been told to avoid a large number of potential triggers and her son's bedroom had been left very bare. This, though, had had little or no effect on his asthma: his bedroom had been gradually brought back to normal, with no harmful effects.

As with all potential triggers, the presence of pets could provoke asthma in some people but not in others. The parents of one young child had to get rid of some rabbits and a hamster almost as soon as they had bought them because they set off their son's asthma. Other parents, though, refused to give up a cat despite medical advice because they were certain that it was not a factor in their own child's asthma. Two respondents pointed out that it was not just a question of getting rid of any pets they might already have: their children wanted to have a pet and it hurt the parents not to allow them to have one.

In cases where a household member smoked, [less than a quarter of smokers gave] up smoking because it might make the asthma worse. However, many parents of asthma sufferers said that they did not smoke if their child was in the room. Others said that they would not allow visitors to smoke in the house.

Fifteen parents of children with asthma also said they did more housework because of their child's asthma. This typically involved additional cleaning and dusting.

## School

Fourteen of the children attended school. Only three of them had not missed any time off school in the past year because of asthma; the average number of days missed from school because of asthma was 6.6. The reasons given by parents for keeping their children off school included bad wheezing, breathlessness and bad coughing.

Eight of the children had suffered from asthma while at school. However, none of the children suffered any restrictions in the classroom and all were able to take part in sports and PE. In only three instances did children sometimes have to finish early when taking part in sports or PE: the activities mentioned in this context were running and circuit training.

One child did not have any medication at school, six were responsible for their own medication, and in six other cases the medication was kept and supervised by school staff. Most parents said there were a number of other children with asthma at school and the staff were used to handling the medication. In one case, though, this issue caused a major problem. Staff at the school in question said they did want the responsibility for handling or supervising medication; they added that they did not have enough staff to take this on anyway. The child's parents complained that the staff did not realise how important it was for him to take his medication regularly; one staff member had allegedly queried whether he even needed to take any drugs at all. Although this (five-year-old) child's medication was kept by a care assistant at the school, it was then up to the boy's seven-year-old brother to collect the medication each lunchtime and to give it to him.

The parents said that this was a very unsatisfactory state of affairs but they had been unable to find any other solution.

Asthma rarely affected children's relationships with others at school. One child had lost friends in the past because of his frequent admissions to hospital, but this was no longer a problem. Two others were unable to keep up with other children when they were running about. One parent said her son was picked on because of his asthma, though no specific examples were mentioned. With the one exception above, teachers were generally praised for being helpful and caring: only one teacher was said to be a little over-protective.

## Practical effects on carers' lives

Two parents had been taking a lot of time off work [because of their child's asthma] and felt they could not keep up their jobs; one child's aunt had been looking after him during the day but then became afraid she would not know what to do if he had an attack; the father of another young child gave up a job that involved a lot of time away from home and took a less well-paid job in order to help his wife with the care of their daughter. Two mothers wanted to go back to work, now that their children had started school, but they had decided not to do so just yet: they felt there should be someone at home in case there was a problem at school or if their children had to come home during the day.

For over half of the parents, asthma meant that they themselves had occasional bad nights' sleep: most of them consequently felt exhausted the next day. Seven of the parents experienced such exhaustion at least once a week. The mother of a three-year-old child noted that 'the worst thing about the asthma is the sleepless nights': other parents similarly referred to feeling exhausted through lack of sleep.

Six parents said that the asthma sometimes stopped them from going out socially. For most people, this only happened infrequently.

For [some] respondents, taking time off work had resulted in a loss of income: this varied from an occasional day's earnings to a total loss of wages or salary where people had given up work completely. In addition, asthma had involved extra costs. These were sometimes one-off costs such as for non-allergenic bedding, more suitable curtains or floor-coverings, vaporisers and nebulisers. More regular costs included travel costs to hospital [and] extra heating.

Some respondents had received additional income because of the asthma, though the amounts were often small. One parent had previously received a weekly addition under the former Supplementary Benefit scheme, as well as a grant for a vacuum cleaner. Three parents had received small payments from a private health care scheme when their children were admitted to hospital. However, the parents of one child mentioned that they had been unable to obtain private health cover for their daughter.

## Worry

The parents of four children said the asthma did not worry them at all. However, some of them pointed out that there had been times in the past, especially soon after onset, when it had caused them considerable worry; but they had now learned to live with it. The remaining respondents said that the asthma continued to cause them some degree of worry; the parents of two children [said] it was the cause of 'a lot' of worry. Respondents mentioned a large number of reasons for feeling worried. Many parents said they were aware that asthma can kill and had sometimes wondered whether their children would manage to recover from severe attacks.

Many parents said their main worry was whether their children would have further attacks, how serious those attacks would be, and whether appropriate help could be provided quickly enough. A quarter of the parents expressed serious worries about the future. Two parents were concerned how their children would manage once they started school. Five others were worried about possible long-term effects of the medication.

## Effect on family life

The worry caused by a child's asthma frayed many parents' nerves; frequent attacks could lead to tiredness and to short tempers; family holidays were ruined; arguments erupted about appropriate levels of medication; parents disagreed about whether or not to take the child to hospital; and admissions to hospital added to the tensions already present. One mother said the family had to adjust its lifestyle around the asthma, and this caused problems. Other family members sometimes resented the attention the child received and, for one family, the asthma was a further cause of stress in an already tense atmosphere.

However, respondents also said that crises brought families closer together and everyone tried to help out more. One mother said that the asthma had given her family a sense of 'togetherness' and had made them aware of the importance of the family as a unit. Another explained how it made her appreciate her daughter more: it helped her to realise how precious the children were. Several parents found that talking and sharing offered them a means of coping with the worries caused by the asthma: they needed to keep each other going.

Twenty-six of the children with asthma had brothers or sisters. In 11 (42 per cent) of these families, parents stated that asthma did not have any effect on relationships between the children. None of the parents felt that any of their other children 'picked on' the child with asthma. However, three said that one or more of their other children were jealous of the attention given to the child with asthma. The brothers of a young boy objected to him being allowed to get away with misbehaviour without being punished. One young girl was said to be jealous of her brother being able to go to hospital; another child became particularly distressed when her mother stayed in hospital with her sister. The sisters of a young boy who was allergic to horses initially resented having to give up horse-riding: even a few horse-hairs on their clothing could trigger off severe asthma attacks. Additional problems could arise if children shared a bedroom: two parents mentioned that this led to their other child being woken up and not getting enough sleep.

However, in one of these instances a young girl's sister would make a point of listening out for signs of asthma and then calling her parents. In all, nine of the parents said their other children were very understanding towards their brother or sister's asthma. One boy tried to stop other children from making his sister run around too much. Another was said to 'torment her brother less' because of his asthma. Other children generally tried to help out.

## Effects on children with asthma

Only one of the 16 children with an inhaler was embarrassed by using it. Indeed, using an inhaler was often seen by children as something special: something which children who did not have asthma often wanted to do as well!

Eighteen parents felt that asthma affected their children's behaviour in some way, mainly when they were unwell. At such times, several children were reported to become bad-tempered, though two became particularly quiet. One child was said to be very naughty when in hospital, another on coming home after a spell in hospital. The mother of a young boy admitted that she had molly-coddled him a little and that he now wanted his own way. Another mother said that her five-year-old son was allowed to get away with more than the other children because of his asthma.

However, only three children were said to try to 'use' the asthma to their own advantage. One breathed heavily in order not to have to go to school – though his parents said this did not work! The others feigned symptoms of asthma in order to get their own way, though in both cases the parents said this rarely happened now.

## Emotional effect on parents

Three parents were angry that their children should suffer from asthma. Other parents referred to the disruption it had caused within their families, for instance when they had to return home early from holidays. One mother said she became angry if her child showed signs of a cold, especially if they were on holiday, as this could signal the onset of an attack. Another voiced her anger at the exhaustion she experienced when her child had bad asthma. One person said her son wanted constant attention when he had asthma: this prevented her from getting on with other work. One mother said she tried desperately to do everything she could to avoid her daughter having to go into hospital – and felt angry when she nonetheless had to be admitted.

Two parents said they felt guilty because they might themselves have contributed to their children's asthma. One said she had started smoking two months before her daughter was born; in the other case the child was born prematurely and was admitted to a special care unit. In neither case, though, had these factors been formally identified as causes of asthma. Two other parents felt guilty that they could not prevent their children from getting asthma. Another felt guilty when the family was on holiday and everyone except her daughter were enjoying themselves. Three parents mentioned the effect on their other children. One parent said he had felt guilty in the past that his Christian faith was not strong enough for his son's asthma to be healed.

The majority (29) of parents felt confident in handling their child's asthma. Three, though, said they sometimes felt unsure what to do for the best when their child had a bad attack. One of these felt unable to do much herself and tended to panic, as did one of the other parents. Another commented that only a doctor could really know what to do: she herself relied on guesswork. An issue mentioned by several parents concerned the difficulty they experienced in deciding whether or not to seek medical help. Many doctors had themselves suggested that parents should seek medical assistance if they were in any doubt. But although most parents preferred to err on the side of caution, they did not want to be criticised for wasting doctors' time.

Asthma often imposed a considerable emotional strain on families. One mother stated that 'last year was just a nightmare' and she felt she had simply been 'working on overdrive': she had seen a doctor herself because of the strain she was under. Another said 'you live your life perpetually tired' and 'you never have a rest from an asthmatic'. When the other children also fell ill, she felt she just could not cope. A third noted that 'anxiety gets the better of you'. She felt very frightened when her two-year-old daughter had attacks and she stated that asthma 'affects you in some way most of the time'. The strain caused by asthma compounded the problems of one child's parents and brought them close to splitting up.

When they were at their wits' end, parents wanted someone to talk to, someone who could sit and listen while they aired their grievances or anxieties. This should be a professional person: they felt that other parents, for all their understanding and helpfulness, might not preserve the same degree of confidentiality.

The physical dimension of asthma does not fully account for its overall social impact on the lives of sufferers and their families. It is only through taking full account of the various emotional and practical aspects that make up a person's life that the impact of a condition such as asthma can be comprehensively assessed.

This article is a heavily edited extract from a report, *The Social Impact of Asthma*, commissioned by the Sheffield Asthma Society; the research was carried out by Andrew Nocon and Tim Booth in the Department of Sociological Studies at the University of Sheffield, and published by the Department in 1990. The original report also covers the social impact of asthma on adult asthma patients. Andrew Nocon is now at the Social Policy Research Unit, University of York.

# 14
# Coping with migraine

## SALLY MACINTYRE AND DAVID OLDMAN

The main emphasis in the following accounts is on the acquisition of our knowledge of migraine. In these two accounts we introduce the idea of knowledge as developing in a series of discrete *stages* concerned with experiencing the complaint, identifying it as migraine, and finally acquiring a repertoire of methods for coping with it. All migraine sufferers pass in turn through these stages. The forms of the repertoire of coping may change over time through a series of *phases*, each phase characterised by an emphasis on one or another cell in a typology of treatments. Shifts between these phases do not have any necessary sequence.

### Sally Macintyre's account

The first stage of my career as a migraine sufferer we characterise as being an anomic stage. My first migraine attack, which I distinctly remember, occurred when I was twelve. During the following five years I had further attacks ranging in frequency from every six weeks to six months. I was unable to name, predict or account for these experiences, and did not possess the appropriate vocabulary with which to describe them to others. I did not know what these attacks were or what they implied. Was I 'just tired', developing a serious illness, about to have a stroke, epileptic, or mad? I had no means of predicting attacks and I had no means of establishing how best to cope with them when they happened. They were thus inexplicable, unpredictable, not amenable to rational means of coping, and apparently alien to everyone else's experience.

The second stage was an identificatory stage, occurring when I was seventeen and lasting for several months. The trigger for this stage was my collapsing in public during an attack. Having been trying for five years unsuccessfully to explain to others that I had 'funny turns', this public manifestation forced a recognition of this account and the process of diagnosis was set in motion. After a number of diagnostic tests arranged by my GP I was admitted to a hospital in London for investigation. The whole of this identificatory stage was characterised by negative diagnosis, i.e. identifying and eliminating what I had *not* got. Thus, the tests I underwent were designed to examine the possibilities of a brain tumour (skull X-rays, angiogram, radioactive tracing tests), epilepsy (EEGs) and other CNS disorders (reflex tests, lumbar puncture). I was finally told, 'Well, you'll be relieved to hear that you haven't got a brain tumour after all – it's only migraine.'

Immediately after the diagnosis my emphasis was on the physicalist/ameliorative aspect of migraine. I accepted myself, and was so accepted by others, as a basically normal person who periodically experienced transient physical disturbances. These disturbances were regarded as being separable from me as a social being with a particular biography, personality and social environment: I was merely a host for occasional physical disturbances. The propensity to attacks was regarded as a morally neutral matter, a definition which I suspect was enhanced by the fact that the diagnosis was conducted through the high technology and high prestige of a neurological department, rather than, for example, a psychiatric department. Coping consisted of handling the attacks, once they occurred, with Cafergot-Q, and learning how to recognise the onset of an attack and how to judge the most efficacious dosage. My knowledge about these techniques derived only secondarily from my GP, mainly stemming from personal experience and trial and error.

On arrival at university my attention shifted to the 'personal/social' and 'preventive' cell. The student health service doctors were oriented towards patients as 'social beings in their total environment'. Rather than providing repeat prescriptions of Cafergot-Q, these doctors recommended recognition and avoidance of stressful situations, a reduction in ambition and competitiveness, and mild sedation at the onset of an attack. The prevailing etiological theory was that migraine was typical of over-conscientious, neurotic and intelligent women; role conflicts (e.g. degree versus marriage); and stressful life events (exams). I was redefined from a blameless, passive host to an active producer of migraines. I learnt and developed strategies for coping with the problem of being a 'migrainous person', mainly by stressing the assumed flattering correlations (conscientious, intelligent, sensitive), avoiding situations in which an attack would be disruptive, and exploiting the definition of myself as neurotic.

This phase of regarding migraine as a personal attribute reached a crisis when I moved to another university for a year and registered with the student health service there. My new GP believed that migraine was the result of deep-seated personality conflicts. When I declined to enter a course of psychoanalysis he refused to provide any further advice or chemotherapy. He variously informed me that my migraine resulted from my not having a boyfriend, sublimating my desire for children for postgraduate studies, and having over-strong internalised guilt and achievement-strivings. When I became depressed lest all these analyses were true, the migraine was attributed to depressive tendencies. These theories were to me highly unwelcome and on one level I rejected them. On another level I suspected that they might be true.

During this time I experienced an attack while on the top of a London bus, and found the experience of social and mental incompetence in such a situation to be deeply disturbing. I developed a fear of having an attack, which after a few months developed into acute anxiety states about travelling by public transport, eating in restaurants, attending seminars and other public meetings. My GP felt that my agoraphobia confirmed his previous character analysis of me, and attempted to refer me to another psychiatrist. When I was unable to keep the appointment, my plea that agoraphobia had prevented me from travelling across London was rejected as a rationalisation.

An acquaintance commented on my rather sorry state at this time, and when I explained the situation arranged for me to see her GP husband. He prescribed Valium. I began to conquer the phobias, started to eat properly again, found the frequency and severity of migraine attacks reduced, and ceased feeling panicky about the possibility of having attacks. I sought out information about the physical correlates of attacks, learned to stop eating certain foods, and wore dark glasses in bright sunlight. Over exams the GP put me on the Pill, which I found made a great improvement in the attacks previously correlated with the two days before a period. I thus moved out of the 'personal/social' phase back into a 'physicalist' phase, but this time one with the main focus on prevention. Having obtained what to me was satisfactory evidence that physical prophylaxis 'worked', I totally rejected the psychoanalytic interpretations of my previous GP, which I had in any case found injurious to my self-image.

When I moved to another part of the country I registered with a group practice and discovered that the practitioners espoused widely differing theories about migraine and its proper treatment. While registered with one doctor I continued regularly to consume Valium with his approval. He was interested in migraine, would discuss various new theories about it and tried out some of the new prophylactic drugs on me. When he left and I applied to another doctor for a repeat prescription I was scolded for taking dihydro-ergotamine and was refused further prescriptions. The next doctor spent six months weaning me off Valium; the fourth partner in the practice said that he himself was a sufferer, and found that Valium was the best way of managing it.

I registered with a new practice, and informed the new GP of the regimen I preferred. I now regard myself as an 'expert' patient, knowing exactly what I want and using the GP partly as a resource to supply me with those drugs that I want, but which are on prescription.

### David Oldman's account

The first significant point about my own career as a migraine sufferer is that I cannot remember my first attack. Fairly regular attacks began somewhere around the age of nine, but the anomic and identificatory stages took up no more than an hour or two of my life. My mother had experienced frequent attacks during childhood and adolescence and was presumably able to normalise my first encounter with the complaint. I have a dim recollection of my mother prescribing by her actions what became for me the standard organisation of an attack – bed, a darkened room, hot-water bottle, bowl within easy reach for the attacks of vomiting, and Lucozade as the only liquid I could tolerate. So, from the start I not only had the complaint identified, but was also given the elements of a therapeutic routine which changed little for twenty years.

The imposition of identification and routine has not necessarily been as helpful as one might expect. If it is done early in life it may prove very hard to alter, and may take on a ritualistic quality which may even hamper the possibilities of more effective

prevention and relief. I sweated my way through every attack in childhood surrounded by at least two hot-water bottles and never quite managed to convince
myself that I suffered less when chilled – a 'fact' to which I now subscribe. More
seriously, on four occasions in thirty years of attacks I have been caught in situations
in which it was impossible to withdraw from ongoing social routines. In three cases
I was able to get by, with much distress but not necessarily any more than I would
normally have felt in the comfort of my own bed. Indeed, on the two occasions when
I started an attack on top of a Scottish mountain, the effort of walking at least six
miles to safety distracted me from the pain. Occasionally I have wondered whether
withdrawal during an attack is either necessary or beneficial.

The very imposition of routine during my school years contained the seeds of
liberation. My attacks were then almost invariably associated with the relief of tension *after* two classes of event – exams and rugby matches. The frequency and
unpredictability of rugby matches made them loom largest in the production of
migraine. I suddenly found myself in a position of control, for when I left school I
stopped playing rugby and reduced my migraines to two attacks in five years!

Over the past thirteen years, during which period I have been regularly employed,
residentially stable and suitably married, my relationship with the medical profession
has been one in which I am invited to speculate on the causes and consequences of
migraine as a 'normal' member of society – indeed, one of rather high status. Provided that I remain within the boundaries of legitimate migraine pharmacology I can
discuss the effects of drugs and even request some rather than others. My current diet
of dihydro-ergotamine and Migril resulted from an egalitarian discussion with my
GP. The fact that I top this up with Stemetil and Valium for an actual attack is
unknown to him, and is only possible by 'borrowing' these drugs from friends and
relatives.

These ways of coping are not merely the result of achieving a 'normal' social status
in the lay sociology of the GP, but are also a result of a definite attempt on my own
part to 'medicalise' migraine given that, over the last thirteen years, I have lost the
power to correlate my attacks with features of my own life style. I get about three
attacks a year and if they correlate with anything at all, it is with quite major events
such as moving house or changing jobs – not aspects of one's life that can be stepped
around. I now have no way of avoiding migraine – I can only treat the attacks.

So far, then, my career as a migraine sufferer has been a prolonged attempt to find
improved physical methods of preventing, and particularly treating, attacks. My 'way
of life' has never seemed amenable to change in ways that would affect my migraines.
As a child I had no power over my social routines; as an adult my routines have been
regarded as too desirable to warrant change. The only development in my methods
has been an increasing awareness that I could dictate the physical treatments and, at
the same time, an increasing divergence from accepted and acceptable pharmacology.

### Discussion – the development of personal theories of migraine

The most striking difference between our two accounts is the different length of time
it took us to pass through the anomic and identificatory stages – $5^{1}/_{2}$ years compared
with at most a few hours. We attribute this to the respective absence and presence of
fellow-sufferers or 'wise' persons in our immediate social environments. We suggest

that it is not surprising that migraine 'runs in families', if the quickest identifier is a fellow-sufferer. Subsequent to her own diagnosis, Macintyre 'identified' classical migraine in her brother and sister.

When fellow-sufferers are available as identifiers, symptoms may rapidly be interpreted and named as being migraine, and we suggest that the learning process may be a didactic one of imparting received wisdom both about etiology and coping. In the absence of a pool of fellow-sufferers such symptoms may have to be interpreted by the medical profession. Such medical identification may rely more on the negative diagnosis described above – the successive elimination of alternative and more serious diagnoses – and may present the sufferer with fewer practical recipes for coping. Given this lack of practical advice or the outlining of etiological theories, the sufferer may then more actively search for knowledge from which to construct useful theories, and his knowledge may differ from that of a sufferer socialised by fellow-sufferers.

Another consequence of our differing experiences of identifying migraine is that it appears that Macintyre found the 'anomic' stage deeply disturbing and that this has left a greater residue of anxiety about the topic than that experienced by Oldman, with his relatively unproblematic and matter-of-fact introduction to migraine, mediated by 'wise' family members.

In general, Macintyre's experience more closely approximates the models of illness behaviour posited by medical sociologists than does Oldman's – an initial period of disorganised symptomatology, a 'trigger' for seeking medical help, diagnosis and treatment offered by the medical profession, and reappraisal of doctors' actions.[1,2,3,] We suspect that it is Macintyre's experience which is atypical, and that the experience of illness behaviour, diagnosis and coping, without contact with the medical profession, is a more ubiquitous and frequent phenomenon than is often implied in the medical sociological literature.

## References

1. Rosenstock, I. M. 'Why people use health services', *Milbank Memorial Fund Quarterly*, Vol. LXIV, No. 3, Part 2 (1966).
2. Mechanic, D. *Medical Sociology: A Selective View*, Free Press, New York (1968).
3. Stimson, G. and Webb, B. *Going to See the Doctor: The Consultation Process in General Practice*, Routledge and Kegan Paul, London (1975).

Sally Macintyre is Director of the MRC Medical Sociology Unit at Glasgow University. At the time of writing this article, David Oldman was a medical sociologist at Aberdeen University. This is an edited extract from a chapter with the same title which originally appeared in the book *Medical Encounters*, edited by A. Davis and G. Horobin and published by Croom Helm, London (1977).

# 15
# Coming to terms with diabetes

## DAVID KELLEHER

The study of people with diabetes reported here is not a study of a group of people who are peculiar in themselves; while attempting to describe some aspects of the social life that such people experience, this study does not assume that the illness dominates their lives. It is a study of a group of people with an impairment which makes them chronically ill, there is no cure; but in many ways they are very ordinary people, normal people managing a problem.

> I'm the same as the next. You know what I mean, I class myself the same as everyone else, even though I take injections, injections to keep yourself alive, I suppose. But I ain't no different from anyone else. (Mrs A, aged 23)

So the problem has a physical basis but it is also only one of the identities that people with diabetes present to the world of others.

The following conceptual categories have been developed to describe the strategies for living with diabetes among patients in this study: those who manage their diabetes and treatment regimen without altering their life-style are described as 'coping'; those who manage their diabetes and treatment regimen by minimizing the importance of it, but who also make changes in their life-style are described as 'adapting' to their diabetes; while a third group manage their diabetes by continually worrying about it.

The people in this sample of thirty diabetics were all aged over 17 and living in London. The respondents were interviewed once and in all but three cases interviews were conducted in their own homes. The interviews were semi-structured and tape-recorded. Where appropriate the views of another member of the diabetic's family were sought and observation in waiting rooms and in consultations has also been carried out.

### Being in control – 'coping'

The two central criteria used to differentiate those who were in control of their diabetes from those who were not, were:

1. the degree to which they followed medical advice, and;
2. whether they applied it in a variety of situations without restricting their lives in the process.

Respondents [were] asked what they did if a urine test they had made showed positive signs of sugar; what they did if they were ill with colds; whether they changed their diet or treatment if they were planning to do something energetic; or if they changed their treatment for any other reasons. On the basis of the answers to these questions, and any other volunteered statements relating to their making decisions about altering their treatment, they were classified as being either high or low in terms of being in control of their diabetes. Those who said they ate only a limited range of foods, for example, were said to be low in control. Those who said that they altered the timing or amount of their injections or the timing of meals to accommodate a change in their work or social life were said to be high in control. Only six of the thirty were classified as high in control.

One very determined young woman with a family to look after, Mrs B, was gradually reducing the amount of insulin she took because she said she was always going 'hypo', that is, getting the feelings of weakness and confusion resulting from having too low a blood sugar level,

> I've told the doctor I'm down to one [unit] and I still go hypo. I think I should cut out the insulin, just the evening. And he said: 'Well let's see how you go. Come back and see me in three months' – which to me, hypos for three months, is not good enough. I've got two babies to look after.

She had had a number of problems with her diabetes and as a teenager she had been reckless in her attitude to eating, but since having two children she felt her diabetes had improved in a way that, according to her, medical authorities seemed to doubt. She was in fact the person in the sample who knew most about diabetes from the medical viewpoint. Another person who was high in control was a very active man aged 76, Mr S, who carefully kept a chart of the results of his urine tests and then altered his diet if the tests showed positive. He said he had read up about diabetes in 'The Home Doctor'.

A further example of someone who was high in control was an insulin-dependent man in his thirties, Mr Y. He had a physically demanding job and he did not calculate his extra insulin needs very carefully. He either ate a Mars bar between meals if he felt his blood sugar was going low or gave himself extra insulin if he was going out for a drink and a meal with friends. Nevertheless he did make adjustments and in the casual way that fitted his 'macho' image of himself. Thus 'coping' with diabetes in this study meant attempting to control the disease, insisting that it fit in with daily life rather than dominating it.

## Adapting to diabetes – 'normalizing'

An alternative way of managing diabetes was followed by nine people who were not high in control but did regard themselves as healthy. They had given up some social activities such as eating out or going to some of the places they used to frequent but they appeared not to be concerned about these restrictions and accepted them as part of their 'normal' life-style. They accepted as normal the symptoms they experienced and did not make a great effort at controlling their diabetes to eliminate these symptoms.

Mr L accepted the fact that he felt very thirsty in the evenings and drank a lot of water and then had to get up in the night to got to the lavatory as part of what it is to have diabetes. His involvement with his work and his enjoyment of the food his wife cooked for the family also meant that following a diet was something in the back of his mind rather than dominating his thinking, although he did make the effort to avoid sugary drinks by taking his own drink with him to work. He also did not take his daily tablet because he had been told to take it with his breakfast and he did not usually have breakfast. However, his wife was less than happy with this strategy for handling his diabetes, especially when she was also disturbed at night.

Mr J, another respondent who saw himself as fit and healthy, described his eating habits:

At home here just cabbage, carrots, lettuce, tomatoes.

He said he had cut out rice, only drank Pils lager, did not eat café food because it was 'all greasy' and refused drinks from friends because he did not want to get 'his system upset'. He worked as a street cleaner and said his diabetes caused him few problems unless he rushed about at work, which made him break out into a sweat, which was possibly an effect of his diabetes. He accepted the restrictions and the symptoms but said he did take his tablets and did test his urine three times a week.

Another example of a man who normalized was Mr N who said that his diabetes did not trouble him much and he did not bother much about his diet although he had had a breakdown just after he had been diagnosed diabetic. He then went on to say:

I'm not one of those who ignores everything. It's a thing if you want to keep it under control, you've got to, you know, which I do.

He had given up his place in the pub darts team because he thought he was going out too much. Mr N is an example of someone who tried to hold his diabetes at arm's length. By controlling his life-style he was able to manage his diabetes in a way that kept it out of his mind most of the time. He did not check his blood sugar level but did check his weight carefully, which was perhaps a less threatening part of the regimen. He said that in other people's homes he refused food if it had too much sugar in it on the grounds that he was diabetic.

These nine people who accepted some restrictions on their lives without seeing them as restrictive saw themselves as healthy and managed their diabetes without worrying or agonizing about it. They accepted it as 'normal'; they did not make precise efforts to manage it by using the system of exchanges of foods so that they could continue to eat a varied and interesting range of food. If they did test their blood sugar levels they were more likely to do it as part of routine compliance rather than as a way of gaining information which they themselves would use in planning their eating activities. But neither did they complain about its effects on their lives. They achieved their own balance. Such people were not on the whole regarded by doctors as difficult patients but they are quite an important group to consider when trying to assess how diabetics perceive and manage their diabetes. What they mean when they answer doctors' enquiries by saying they 'feel fine' perhaps needs to be explored further.

## Worriers and agonizers

Half (fifteen) of the sample had difficulty in accepting [their diabetes] as a normal part of their life, either by giving it a low priority in their life (normalizing) or by being on top of it in terms of feeling confident enough to make adjustments in the treatment according to what activities they were planning (high control). Twelve of the fifteen (80 per cent ) regarded themselves as unhealthy. Not surprisingly all but one of the five newly diagnosed diabetics were in this category of seeing themselves as unhealthy.

Typical examples of the worriers included a woman of 75. She said she kept to a pretty restricted diet of salads and boiled fish but would not explain to people that she was diabetic because:

I mean they think it's a terrible thing.

She said she checked on the blood sugar level of her urine but wouldn't alter her diet because:

I wouldn't do it myself, no. No because it's one thing I'm not very clever regarding that.

A man of 58, Mr H, was being treated by diet only and had been diabetic for four years. He tried to keep to a diet and had given up going out to restaurants where he had previously enjoyed eating cakes or pastries. He tried also to get his wife to 'barbecue' (grill) the meat to reduce the fat on it. Overall he felt he was not managing the diet very successfully and he sometimes got up at one or two o'clock in the night to raid the fridge. He thought about his diabetes constantly and was concerned that there was no cure,

in this case you cannot get rid of what is wrong with you and it is always with you.

He was in the process of slowly withdrawing from the running of his shop and handing it over to his son.

These two people were not in great pain or severely disabled by their diabetes but they were worried about it and aware of the effect it was having on their lives and on themselves. Mr H, in particular, thought he had become both irritable and someone who worried over problems without taking action to deal with them. The role of diabetic was high in his hierarchy of roles and had salience across many other roles. The five people who were classified as 'agonizers' were in a similar position to the 'worriers' in that they were unhappy about their diabetes and it remained a problem for them in their everyday life. They were different from the worriers in the degree of their concern about it. A number of them spoke about being depressed about it. One woman, Mrs E, was several times in tears during the interview. She found it difficult to keep to the diet and felt hungry after meals but in spite of the diet she was still putting on weight. She was an insulin-dependent diabetic and found the business of injecting herself a strain, she hated doing it.

Before I never used to take an injection in my life so I'm very very much scared about needles ... I manage to do it, but I don't feel alright with it. But I still manage to do it, and worst of all, two times a day, which is so difficult.

The idea that she had an incurable disease worried her a great deal, she compared it to TB which she said was thought of as a terrible disease but she felt diabetes was worse.

Another woman, Mrs D, was also in a depressed state. She lived in council housing with her unmarried daughter and the daughter's three children and was supported by social security payments. Her physical health also seemed poor and she, like all the agonizers, thought of herself as unhealthy. She said she found it difficult to keep to a diet because it was expensive and because the children did not like salads. Her sight was poor and she said she had difficulty in crossing roads because of this, consequently she did not go out very much. She said:

I don't mix with anyone, just the family.

Her blood sugar level was not well controlled and she had a number of other symptoms besides being overweight and having poor eyesight. Her poor economic circumstances did not help her to feel able to manage her diabetes, which remained a source of worry for her, restricting her activities and encouraging her to see herself as a sick person. Towards the end of the interview she said:

I do get irritable at times. It's a terrible feeling. I was never miserable, always happy, you know. I can sit here now with the family and not say one word some days, just sit there with the hump for no reason at all.

## Conclusion

Coping is a word much used by health-care professionals who are keen to find examples of coping strategies which can be taught to people who have not developed them themselves. As it is used in this study, however, coping has referred to the kind of behaviour and meaning which some people have constructed around their experience of having diabetes; they see diabetes as a practical but manageable problem; but, as an experience, it is not something which can easily be taught to others.

Those who coped with their diabetes were in a minority, being characterized by having a basic knowledge of how treatment works and the determination to apply that knowledge. They were prepared to alter their treatment regimen rather than reduce their social roles, their engagement with others in the social world. The role of being a diabetic was for them a less salient role in their identity than being a husband, a wife, a worker, or a mother; they did not deny the reality of their diabetes but, by trying out alterations in their medication and exploring the boundaries of their own reactions, they achieved a sense of control. They did not deliberately take risks, but attempted to apply the principles of diabetes care that they had learned from medicine, and were sometimes likely to be labelled as 'difficult' patients because they felt that their own knowledge of diabetes, gained by experience, was more appropriate than the doctor's generalized scientific knowledge.

From the evidence of this sample, however, more diabetics manage their diabetes by adapting to it rather than by coping with it. The adapters have minimized diabetes as a practical problem but it remains a problem at the cognitive level and the meaning they give to their diabetes is only relatively stable. Those who have accepted that they have diabetes but have altered their social relations and level of engagement in social life, and who, in some cases have accepted the continuance of some symptoms, are described as being normalizers. In their day-to-day living there is an element of denial that their diabetes causes significant problems as they attempt to achieve a normal but restricted life. They do not take on the diabetic role in public, but backstage in their lives the spectre of it remains. They have constructed a place and a meaning for diabetes in their lives by reducing their roles in situations where they feel their claims to being normal are vulnerable.

Those who constantly worry or agonize about their diabetes find that it interferes with their other roles, and their health ceases to be a taken-for-granted resource or springboard from which they can manage everyday life. For these people diabetes achieves a dominant place in their identity; it remains a problem at both the practical and cognitive level.

In summary, the experience of chronic illness, for some, is one of existential insecurity, as the British Diabetic Association poster showing people walking a tightrope across Niagara Falls suggests; for others it is much less stressful – the physical disruption of the metabolic system is managed and so is the disruption of the person, the self. It is with describing variations in experience such as these that the present [article] has been concerned.

Those responsible for the care of diabetics are already concerned about improving the level of knowledge that diabetics have about their diabetes; the evidence of this study suggests that important though this is it will not be sufficient. It might also be helpful if doctors were able to distinguish those who are high in control from those who deal with questions by normalizing the restrictions they impose on their lives and the symptoms they push to one side. It could also be helpful if doctors gave their attention in consultations not only to the practical problems of managing diabetes but to the cognitive problem of what having it means to an individual. Those described here as worriers or agonizers need support and reassurance with regard to the particular problems they face. In sum, the strategies adopted by patients relate to a broad psychosocial terrain, and this needs careful consideration if the experience of living with diabetes is to be at the centre of medical management.

David Kelleher is a Reader in the Department of Sociology at the Guildhall University in London. This article is an edited extract from his chapter 'Coming to terms with diabetes: coping strategies and non-compliance' which appeared in *Living with Chronic Illness*, edited by R. Anderson and M. Bury, published by Allen & Unwin, London (1988). David Kelleher has also published a book, *Diabetes*, in 'The Experience of Illness Series', Routledge, London (1988), and is the editor, with Jonathan Gabe and Gareth Williams, of *Challenging Medicine*, Routledge, London (1994).

# 16
# Living with HIV and AIDS

## NEIL SMALL

### Introduction

The way HIV and AIDS is talked about is not something neutral. It is, for many, a part of the problem and an aid to the virus. Particularly powerful is the way terms are run one into the other. HIV/AIDS is presented as if two things were one and the same. They are not. AIDS is equated with death in a way that superimposes one term on the other. This article argues for a different way of talking, which recognises that the challenges of living with HIV and of living with AIDS are different. Further, and most important, in the way that we talk about and respond to AIDS, we must make space for the experience of living *with* AIDS rather than dying *from* AIDS.

HIV is a global epidemic and, just as the virus is transmitted across national boundaries, so too are images of HIV-positive people and people with AIDS. Of particular importance has been the way responses to the epidemic in the USA have impacted on other countries. There are many examples. Film star Rock Hudson seeking treatment in France and then returning to the USA to die offered an image of the person with AIDS as 'wasted', hollow cheeked and emaciated. The publicity around the diagnosis and the deaths of celebrities and the portrayals of HIV and AIDS in popular culture, including Jonathan Demme's 1993 Oscar-winning film 'Philadelphia', have imprinted aspects of the US experience on the worldwide epidemic.[1]

In talking about living with HIV and AIDS this article will refer to academic literature from the UK and also from the USA, but will seek to concentrate on the growing body of autobiography that is informing us about those things that change and those that stay the same after you find you are HIV positive.

### The public and private worlds of HIV and AIDS

One of the paradox's of HIV and of AIDS is that they have a very high public profile. They are much discussed phenomena. But at their centre is something that for many people is intensely secret. For this is not just an individual's illness and part of a worldwide epidemic; it is also something for which people are stigmatised. It is linked, in the public eye, with a series of accompanying characteristics, all of which are subject to social disapproval. Male homosexuality, injecting drug-use, prostitution, promiscuity, prisons, are all assumed to sit in close proximity to HIV infection. To be HIV positive, in the view of much of the public debate, is evidence of complicity because of an assumed involvement in one or more of these activities. These are the guilty as well as the infected. (There are 'innocents' in this public view of the epidemic; children born to HIV-positive mothers who in turn become positive, those infected during blood transfusion and those haemophiliacs who contracted the virus before the routine screening and treatment of the blood they received.)

The second paradox is that the high public profile of the epidemic sits alongside a considerable public ignorance about its origins, its transmission, its progression and its prevention. It is as if the very way we have chosen to talk about the epidemic gets in the way of us hearing properly about how to respond to it. It becomes a problem for *them* and not for *us*. Out of such evasions the epidemic spreads.

What this means for people seeking to live with HIV and with AIDS is that they not only have to cope with the impact of the virus, but also with ignorance and hostility. Consider Amanda Heggs, a person living with AIDS, writing in 1989:

> Sometimes I have a terrible feeling that I am dying not from the virus, but from being untouchable.[2]

Others do not feel eligible to seek help because they do not associate themselves with the public image of people with AIDS. Alan was diagnosed as having AIDS. He lived with his wife and child in a city in the north of England. He felt a considerable need for information and support after his diagnosis. Although the hospital offered some help, he wished to meet others who had AIDS and others involved in caring for partners with AIDS. There was an organisation nearby which could have met these needs, but Alan identified it as somewhere for gay people, not for him.

> It's for people who are, you know, people who are . . . well that's their life. My life's here at home. I'm not like that and I don't really want to associate with them.[3]

Identifying the epidemic with certain groups of people means, for others, that they can rationalise not changing their behaviour. A man in an Edinburgh pub sitting with his girl friend says:

> Condoms? Well, yeah, I use them. But not all the time. Who the hell does? Anyway, if only one woman in 250 has got it, they're not bad odds are they?[4]

The idea that HIV and AIDS can affect anybody has been difficult to communicate effectively. Tony sums up his thoughts:

> I think generally people think if you have got AIDS or you're HIV positive you've got to be full of spots and look right weird. I think a lot of people still don't understand, you know, that people are just normal with it. I mean, I must admit prior to my getting it, when it was ever mentioned on television or through the media or anything like that, I used to think, 'Oh, you would be able to tell if somebody's got that.' But you can't. Unfortunately I've proved it myself.[3]

If stigma, evasion and denial are important features of the epidemic, there are also much more positive features to report. The dominant public reaction has been countered by individuals who have spoken out on behalf of the rights and needs of those people infected and affected by the epidemic. There has been a major achievement in reducing the spread of HIV amongst gay men.[5] Many people have entered into collaborations with scientists and, in so doing, have speeded the growth of knowledge about patterns of virus transmission and have aided experimentation and innovation in treatment. Others, sometimes the same people, have confronted the prejudice evident in reactions to the epidemic. In so doing they risk vilification, but contribute to the necessary realisation that it is not 'others' who are at risk, but everybody.

For those living with HIV and with AIDS anxieties can be raised when the politics of the epidemic appear to come into conflict with what they see as their lifeline to doctors and hospitals. Nigel moved from London to the north of England and then became ill. He felt vulnerable because he was 'on strange ground and I need all the help I can get.' But activists criticising the care he was offered raised his levels of anxiety. 'They were asking sick people to join in criticism of hospital authorities'. He shared some of their concerns, but his agenda was much more focused on the short-term need to overcome his illness, and for that he felt he had to have confidence in those treating him.[3]

Some HIV-positive people, people with AIDS and those close to them, have acted to care *for* and to care *about* others, to do something at the level of the individual and to do something about the social context of the epidemic. Examples include the development of 'buddying', of self-help groups, of organisations including the Terrence Higgins Trust and the London Lighthouse, and of activist groups such as ACTUP. In the USA, and influential in many countries, are the examples of Gay Men's Health Crisis and of the Names Project. One commentator identified the AIDS epidemic as:

> . . . the only epidemic in history in which relatively large numbers of people have actively assisted the dying over a prolonged period of time. It is even more distinctive because it represents an epidemic where the dying themselves also provided help to others and where helping others was viewed as a way to prolong their own lives.[6]

For some of those involved, such a mobilisation of care can be life enhancing. People see that it is possible to reclaim power over their own lives.[7] One member of the self-help group Frontliners says:

> I am not suffering with AIDS, I'm living with AIDS . . . It's not necessarily the quantity of your life, it's the quality that matters.[8]

For others the gains are more modest, but no less valuable. Juan came from Spain. He was living by himself in London. He tells how he sought out places that would accept him, that would stop him feeling so alone.

> I went to the Terrence Higgins Trust. I think they were so beautiful to me in there, even though I was an AIDS patient. The people were so nice. I spent one afternoon, two hours, talking about the illness. This person he had as well exactly the same virus and more or less exactly the same things as I had with my legs.[3]

## HIV and AIDS are not the same thing

The different ways individuals live with the virus is, in part, conditioned by the physical manifestations of being HIV positive or of having AIDS. To be diagnosed HIV positive does not automatically mean that one has any symptoms of HIV-related illness. To be diagnosed as having AIDS involves a medical judgement about the state of an individual's immune system, but also includes outward manifestations of ill health. The needs of someone who is HIV positive and their ability to live in the world, are thus shaped in very different ways from those of someone with AIDS. To try and live as if nothing had happened, or to be preoccupied with keeping healthy, are possible when you are HIV positive.

> I had grown accustomed to life under the sign of the plus. It was my cross to bear and I bore it without boring others. My cell count hovered in the upper two hundreds, I suffered occasional fungal flowerings, but in every other aspect my life was uninhibited by anything more serious than a condom.[9]

When you are living with AIDS the same is true for periods of one's life, sometimes long periods, but these are interspersed with times when one is having to be helped to cope with sickness. The balance between the two sorts of life varies. Paul Monette, writing about his own life with AIDS, tells how

> One of the cruellest ruses of the virus is letting you think the good times are the real times.[10]

The advances in treatment and care that are evident now mean that many people will live longer with AIDS. In the past, AIDS was a syndrome manifest via a number of episodic, serious and often worsening illnesses that had to be treated in hospital; now it has become a chronic illness. For much of its duration it can be managed in an outpatient setting. But at the same time HIV and AIDS are becoming more identified with poverty. Both in its worldwide distribution, and in the changing picture of infection in western countries, we can see a shift towards lower-income groups, towards women and towards people of colour.[11,12]

The consequences of these crucial changes in the pattern of the epidemic will impact profoundly on who lives with HIV and AIDS and what course their life is likely to take. The essence of living with AIDS in situations of economic adversity is to struggle for survival. In this respect it resembles living with any serious and life-threatening condition, which can be seen as a situation in which one has to reconcile issues of personal loss and personal resolve, and is therefore about survival. Further, surviving with any serious illness is, for many people:

> . . . a profoundly social phenomenon . . . More than a matter of simply individual luck or will, survival has always been contingent upon the most basic requirements of human existence, the most basic structures and values of human society. Food and shelter, work and rest, family and friends.[13]

The specific circumstances of living with AIDS include the possibility that society at large may act to the disadvantage of this group, and further, that economic adversity may make the possibility of improvements in treatment an irrelevance for affected people in many parts of the world.

I will conclude this section with Ian's words as he separates HIV and AIDS, as he contemplates his death and as he considers the stigma he sees attached to his diagnosis.

> HIV means you are going to live. AIDS means you're dying. That's the way I look at it. HIV you can go on for years, but once you are full blown, you know, you are on a downward trek, there's no if's and but's about it, you're on your way out. It's such a futile thing. What can you do? ... When you read in the paper about the amount of people who have got it and the amount of people who are dying from it ... I think things are going to be very hard ... People think its cancer. Well, that's what we tell everybody officially.[3]

## What changes and what stays the same?

For some people diagnosis changes everything; for others there are times when it can seem to impinge very little. Novelist Harold Brodkey decided 'to try to go ahead and have AIDS, live with AIDS for a while'. But he still saw becoming ill and being diagnosed as 'how my life ended and my death began'.[14] There is a clash between a sense of certainty in terms of one's death and uncertainty about how one will be able to live from day to day. Novelist Edmund White, who found he was HIV positive in 1985, reflects on those around him who live with AIDS:

> The person with AIDS ... sees through necessity to the end of all needs – death. This vision neutralizes everything that is cosy, familiar and automatic. Someone once said that we couldn't go on living if we knew the moment of our death. AIDS gives us that tragic certainty. If we go on living, it's either courage or purest folly.[15]

John MacLachlan stresses:

> The uncertainty which seeps into every aspect of my life, from the mundane to the profound, is not insurmountable. It just reminds me, all the time, how strange the business of living is.[16]

As others have done, John MacLachlan talks about how his diagnosis did not mean that everything else stops:

> The day-to-day world doesn't stop just because you're hurting. A letter from the council says my poll-tax rebate runs out next month. I have to reapply.[16]

One poignant testimony from an HIV-positive woman in the USA underlines the recognition that there will be other, more fundamental, existing obligations that will continue:

> I'm not telling my mother about the HIV yet. I'm hoping that by the time I need her to take care of us she will love the baby so much that she won't put us out.[17]

The problem is the same for Susan in Scotland:

> I've got things planned just in case ... I've got care provision planned for them, which was a big battle, you know. Social Work Department was coming 'Wait till you're ill'; I was going 'No danger am I waiting till I'm ill.' I'll have enough to worry about when I'm ill, to use my energy up to get better, without having

to put up with all this getting childcare for my kids. Not just any childcare, I want somebody that's going to love them as much as I love them.[18]

Some concerns are more to do with the problems in pursuing the interests of the past. A year after his first admission to hospital Bill was feeling quite good.

I run about, I go and watch my local football team, I try and play myself, but . . . there's just the odd day when I feel really tired. There are days when I just can't seem to get going, when I can't get out of first gear. But generally, yes, I'm well. I wouldn't say . . . yes. I suppose I am enjoying life again.[3]

But Bill is aware of the precariousness of his health.

I go for check ups and to have little things that I felt were going wrong put right. I rang [my doctor] last Monday. He said 'Don't worry. I don't envisage anything going really wrong for some considerable time.' So obviously he knows something that I don't, you know as regards . . . if my blood's OK and everything.[3]

Sometimes the reaction to diagnosis is surprising. When Jane spoke of what being diagnosed HIV positive had meant for her, she said that 'it was the best thing that could have happened to me.' She went on to explain that she had repeatedly tried to give up drugs, nothing had worked until now – the shock of the diagnosis had provided the impetus to try again, and she was confident of success. Her rationale for the diagnosis being good news was that the drugs would have killed her more quickly, and more surely, than HIV.[3] Likewise Peter heard his diagnosis and felt some relief. His symptoms had been so dramatic that he had felt he would die that night. Now 'at least I had some time.'[3]

What stays the same, as HIV and AIDS spreads, and as the characteristics of those living with these conditions changes, is the reality of an epidemic that is not just a health issue. It goes beyond issues about type and availability of medicine. It raises issues about access to health and social care, about suitable housing, about social injustice, human rights, and the search for health education that reflects the needs of those at whom it is targeted rather than the prejudices of those who devise it.[19]

## Carrying on living with HIV and AIDS

How one lives with HIV and AIDS is a mixture of what the individual chooses to do and what they are allowed to do. One has choices, but the scope either to envisage them or to realise them is shaped by the characteristics of the illnesses associated with AIDS, by the possibilities for care and treatment, and by the social reaction to the epidemic. To argue that a person's life with HIV or with AIDS is shaped by a mixture of the personal, the biological and the social is to risk sounding trite. All of our lives are shaped by such forces. But living with HIV and AIDS involves adding intensity to this commonplace. There is an intensity generated by the vehemence of the symptoms associated with AIDS. There is an intensity in the social context – both a destructive hostility and a realisation that there is real fellow-feeling, support and resistance. There is, finally, an intensity generated by the individual and social encounter with mortality that diagnosis and symptoms engender.

## References and notes

1. Discussed further in Small, N. 'Dying in a public place', in Clark, D. (ed.) *The Sociology of Death, Sociological Review Monograph*, 40 (1993).
2. Amanda Heggs, quoted in *The Observer*, Review of the Year, 31 December (1989).
3. Between 1989 and 1993 Neil Small was involved in research into aspects of AIDS, which allowed him close access to the lives of a small group of people living with AIDS and to those most intimately caring for them. Many of these people's reflections on the challenges of living with AIDS were tape-recorded; the words of some of those who were enthusiastically supportive of such use being made of their experiences are quoted in this article. Names have been changed.
4. Quoted on p. 10 of Dalrymple, J. and Kingman, S. 'AIDS, and the ostrich position', the *Independent on Sunday*, 15 July, 8–10 (1990).
5. King, E. *Safety in Numbers*, London, Cassell (1993).
6. Quoted on p. 8 in Chambre, S. M. *Volunteers and AIDS Organisations: Responses to a Public Health Emergency*, Centre of Business and Government, Washington, D.C. (1989).
7. Spence, C. *AIDS: Time to Reclaim our Power*, Lifestory, London (1986).
8. Quoted on p. 113 of Silverman, D. 'Making sense of a precipice: constituting identity in an HIV clinic', in Aggleton, P., Hart, G. and Davies, P. (eds) *AIDS: Social Representations, Social Practices*, Falmer, London (1989).
9. Moore, O. 'My days as an acronym', *The Guardian Weekend*, 16 April, 10 (1994).
10. Quoted on p. 302 of Monette, P. *Borrowed Time*, Collins Harvill, London (1988).
11. World Health Organisation, *Global Programme on AIDS*, Geneva (1992).
12. Drucker, E. 'Epidemic in the war zone: AIDS and community survival in New York city', *International Journal of Health Services*, 20(4), 601–615 (1990).
13. Quoted on pp. 583–584 of Krieger, N. and Margo, G. 'The politics of survival', *International Journal of Health Services*, 20(4), 583–588 (1990).
14. Quoted on p. 6 of Brodkey, H. 'My life, my wife and AIDS', *The Guardian Weekend*, 19 March, 6–16 (1994).
15. Quoted on p. 7 in Mayes, S. and Stein, L. *Positive Lives. Responses to HIV*, Cassell, London (1993).
16. MacLachlan, J. 'When you ache for life it's worth taking risks', *The Observer*, 13 January (1991).
17. Quoted on p. 205 in Simpson, B. J. and Williams, A. 'Caregiving: a matriarchal tradition continues', in Kurth. A. *Until the Cure*, Yale University Press, New Haven, 200–211 (1993).
18. Quoted on p. 19 in Littlewood, B. 'Life, love and HIV: the women's symposium on HIV and AIDS', *Critical Social Policy*, 40, 5–23 (1994).
19. Quoted on p. 239 in MacGuire, F. 'Women do not get AIDS they just die of it', *Health and Social Care*, 1, 239–250 (1993).

This article has not been published previously. The author, Neil Small, is Senior Research Fellow in the Social Policy Research Unit, University of York. He is the author of *Politics and Planning in the National Health Service*, Open University Press, Buckingham (1989) and *AIDS: The Challenge. Understanding, Education and Care*, Avebury, Aldershot (1993). He is currently engaged in research into the care of the dying.

# 17
# Pride against prejudice: 'lives not worth living'

## JENNY MORRIS

In May 1990, a 31-year-old man, Kenneth Bergstedt, petitioned the Las Vegas courts for permission to 'end his painful existence'. The press reported that he was 'a 31-year-old quadriplegic hooked to a respirator for more than 20 years' for whom 'life was no longer worth living'. A psychiatrist backed up his application by telling the court that 'The quality of life for this man is very poor, moderated only by momentary distraction, but forever profaned by a future which offers no relief.'[1]

This case is but one of an increasing number which have occurred in the USA over the last few years. The first one to be taken up by the disability movement was that of Elizabeth Bouvia, who had cerebral palsy. Dr Paul Longmore, a historian who is also disabled wrote:

> A 26-year-old woman, attractive and educated, checks herself into a hospital psychiatric unit announcing her wish to commit suicide. She reports that she has undergone two years of devastating emotional crises: the death of a brother, serious financial distress, withdrawal from graduate school because of discrimination, pregnancy and miscarriage and, most recently, the breakup of her marriage.
>
> She also has a serious physical disability, which she says is the reason she wants to die.
>
> Three psychiatric professionals ignore the series of emotional blows, concluding that she is mentally competent and that her decision for death is reasonable. They base their judgement on one fact alone – her physical handicap.[2]

The judge who heard the Bouvia case pronounced '. . . she must lie immobile, unable to exist except through the physical acts of others' and expressed the hope that her case would 'cause our society to deal realistically with the plight of those unfortunate individuals to whom death beckons as a welcome respite from suffering'.[2]

A key question for the American courts in these cases has been whether the person petitioning for 'assisted suicide' is taking a rational decision, that is, whether their wish to die is determined by emotion or impulse, or whether it is a reasonable judgement based on a realistic assessment of their situation.

As disability activists like Paul Longmore and Mary Johnson have pointed out, this assessment is made by people who often have no experience of disability, are certainly not disabled themselves and who find it inconceivable that someone who is completely (or almost completely) paralysed and who may have to use a respirator even to breathe, can experience a life which is worth living.

It seems to be relatively easy for the non-disabled world to judge that people who require physical assistance to such a high degree are making a rational decision when they say they want to die. It has been left up to other disabled people to examine the social and economic context in which such decisions are made. The case of Larry McAfee, whose case hit the American press in 1989, illustrates the way in which it is not the physical disability itself but the social and economic circumstances of the experience which can lead to a diminished quality of life.[3]

McAfee was aged 34 when a motorcycle accident resulted in complete paralysis and the need to use a ventilator. His insurance benefit (of $1 million) enabled him to employ personal care attendants in his own home for a period after his accident but when this ran out he was forced to enter a nursing home. He decided life wasn't worth living and tried turning his respirator off but couldn't cope with the feeling of suffocation. So he petitioned the courts to be allowed to be sedated while someone else unplugged his breathing apparatus.

In the event, he acquired a delay mechanism which would allow him to turn off the respirator himself and still allow for sedation, and the court ruled that he could not be stopped from doing so. Throughout the case and the publicity accorded to him, the general assumption was that McAfee's decision was a rational one based solely on the extent of his physical disability.

Yet when, as a result of the publicity, McAfee received an outpouring of support from disability activists, he decided to delay the decision to take his own life. What he really wanted was to live in his own home and to get a job. A disability organization arranged for him to receive training in voice-activated computers and he received tentative offers of employment. However, at this point, his Medicare benefits (the more generous part of the American health benefit system) ran out and the less-generous Medicaid would not pay for his place at the nursing home which was equipped for people who use a respirator. The Georgia Medicaid regulations did not allow Medicaid benefits to be used on home care but McAfee, together with disability activists and organisations, tried to get a waiver to the regulations to allow him to hire care attendants in his own home.

The type of nursing home which was equipped for McAfee's needs cost between $475 to $650 per day (a level which could be paid by Medicare but not Medicaid). McAfee calculated it would cost $265 per day to pay for attendant services in his own home but Medicaid paid only $100 per day for residential care. The Georgia Department of Medical Assistance therefore rejected his proposal. McAfee was then admitted, temporarily and on a voluntary basis, to a psychiatric hospital. Anyone in his situation must be extremely depressed and upset.

The social and economic context of Kenneth Bergstedt's desire to die is also clear. His case was brought into the limelight when his 65-year-old father presented the Las Vegas court with an affidavit from his son that he 'had no encouraging expectations to look forward to from life, receives no enjoyment from life, lives with constant fears and apprehensions and is tired of suffering'.[4] But were these feelings about his life a result of his physical disability or a result of the situation in which he lived? Bergstedt was being looked after by his father who was disabled himself (he had lost a leg in an industrial accident), had high blood pressure and was scared of getting cancer or having a heart attack. Bergstedt was said to be worried that if anything happened to his father he would either die if left on his own in an emergency or be forced into residential care. The court ruled that Bergstedt's wish to die was rational given the level of his physical disability, with no consideration as to whether, if the context in which he experienced his physical disability were changed, his attitude to dying might have been very different.

The question is, in such a context, is the wish to die a so-called rational response to physical disability? Or is it a desperate response to isolated oppression? As Ed Roberts, head of the World Institute on Disability, said, 'It's not the respirator. It's money.' He explained, 'I've been on a respirator for 26 years and I watch these people's cases – they're just as dependent on a respirator as I am; the major difference is they know they're going to be forced to live in a nursing home – or they're already there – and I'm leading a quality life'.[5]

In America, the debate is couched in terms of civil rights. Elizabeth Bouvia received the help of the American Civil Liberties Union lawyers who were intent on winning for her the legal right to assisted suicide.[2] It is also couched in terms of humanitarianism, of concern for the individual and their quality of life.

In Britain, where such cases rarely reach the courts, public opinion has also been concerned with the issue of quality of life for physically disabled people. There has been a similar willingness to accept that a high level of paralysis necessitates an unacceptable quality of life. One example of this involved James Haig, who was tetraplegic as the result of a motorbike accident. During the year following his injury he tried to adjust. Journalist Polly Toynbee wrote in *The Guardian*, 'He tried writing but football had been his great interest before the accident and he found he could not adapt. He was told he could never have any kind of job.' She wrote, 'He looked down at his immobilised and wasted arms and legs. "Suicide is the sensible answer for someone like me," he said'. Toynbee invited the reader to agree with Haig, arguing how wrong it was that it was against the law for anyone to help Haig in his wish to kill himself: 'What Arthur Koestler could do for himself, with dignity and, one hopes, without pain, or panic, the law forced James Haig to do to himself brutishly and cruelly.' Haig set fire to his bungalow and died in the flames.[6]

Steven Bradshaw, director of the Spinal Injuries Association and himself tetraplegic, responded to Toynbee's article. 'We are concerned that she has . . . suggested that suicide is a logical response to tetraplegia.' He could also have pointed out the inappropriate analogy which Toynbee drew between Arthur Koestler who was terminally ill and was merely choosing the form of his death which was inevitable soon, and Haig, who was not ill, who could have lived for 50 more years and whose decision was not about the form of his death but a rejection of his life.

Instead of encouraging the idea that physical disability in itself means an unacceptable quality of life, why didn't Toynbee ask why our society causes young men to think that if they can't play football then life isn't worth living? Or ask why Haig had been told he would never work again?

A liberal humanist approach to euthanasia may insist that individuals should be able to choose the manner and time of their death; that if someone genuinely feels that their life is not worth living then they should not be forced to endure pain and suffering and unhappiness. But individuals do not exist within a vacuum. We are all influenced by the values of the society in which we live. Our society not only values physical ability and perfection; it devalues and discriminates against those who do not conform to the physical norm. The prejudices against disabled people do not just exist out there in the public world, they also reside within our own heads, particularly for those of us who become disabled in adult life.

Given the level of prejudice against disabled people, we cannot realistically expect non-disabled journalists or the medical profession, or the legal profession, to mount a challenge to the assumption that a physical disability means a life not worth living. We have to challenge it ourselves. We have to question the way in which, while it is commonly assumed that a non-disabled person who is not terminally ill but who commits suicide, does so while 'the balance of their mind is disturbed', the suicide of a disabled person is often treated as rational behaviour. No mental disturbance or emotional trauma is deemed necessary to explain the rejection of life by a disabled person. Instead their physical disability is taken as sufficient grounds to want to die.

## References

1. p. 16 in Johnson, M. 'Unanswered questions', *Disability Rag*, September/October issue (1990).
2. p. 195 in Longmore, P. 'Whose life is this anyway?' In Maddox, S. (ed.) *Spinal Network*, Sam Maddox, Colorado, USA (1987).
3. pp. 11–12 in *Disability Rag*, July/August issue (1990).
4. pp. 18–19 in Johnson, M. 'Unanswered questions', *Disability Rag*, September/October issue (1990).
5. p. 21 in *Disability Rag*, September/October issue (1990).
6. Toynbee, P. *Guardian*, 25 April (1983).

Jenny Morris is a freelance writer and former lecturer, who broke her back in a fall. This article is an edited extract from Chapter 2 'Lives not Worth Living' in her book *Pride Against Prejudice: a Personal Politics of Disability*, published by The Women's Press, London (1991).

# 18
# The stigma of infertility

## NAOMI PFEFFER

The recent controversy over the new methods of overcoming involuntary childlessness has focused on the ethical aspects of the techniques. A focus on ethical considerations effectively excludes any discussion of the social and historical context of the condition of infertility. Consequently, none of the many different and often opposing reasons given for the recent interest in new techniques to overcome infertility can be challenged persuasively. Furthermore, this absence of a social and historical context has had an unfortunate consequence for infertile men and women, which is that in the course of considerable public exposure given to infertility, the stigma of infertility has been compounded. Providing a social context has therefore another and to me a more important purpose; that purpose is to deconstruct the stigma of infertility.

Besides their involuntary childlessness there is one characteristic which the infertile are said to share, that of desperation. The word desperation or some such synonym appears so frequently in conjunction with infertility that sometimes it appears that what troubles infertile men and women is not the absence of a child as such but some form of emotional disorder related to their failure. Desperation combined with infertility appears to produce a particularly potent mix; one that forces fecund women to lease their womb, sends infertile men and women scouring the world for orphans to adopt and incites some doctors into developing new techniques that subject people to many indignities.

Does infertility lead inevitably to unremitting desperation? Infertility is a very negative experience and at times most infertile men and women probably will feel desperate. But desperation is only one of many different emotions that infertility can arouse, and not all of these are negative. There are positive aspects to childlessness which are rarely mentioned, or which are glossed as selfishness. Furthermore, desperation may not be a result of the condition of infertility but of the insensitive and humiliating treatment sometimes received at the hands of medical and other authorities, the very people who claim to be interested in rescuing the infertile from desperation. Focusing on desperation to the exclusion of all other emotions serves not to explain but to make a caricature of infertile men and women.

Physical infertility is not synonymous with involuntary childlessness. It is generally forgotten that some men and women are childless because of social and not physical impediments.[1] The litmus test of physical fertility is conception and the safe delivery of a live baby. With few exceptions, no one knows in advance of trying to conceive whether they are fertile or not. Those people rendered sterile by their genes or through disease may not in fact want children; indeed, they may regret the loss of their fertility as a potential but they may not grieve the absence of a child. It is in the attempt to conceive that one discovers whether one is fertile or not. The decision to embark on parenthood, to undertake a major change in social status, antedates the attempt to conceive, particularly today when more effective means of fertility control are available. This decision is the result of processes that are shaped by social and historical forces, the impact of which are shared by the fertile and infertile alike; there is nothing peculiar about the motivation for parenthood of those who later find themselves infertile.

Scientists and doctors do not agree about what is the normal length of time it takes to get pregnant. Hence infertility is a self-imposed definition. At some point during an attempt at conception, frustration is acknowledged; a problem emerges that may require some sort of solution. Not everyone who acknowledges a fertility problem takes that problem to a doctor. Indeed, seeking medical advice is only one of the many options available. These options include denial, applying for a child to adopt or foster, changing partner, finding a new job, moving home, going on a long holiday or grieving the loss of a potential relationship, that of parent and child.[2] The choice of options is shaped by social factors such as class, gender, race, age, marital status, education, social isolation, etc., none of which feature in the discussion about the needs of the infertile.

There is no evidence that the involuntarily childless who take their problem to a doctor are more desperate to have a child than those men and women who choose other solutions to their childlessness. The only factor that distinguishes them is their decision to seek a specifically medical solution to their infertility. It is often claimed that the problem of infertility is growing in scale so that it sometimes appears as though the cumulative desperation of the infertile threatens to engulf the fertile majority. It may be that the number of people seeking a medical solution to their infertility is on the increase, but as statistics are not collected on such issues (and would be very difficult to collect) we have no way of knowing this for sure. Nevertheless, we cannot assume that once in the surgery these people will countenance uniformly the whole panoply of invasive investigations and treatments on offer. There is copious evidence which shows that not all patients concur with their doctors' recommendations.[3,4] Men and women have clear limits beyond which they will not venture. Some will not consider artificial insemination using donor semen, others refuse in-vitro fertilization whilst yet others reject adoption. Such limits are not evidence that some people's motivation for parenthood is insufficiently strong. Rather, these limits highlight the real social differences that exist amongst infertile women and men.

Fleshing out the real and complex experience of infertility leads us to ask who benefits from the pervasive caricature of the infertile as desperate people. Not the infertile themselves, who cannot be helped by the reduction of a complex set of changing emotions and needs to a single negative word. Infertile women are not, I suggest, helped by a description of any distress they may feel as that of a 'barren woman's suffering' (p. 47).[5] These words are Robert Edwards's, the embryologist who, with his collaborator the gynaecologist Patrick Steptoe, pioneered the technique of in-vitro fertilization and embryo transfer.

Who then benefits from this caricature? There is a false assumption frequently made that professionals and their clients share the same goals. In this context, the professionals are the gynaecologists and embryologists and their clients are the infertile men and women who seek their help. For both, the aim is indeed the birth of a child, but their reasons for wanting this child clearly differ. Gynaecologists and embryologists who champion these new techniques have made their views known through articles in newspapers and television documentaries which portray them in heroic terms. We know that these doctors and scientists want to be able to continue to offer in-vitro fertilization and embryo transfer. These professionals have claimed that the new methods for assisting reproduction are indispensable in their endeavours to help their infertile patients. And we know from opinion research that a majority of the population of Britain wish them to be allowed to do so.[6] What we do not know is if this same desire is shared by the majority of men and women who are infertile, most of whom will *not* undergo in-vitro fertilization and embryo transfer.

Little information is available on what infertile people in general want. One survey (the only one of its kind and a little out of date) may provide us with some clues. In 1977, the members of the National Association of the Childless, a voluntary organization which offers support and advice to the infertile, were asked to state the single thing that they felt would most improve the medical treatment they had received. Admittedly, this survey was conducted before the birth of Louise Brown, the first test-tube baby. Nevertheless, its findings are of interest. Only 2 per cent of the respondents stated that more up-to-date techniques would have been beneficial. Of much greater importance to these infertile men and women were improvements in both the organization of the clinics they attended and in the attitude of the doctors they saw. Specifically, they complained about the length of time it took to reach some sort of diagnosis of their condition. This delay was caused by the infrequency of clinics which meant long gaps between each appointment, and when they did see a doctor, many complained of how difficult it was to get an adequate account of their problem. These difficulties in communication were compounded by patients rarely seeing the same doctor throughout the course of a treatment.[7]

These findings have an all-too-familiar ring about them; many patients, whatever their condition, level similar criticisms at their doctors. But in the recent debate about new approaches to the treatment of infertility, these well-rehearsed complaints have disappeared; the hearts and minds of even the most intransigent critics of doctors appear to have been won over. It is now common currency that those same doctors whose attitudes in the past provoked the complaints that I cited above are today concerned solely with the interests of their infertile patients. This is, I suggest, a simple and naïve rendering of an institution as complex as medicine.

## References

1. Porter, M. 'Infertility: the extent of the problem', *Biology and Society*, 1, 128–35 (1984).
2. Woollett, A. 'Childlessness: strategies for coping with infertility', *International Journal for Behavioural Development*, 8, 473–82 (1985).
3. Stimson, G. V. 'Obeying doctor's orders: a view from the other side', *Social Science and Medicine*, 8, 97–104 (1975).

4. Cartwright, A. *Patients and Their Doctors*, Routledge and Kegan Paul, London (1967).
5. Steptoe, P. and Edwards, R. *A Matter of Life*, Hutchinson, London (1980).
6. *The Times*, 11 October (1982), p. 2.
7. Owens, D. and Read, M. W. The Provision, Use and Evaluation of Medical Services for the Subfertile: An Analysis based on the Experience of Involuntary Childless Couples, SRU Working Paper 4, University of Cardiff, Cardiff (1979).

Naomi Pfeffer is a social historian and Senior Lecturer in Health Studies at the University of North London. She has written extensively about the medicalization of infertility, contraception and assisted conception, most recently *The Stork and the Syringe: A Political History of Reproductive Medicine*, Polity Press, Cambridge (1994). This article is an edited extract from her chapter 'Artificial insemination, in-vitro fertilization and the stigma of infertility' which appeared in *Reproductive Technologies: Gender, Motherhood and Medicine*, Stanworth, M. (ed.), Polity Press, Cambridge (1987).

# 19
# Hard-earned lives: experiences of doctors and health services

## JOCELYN CORNWELL

People in the study [of families in the East End of London] rank medicine superior to ordinary commonsense and doctors as more important than social workers (who are on a par with themselves and other ordinary folk) because medicine has to be learned and because it treats problems which are beyond the capabilities of the ordinary person to treat. When this frame of reference is applied to the health service they distinguish between its different parts according to the type of problem the service treats. Thus the service for which they have the greatest respect is the hospital service because it deals with 'real' illness; GPs are positioned lower down the hierarchy because their province is, first and foremost, 'normal' illness, and to a lesser extent 'real' illness in the sense that they supply the referral to a specialist; at the bottom are the community services (school health; mother and baby clinics; child health clinics; health visiting) and the maternity services (ante-natal clinics and classes and the obstetric service), which deal with health problems which are not illness.

To a certain extent, the hierarchical approach to the health service accurately reflects people's experience of being patients in the local health service. They preferred large hospitals to small hospitals, and teaching hospitals to other hospitals, because they believed – with reason – that the staff in these hospitals were better trained and the hospitals were better equipped. William Cox, for example, had twice been treated for a knee injury, the first time in St Leonard's Hospital in Hackney, and the second time at the London Hospital, Whitechapel. At St Leonard's, he had a painful operation performed on his knee without local anaesthetic; at the London the same operation was performed with a local anaesthetic. On the basis of this experience, William and his family had concluded that the London is the better hospital of the two and had generalized this observation to all teaching hospitals and to larger as opposed to smaller hospitals.

The idea that general practice is less prestigious and less important than hospital medicine is confirmed for many people by the shabbiness of many of the local surgeries and by the difficulty they have in seeing the doctor. This is how Kathleen Read described the difference in her feelings in anticipation of a visit to the local surgery compared with a visit to an out-patient clinic in hospital:

> If it's just an ordinary GP now, I hardly have to go up there, I only have to go for me tablets, I take no notice. But if it's to go to the hospital for anything or other, although you've got confidence in them, I still get awful butterflies. Although I'm discharged from the Chest Hospital, I can ring them up for an appointment on that morning, although I know everybody up there I still feel sick as a dog. I can't eat, which is ridiculous really, I suppose, unless it might be fear of the outcome of what you're going up there for, I don't know. But the actual doctors and that, I still get the colly wobbles, hospital-wise anyway, not so much me GP.

The most common complaint about general practice arrangements was that the local GPs do not work an appointment system, but see their patients instead on the basis of first come, first served. For patients this can mean waiting anything from a few minutes to a couple of hours to see the doctor and not being able to predict in advance which it will be, something which is especially irksome for women with young children. People complained that the waiting rooms were also often uncomfortable and unpleasant, and said they were afraid of catching something while they waited to see the doctor.

The complaints about some of the community and maternity services were very similar to the complaints about general practice. The women (for it is women who use these services in the main) complained that it was difficult to get appointments at the Family Planning Clinics and they were kept waiting for long periods at antenatal clinics. Underlying their complaints was the feeling that the staff who ran the clinics were not interested in their patients. This was Sharon Berthot's description of her visits to the ante-natal clinic at the London Hospital:

> I hated it. You sit up there for hours, four hours sometimes we'd be up there at the London. You'd get up there at quarter to one, by five o'clock you're just walking out of the place.
>
> JC: What did they do to you in the clinic?
>
> Not a lot, waiting time really. I mean by the time you, all right you had your blood pressure taken, you used to have to give a urine sample, you was weighed. The actual time that you spent with the doctors must have been five minutes. So I mean you had about ten minutes actually doing anything, and all the rest was waiting time. I can understand why people don't go. All those mothers crammed together into a little space, all waiting to do the same thing. Oh, it was horrible.
>
> JC: Did you get anything out of going to the clinic? Did you talk to the doctor, or ask questions?
>
> He didn't seem to have time, to be honest. I mean, they'd come in and they'd say, 'Oh, yes, Mrs Berthot, how are you?' and you'd go, 'Uh'. 'Yes, well you're doing fine, we'll see you in a fortnight's time.' 'Yeah, yeah – I'm fine.' It was like that. They really didn't have the time. I suppose if there was anything really wrong with you, you'd push it. But I suppose, I mean they've just had so many cases of morning sickness and feeling dizzy that they just don't want to know anymore. That's the way I found it.

It is clear that people's experience as patients in the local health services partially accounts for their attitudes towards different parts of the service, but it does not entirely explain them. For example, it does not adequately explain their hostility towards the maternity services. Most of the ante-natal care they receive and the majority of their babies are delivered in hospitals, and in every other instance they are respectful of hospital medicine.

The women in this study regard the different stages of the reproductive process as potential health problems but not illness, and in their view the proper way to manage them is by learning from experience (one's own and other women's) and using commonsense. They believe that the experience of childbirth is different for each woman and varies from one pregnancy to the next, which makes it impossible for anyone else to instruct them in how to cope with it. Only two of the women – Sharon and Jackie – attended relaxation classes before they had their first baby, and in both their cases something unusual happened during their labour. Sharon's baby was delivered unusually quickly, and Jackie's turned into an emergency when the baby showed signs of distress. Both women felt the classes were of no help in coping with what had happened, neither went back to the classes with subsequent pregnancies and neither would recommend the classes to other women:

> So there's me, sitting and taking it all in and, as it turned out, it just didn't happen that way. I mean, they tell you it does take a long time, your first baby and all this, and not to go to the hospital too soon because you won't be very pleased by waiting hours in the hospital. And at first you'll just have these niggly pains, maybe a back ache, then you'll have a show and then they said like, just get prepared for it. Get your suitcase ready and potter about indoors. When the time comes, like, say they're coming every twenty minutes, then go to the hospital. Fine, fine. They didn't tell me it could go completely wrong and sometimes it just doesn't happen that way. They don't tell you that. So there's me waiting for them to come every twenty minutes and the poor little sod was nearly born in me mother's bed.

Most of the women had not talked to their mothers or sisters about childbirth and were often totally unprepared for their first experience of it. However, once they had one baby, in their view they were as knowledgeable about the whole process as anyone else; certainly as knowledgeable as the medical and nursing staff who delivered their subsequent babies. It is significant therefore that seven out of the ten women in the study with more than one child described head-on clashes with the staff during the delivery of babies other than their first born:

> I know it's different, isn't it, after you've had the first one. You know the second time what's going on. So I woke Paul up and we got to the hospital about six o'clock. Of course I walked in, I says, 'Oh, here's me card'. She goes, 'You're not in strong labour yet, you can have a bath'. I says, 'I ain't getting in a bath, I'm going to have it soon'. 'No, no, you've got plenty of time.' You know, they won't listen. I said, 'No. I know that it's going to happen fast.' And of course by the time I go into what they call strong labour at six-fifteen and she was born at six-thirty. And the doctor wasn't even there because she hadn't called him. She'd run a bath and was expecting me to get into the bath.

I was in for bed rest and I started getting pains in me back, and I thought, this is it. So I called up the nurse and she said 'Come up here', she said, 'you're only in for bed rest'. 'I don't care what I'm in here for', I said, 'my pains have started'. So she gave me an injection. She said I'd be all right after a sleep. So that was like on the Saturday night and I had a little couple of hours kip and something woke me up again. I rang the bell again. 'Nurse', I said, 'they definitely are labour pains I'm getting in me back'. 'No', she said, 'you're not down to have him yet'. I said. 'I ain't got a date for when'. And the girl in the next bed said, 'Oh, isn't it ridiculous. You'd think they'd take you down there and get you prepared.' And about, what was it? Half past seven, I held on to that bell. I said, 'If you don't hurry and get me down there I'll have it in this bed'. 'Oh, my God', she said, 'the head's there', and the next thing it was like panic stations.

These were the only situations in which anyone – man or woman – said that they knew better than the medical staff, and although there were other situations in which people described themselves having arguments with medical staff, these were the only occasions on which it was the patient who did the arguing. At other times it was a relative of the patient who was said to have tackled the doctor, usually after the incident in question had blown over. The justification the women gave for their behaviour was the same justification they gave for their attitudes towards social workers. To them, the knowledge that was required in this particular situation was commonsense knowledge based on personal experience.

The point we return to in commenting on accounts of doctors and health services in general, is the significance of the images of medical practice and the medical profession which dominate them. The interviews show that the positive image of the medical profession overrides memories of 'bad' doctors, wrong diagnoses, prescriptions that are unwanted and do not work, to make 'all doctors', in hospital and in general practice, 'good doctors'. The theme of doctors' power, and of the social distance between doctors and patients created by it, is constant.

This extract comes from Jocelyn Cornwell's book *Hard-Earned Lives* (Tavistock Publications, London, 1984), which arose from her long-term sociological study of families in London's East End. She is currently a project manager in the Health Studies Department of the Audit Commission in London.

# 20
# 'Some bloody do-gooding cow'

## TONY PARKER

**An interview with Mrs Williams**

Her blue eyes blank with cataract, she sat in an old armchair with her two rubber ferruled sticks leaning against the arm of it and a pink ribbon in what remained of her wispy grey hair. When she heard the front door close she leaned forward slightly, listening.

'Has she gone dear, that young woman? There's just you and me here is there? I can about make out your shape if you're right in front of me, but I couldn't tell you what you look like. Are you a young man dear, you sound as though you are? Well that's young to me. I'm eighty-seven, so to me you're no age at all are you, goodness I've got grandchildren your age nearly.

And who are you dear, who are you from, what have you come to see me about? It's not that thing they call meals on wheels, is it? Because if it is, I don't want to sound rude dear but I don't want anything to do with it, you're wasting your time.

I was left a widow when I was thirty, with five children to bring up: the eldest girl was twelve, then there were four boys, the youngest of them one year old. My husband worked on the railway, they came and knocked on my door one day and said he'd been run over by a train.

In those days there wasn't the social security and the other things what there is nowadays, so I just had to get on with it. I took people's washing in for them, I went and did cleaning in shops round about, I went on Sundays to help them if they wanted things carrying. I did everything that anybody would offer me, to bring money in. I would never tell anyone I couldn't manage, they'd have taken the children off of me if I had and put them in a home. I wasn't going to let that happen.

Being the eldest, my daughter had to stop at home and help me. She didn't get much schooling but that couldn't be helped: with me out at work till all hours there had to be somebody at home to fend for the boys. None of them got much of a schooling either, they had to leave as soon as they were old enough and get jobs. Things were very hard in those days.

Not being an educated person I couldn't get a regular job myself either: not until I was well past forty, then I was a cook at a road-haulage depot canteen in the docks. I got that job about the time when my youngest boy was old enough to leave school and earn his keep, which was when I didn't really need a steady job any more. But I took it and I stayed there more than twenty years. When I left they gave me a big party and a clock and there were speeches and they said 'Our dear Mrs Williams'.

After that I lived with my married daughter for a while. But her and me have never really what you might call got on. Her and her husband, they're very interested in one of these religious things, they go out knocking on people's doors and giving them leaflets and trying to convert them to their way of thinking. They say they're doing the Lord's work but I don't hold with it myself.

She told me one day she'd seen they were building these flats and she'd been and inquired off of the GLC if they had any old people's accommodation in them. The GLC told her yes they had, there were these ground-floor flatlets and if I'd like one they'd see what they could do. So that's how I got this place, and I've been here ever since.

What I live on is my state pension, but I don't like it because I don't like having to have charity. Now and again one of my sons will come over to see me and when he's gone there's a five-pound note left on the table: it makes me cross, but I think it'd make them cross if I gave it back to them so I use it for the electric because that's such a terrible expense now. This flat is all electric and it eats more money than I eat food. I used to have a gas stove for doing my cooking on, but as my eyesight started to go I couldn't tell when I wanted to turn the gas down if I hadn't turned it out. Sometimes it would be on and I hadn't lit it, and there was matches with a chance of a dangerous explosion, so they came and turned me into all electric. I think it was from the social, some bloody do-gooding cow interfering like they do: I can't stand these people knocking on your door saying they've got some form or another that's got to be filled in, how much is your rent, what do you do about your washing and all the rest of it. You're not from the social people are you dear? No I thought not, you don't sound like you are.

There's a lady comes in on a Tuesday and a Friday, she's one of the what they call home helps. Her name's Matty, she's been coming for seven years, and if it was left to me she might just as well not bother only the problem is I don't know how to get rid of her. All she does is as soon as she comes she says she'll put the kettle on and make a cup of tea. And then when she's done that, she sits and chats for two hours. She used to be very good, but now she doesn't do a blind thing except have a quick run round with a duster, ask me if I want any shopping bringing in, go and get it, and then she's off and I don't see her till next time. Once in a while she'll take my washing to the launderette, but it's God's honest truth that's all she does mostly, spends all her time talking to me. Not talking with me, or letting me talk to her: that wouldn't be so bad, but talking to me all the time, do you know how I mean? A lady came from somewhere once and asked me was everything all right, was I satisfied with the home help. I said I was. Well you have to don't you when it's somebody's job, you can't complain about them because they might lose it and nobody wants to put somebody out of work do they? I mean not except this Tory government we've got, they enjoy doing that, they're wicked; but nobody else would.

There's somebody called a voluntary visitor or something, she comes in as well. I think she's an old age pensioner who's got nothing else to do with her time, she comes about once a month. I don't know her name; but she's another of them, she wants to tell you what she's been doing, her ideas about this that and the other, she's another one gets on my nerves. Apart from her, that's the lot for my visitors. Mr Cross might call in now and again and make me a cup of tea if he happens to be passing, but no one else.

A typical day for me would be that I usually wake up about six o'clock, and I have my wireless on the table by the bed there and listen to that till about half past eight or nine. Then I get up and get dressed. I've got this very bad rheumatism in my hips and arms, so usually it'll take me an hour and a half to two hours to get dressed. I have to keep stopping for a rest. Then if it's the day for the home help she comes, and if it's not I'll make myself a cup of tea and start making my dinner. I don't like these things you get in packets, I don't think there's any nourishment in them: I'd sooner have a few potatoes and carrots with a bit of gravy. I might have a piece of meat, a sausage or something of that sort, or an egg, but not every day. In the afternoon I listen to the wireless again, I might have a doze until it's my tea time. Then I have something on toast as a rule. I like cheese or sardines or a tomato. Round about seven o'clock I'll have a cup of cocoa and a biscuit, then I go to bed and usually I drop off to sleep about nine.

But it's no use us going on talking about that subject, because I don't care what you say, I'm not having those meals on wheels. I think they're disgusting – all that white sauce over everything so you can't see what you're eating. I had one once six or seven years ago. I don't mean to be rude dear but if you go on until you're blue in the face I shan't change my mind. I'm not having them.

Last night I had a dream, I dreamed I was out shopping. I was along the precinct there at Robins Walk, I was walking about and people were coming up and speaking to me and chatting, it was lovely. Then when I woke up and found it was all a dream, I started to cry. It's five years, no it must be more than that now, since I've been along there or anywhere else on the estate.

Sometimes one of my sons will come for me on a Sunday if it's a nice day in the summer and take me out for a little ride in his motor car. There's two of them live near enough to do that. The other two, one's in America and the other one I don't know where he is, I haven't seen him for years. The two that do come, Michael and Charlie, they're good boys but they've got wives and families and children of their own, they don't want to be bothered with an old woman and you can't blame them, not really.

The vicar used to come, but he seems to have dropped off lately. He told me off once for swearing, I do say 'bloody' and that; that might be why he doesn't come. Sometimes the chiropodist comes, she's another one spends all her time talking, I can't be doing with people like that. I don't know why people can't leave you alone; if they don't want me to talk to them, I'd sooner they didn't come and talk to me.

The person I like best is my neighbour next door, the one who goes and gets my pension from the post office for me. She comes and knocks on the door every two weeks for my book. She never says anything apart from 'Good morning' and she's never away more than half an hour because she knows I worry. Then she comes back and comes in and puts the money on the table and says 'Good morning' again, and then out she goes. That's it then, and I don't see her again for another two weeks.

It does get lonely sometimes, and I do sometimes I do have a bit of a cry about it. But I think to myself 'Well Clara' I think, 'Well Clara there's no use crying about it, you're getting to be an old woman now and you can't expect any different.' I used to be such an active person you see, never had a day's illness, brought up all my kids on my own, never asked anything from them since they was grown up and with families of their own. It's not as though I've been used to being a person who couldn't get about until these last years.

One of my boys, Charlie I think it was, he came to me one day and he said him and Michael and their wives had all been having a talk and they all thought it would be a good idea if I had a telephone. He said then if there was ever anything wrong any time, I could ring up and they'd come over; or if I like wanted the doctor I could call him. So they had this telephone put in for me.

It was, it was bloody awful. I said I didn't care if they were paying for it, it was more trouble then it was worth and they were to have it taken away. One thing was they used to ring up and tell me they couldn't come over at the weekend to see me, so they'd rung up for a chat instead. You can understand it, it made things a lot easier for them. But it got to be none of them came for weeks on end – as soon as I heard the phone ringing on a Friday night I knew who it was, it was either Michael or Charlie or their wife to say they were sorry they couldn't come.

The other thing would happen would be you'd be on the toilet or something and the bloody phone would start ringing. It always did it: I knew for sure if I went to that toilet the phone would ring. It was never anybody proper – it'd always be someone like the electricity people ringing up to say they were checking everything was all right, did I have any problems; or the home help woman would ring up, 'It's all right Mrs Williams it's only me, I thought I'd ring up to see how you are since I'm not going to be coming in tomorrow.' I used to feel like shouting I'd been all right till she rang up, why the hell didn't she push off. Only I didn't say push off, I used another word I won't say to you.

And a couple of times, this happened without a word of a lie, this is God's honest truth this is – twice it started ringing in the middle of the night. I switched my light on to see what time it was, and if I hold my alarm clock under the lamp and put my face right to it, I can see what time it is: and both times it was two o'clock. I didn't have my name in the telephone book, so where they'd got my phone number from I don't know: but it was a man, or it could have been a boy even, a young man. In all my life I've never heard anything like it, he said such dirty filthy things, over and over he kept on repeating them. I didn't know what to say so I didn't say anything, I couldn't think. You know you should put the phone down, but somehow at the time when it happens you stand there and you can't move. I nearly fainted with it. I let go of the hand thing, what do they call it, receiver, and I was, I was trembling so much I could scarcely get back to my bed.

I didn't dare put my light out and I don't think I slept any more. But I sort of drowsed off some time though, because the next thing I knew it was daylight and the telephone was making that whirring noise it makes when you haven't got it put down properly. I was very frightened but I didn't tell anybody, I didn't ring up my sons or anything. I wished I had, because the next night I've gone to bed again and the same thing happens, in the middle of the night it starts ringing again at two o'clock. I thought if I didn't switch my light on and didn't answer it, they might think I'd gone away and there was no one here. So I left it, I let it ring and ring. I don't know how long it went on, it seemed like hours but I swore I was never going to answer a telephone again, and I didn't.

Next morning I rang them up, the telephone people at the post office or wherever it is. I said I was an old woman on my own and I was frightened of electricity and they were to come straightaway that day and take it away. I don't remember if they did come that same day or not, but they did cut it off for me there and then until they could come and remove it. I never told them the real reason it was all about, and I never told my sons. I don't know who it was, for all I know it might have been the telephone people – but then somebody told the social I wasn't having the phone no more, so the next thing is they came round to see what was the matter and what it was all about. I never told them either.

That woman from the social, she was another of them, another bloody do-gooding cow. She said how was I going to let anybody know if I felt ill any time and needed help. I said if I did I'd shout; but oh no she said, that wouldn't do, I must have one of their cards to put up at that window there. It had got 'Help Wanted' in big letters on it so everyone could see it and come to help me. That's the sort of thing they do these people, they think up ideas and tell you to do this that and the other, and then they're surprised when you've no time for them afterwards.

What happened you see was that a few days after she'd give it me I did feel a bit queer, so I thought I'll ask someone if they'd go to the doctor for me and get me some medicine. I put the card up behind the curtain there against the window where anyone passing could see it, then I went and lay on my bed and waited for someone to come. Well no one came, did they? I dozed off, I went to sleep, and when I woke up in the morning there was nothing wrong with me so I carried on as normal. Only I'd forgot to take the card down: a day went by, two days, and I'd still forgotten all about it. Then on the third day in the afternoon I'm sitting in my chair having a doze, and there's a hammering and a banging on that door, and people climbing up on the ledge outside and trying to get their hand inside the window and open it. I was frightened out of my life. This is God's honest truth, I thought it was a gang of burglars or something trying to break in and kill me and steal my money.

After that I threw the card away. I thought if anything happened to me I'd sooner lie there on the floor I would for a couple of days, rather than something like that. That's the social for you.'

This interview is taken from *The People of Providence*, a collection of personal accounts about life on a London housing estate, published by Hutchinson (1985). Tony Parker spent five years researching and writing this book and the accounts he has reproduced are taken from his tape recorded interviews with people living in or working on the estate. Mrs Williams is one of the many residents who spoke to him.

# Part 3
# Influences on health and disease

## INTRODUCTION

What factors influence patterns of health and disease? The answers to this question reflect many things: a particular historical or political perspective; the frame of reference provided by an academic discipline; the relative importance attached to biology, individual action or social process. Inevitably, just as the answers reflect these things, so too do the many ways in which the question is posed, and the nature of the evidence considered.

For Frederick Engels, revolutionary communist and close colleague of Karl Marx, the question followed on from his analysis of nineteenth century English society. Cities like Manchester were being dramatically transformed by industrialization, producing explosive rates of urban growth and stark extremes of wealth and poverty. *The Conditions of the Working Classes in England* was first published in German in 1845, but almost fifty years passed before an English edition appeared. In it, Engels set about the systematic documentation of the consequences of this upheaval for that part of the population – the majority – to whom the benefits of industrialization must have seemed far from obvious. In the extract included here, entitled 'Health: 1844', Engels portrays the squalor of existence and the disparities between social classes in death and disease. What marks out his portrait as unique, however, is not the facts themselves (which in large part were culled from official reports) but his repeated stress on the nature of the society which could produce these conditions. The bourgeoisie, 'interested in maintaining and prolonging this disorder', has created these victims and stands accused by Engels of deliberate 'murder'. Although Engels' political conclusions are as disputed now as in the 1840s, his description is generally accepted as a valuable historical document.

J. N. Morris stands in a long tradition of physicians and epidemiologists – indeed, stretching back to the time of Engels – who have demonstrated and drawn attention to the wide disparities in health between different social and occupational classes. In 'Inequalities in health: ten years and little further on', Morris reflects on developments in the decade after the publication of the Black Report on inequalities in health, of which he was a member. Morris argues that the principal conclusions of the Black Report – that the steep gradients in mortality across social classes were primarily related to the 'material conditions of life' – have been borne out by subsequent research. But while Morris accepts that his argument points to a need to mitigate poverty and deprivation and to lessen inequality – and therefore to enter 'the central arena of politics' – he is careful to delimit the role of medicine to the classic areas of public health concern, such as housing and child poverty.

George Brown is a medical sociologist who has written widely on mental illness. In 'Depression: a sociological view', Brown presents an aetiology of a particular condition: depression. Again, emphasis is placed on the social context, including social class. He claims that the connection between the social environment and depression is mediated by a wide range of factors. These can be represented by a causal model consisting of three components: provoking agents, such as major life-events or difficulties; vulnerability factors, for example, the absence of intimate relationships with others; and symptom formation factors, such as the childhood loss of a parent; all of which may influence the type and severity of depression. But despite the convincing empirical evidence that Brown provides of the importance of social class, lifestage and provoking agents in influencing the prevalence and distribution of psychiatric disorders, sociological ideas such as his, which emphasize the current environment, have been slow to influence psychiatric teaching – as he himself acknowledges.

There are many potential reasons why a particular view of the factors influencing health and disease patterns – for example, the sociological view of depression – may fail to make headway in the world. Perhaps one is that the conclusions to which a particular view leads, no matter how well supported empirically, may go against one's intuitive beliefs. A possible example of this is provided by the research of the economists Jean Drèze and Amartya Sen into the characteristics and economic context of mass hunger. Drèze and Sen argue that conventional explanations of famines, often focusing on food supply, are usually misleading. The system of entitlement relations, which dictates whether or not people can obtain food, is much more important. In 'Entitlement and deprivation', they illustrate this with examples of famines occurring in situations where food supply was above average. The policy implications of their work are clear, pointing towards distributional issues.

Where Engels, Morris, Brown, Drèze and Sen all emphasize the broader social context of health and disease, the Medical Services Study Group of the Royal College of Physicians gaze unrelentingly on individual behaviour. Of the 250 deaths examined by them among inpatients in 'Deaths under 50', they conclude that almost 40 per cent can be held as largely to blame for their own death, by choosing to smoke, drink, overeat, ignore medical advice or not comply with treatment, or by taking a more direct path to 'self-destruction' – suicide. The extent to which these patients are held responsible for their own death is indicated by the Study Group's implicit view that the demands placed by such patients on health services are unreasonable and wasteful.

The 'policy' which follows from the conclusions of the Medical Services Study Group is that much more attention should be paid to the advice of doctors, notwithstanding the 'psychopathic' attitude to doctors attributed to many of these patients. Doctors are thereby allotted a potentially central influence in defining and legitimating the existence of disease. Richard Asher, a British physician, describes an entirely different form of self-produced illness: 'Malingering', or the deliberate faking, production or encouragement of illness. The motives for this form of 'illness' are listed as fear, desire or escape and, as Asher observes, the ingenuity of, for example, prisoners-of-war in faking illness is well-documented. However, there is also a 'borderland of malingering', where the purpose is not evident and the motives obscure; Munchausen's Syndrome, which is perhaps the most spectacular example provided by Asher, calls into question the ease with which a dividing line can be drawn between 'real' and 'fake' illness.

Barry Bogin and Peter Laslett are both concerned with the ways in which health alters and is influenced by an individual's life course, but their vantage points and subject matter are very different. Bogin, an American anthropologist, is concerned with adolescence, that period of spectacular biological change accompanying the transition from childhood to adulthood. The human adolescent growth spurt is unique amongst mammals, and Bogin explores what evolutionary advantages this biological trait may confer. In 'Why must I be a teenager at all?' he concludes that adolescence offers maturing boys and girls an ideal opportunity to learn their adult social roles – girls while infertile but perceived as mature, boys while fertile but perceived as immature – and that this in turn has allowed humans to be more reproductively successful than other primates.

Peter Laslett is best known for his path-breaking history of English social structure entitled *The World We Have Lost*. In recent years he has channelled some of his attention towards the present and future, and in 'A new division of the life course', he examines some implications of the vastly increased numbers of people now experiencing old age. Laslett argues that the biological is only one of several dimensions to a life course, and that age has a range of meanings which may be ambiguous and contradictory. He suggests that the historical association of old age with 'dependence and decrepitude' permeates our language, culture and social policies, but has been rendered hopelessly inaccurate by demographic changes, which have resulted in large numbers of active and healthy people beyond the current retirement age. The result is a damaging depreciation of the talents and experience of a large part of the population. Laslett's objective is to displace this dissonant perception of old age, by offering an ordering of the life course in which the period between earning and saving, and dependence and death – what he terms the Third Age – is seen as an era of personal fulfilment.

Finally, in 'Prevention is better. . . .' Helen Roberts, Susan Smith and Carol Bryce combine a number of perspectives on the factors that influence ill-health, to telling effect. They explore one aspect of ill-health – accidents – at one point in the life course – childhood. Where the Medical Services Study Group point to individual behaviour as responsible for a large proportion of the deaths they examined, Roberts, Smith and Bryce argue that individual parents in fact have detailed knowledge of the risks in their physical environment, and undertake a wide range of preventive activities to reduce these risks to themselves and their children. Though not explicit, their analysis also has a social dimension, in that the environmental hazards they discuss are in many ways related to the poor housing and poverty which characterizes the area they are studying. And their conclusion has important implications for health education, which they argue has adopted a misconceived focus on behavioural change rather than environmental change, and in consequence cannot provide much evidence of effectiveness.

The articles in Part 3 represent a wide range of views on what influences health and disease. Some are irreconcilable with others, but some are differentiated largely by the rather arbitrary demarcations of academic disciplines. Overcoming these demarcations would not remove all conflicts of view, but would make the substance of such conflicts much clearer. What is clear is that the conclusions drawn are of much more than academic interest, and have powerful policy implications.

# 21
# Health: 1844

## FREDERICK ENGELS

When one individual inflicts bodily injury upon another, such injury that death results, we call the deed manslaughter; when the assailant knew in advance that the injury would be fatal, we call his deed murder. But when society places hundreds of proletarians in such a position that they inevitably meet a too early and an unnatural death, one which is quite as much a death by violence as that by the sword or bullet; when it deprives thousands of the necessaries of life, places them under conditions in which they *cannot* live – forces them, through the strong arm of the law, to remain in such conditions until that death ensues which is the inevitable consequence – knows that these thousands of victims must perish, and yet permits these conditions to remain, its deed is murder just as surely as the deed of the single individual; disguised, malicious murder, murder against which none can defend himself, which does not seem what it is, because no man sees the murderer, because the death of the victim seems a natural one, since the offence is more one of omission than of commission. But murder it remains.

The manner in which the great multitude of the poor is treated by society today is revolting. They are drawn into large cities where they breathe a poorer atmosphere than in the country; they are relegated to districts which, by reason of the method of construction, are worse ventilated than any others; they are deprived of all means of cleanliness, of water itself, since pipes are laid only when paid for, and the rivers so polluted that they are useless for such purposes; they are obliged to throw all offal and garbage, all dirty water, often all disgusting drainage and excrement into the streets, being without other means of disposing of them; they are thus compelled to infect the region of their own dwellings. Nor is this enough. All conceivable evils are heaped upon the heads of the poor. If the population of great cities is too dense in general, it is they in particular who are packed into the least space. As though the vitiated atmosphere of the streets were not enough, they are penned in dozens into single rooms, so that the air in which they breathe at night is enough in itself to stifle them. They are given damp dwellings, cellar dens that are not waterproof from below, or garrets that leak from above. Their houses are so built that the clammy air cannot escape. They are supplied bad, tattered, or rotten clothing, adulterated and indigestible food. They are exposed to the most exciting changes of mental condition, the most violent vibrations between hope and fear; they are hunted like game, and not permitted to attain peace of mind and quiet enjoyment of life. They are deprived of all enjoyments except that of sexual indulgence and drunkenness, are worked every day to the point of complete exhaustion of their mental and physical energies, and are thus constantly spurred on to the maddest excess in the only two enjoyments at their disposal. And if they surmount all this, they fall victims to want of work in a crisis when all the little is taken from them that had hitherto been vouchsafed them.

How is it possible, under such conditions, for the lower class to be healthy and long lived? What else can be expected than an excessive mortality, an unbroken series of epidemics, a progressive deterioration in the physique of the working population? Let us see how the facts stand.

That the bad air of London, and especially of the working-people's districts, is in the highest degree favourable to the development of consumption, the hectic appearance of great numbers of persons sufficiently indicates. If one roams the streets a little in the early morning, when the multitudes are on their way to their work, one is amazed at the number of persons who look wholly or half-consumptive, pale, lank, narrow-chested, hollow-eyed ghosts, whom one passes at every step, these languid, flabby faces, incapable of the slightest energetic expression.

In competition with consumption stand typhus, to say nothing of scarlet fever, a disease which brings most frightful devastation into the ranks of the working-class. This fever has the same character almost everywhere, and develops in nearly every case into specific typhus. According to the annual report of Dr Southwood Smith on the London Fever Hospital, the number of patients in 1843 was 1,462, or 418 more than in any previous year. Many of the patients were working-people from the country, who had endured the severest privation while migrating, and, after their arrival, had slept hungry and half-naked in the streets, and so fallen victims to the fever. These people were brought into the hospital in such a state of weakness, that unusual quantities of wine, cognac, and preparations of ammonia and other stimulants were required for their treatment; 16½ per cent of all patients died.

In Edinburgh and Glasgow it broke out in 1817, after the famine, and in 1826 and 1837 with especial violence, after the commercial crisis, subsiding somewhat each time after having raged about three years. In Edinburgh about 6,000 persons were attacked by the fever during the epidemic of 1817, and about 10,000 in that of 1837, and not only the number of persons attacked but the violence of the disease increased with each repetition.

But the fury of the epidemic in all former periods seems to have been child's play in comparison with its ravages after the crisis of 1842. One-sixth of the whole indigent population of Scotland was seized by the fever, and the infection was carried by wandering beggars with fearful rapidity from one locality to another. It did not reach the middle and upper classes of the population, yet in two months there were more fever cases than in twelve years before. In Glasgow, 12 per cent of the population were seized in the year 1843; 32,000 persons, of whom 32 per cent perished, while this mortality in Manchester and Liverpool does not ordinarily exceed 8 per cent.

When one remembers under what conditions the working-people live, when one thinks how crowded their dwellings are, how every nook and corner swarms with human beings, how sick and well sleep in the same room, in the same bed, the only wonder is that a contagious disease like this fever does not spread yet farther. And when one reflects how little medical assistance the sick have at command, how many are without any medical advice whatsoever, and ignorant of the most ordinary precautionary measures, the mortality seems actually small.

Another category of diseases arises directly from the food rather than the dwellings of the workers. The food of the labourer, indigestible enough in itself, is utterly unfit for young children, and he has neither means nor time to get his children more suitable food. Moreover, the custom of giving children spirits, and even opium, is very general; and these two influences, with the rest of the conditions of life prejudicial to bodily development, give rise to the most diverse affections of the digestive organs, leaving lifelong traces behind them. Scrofula is almost universal among the working-class, and scrofulous parents have scrofulous children, especially when the original influences continue in full force to operate upon the inherited tendency of the children. A second consequence of this insufficient bodily nourishment, during the years of growth and development, is rachitis, which is extremely common among the children of the working-class. The hardening of the bones is delayed, the development of the skeleton in general is restricted, and deformities of the legs and spinal column are frequent, in addition to the usual rachitic affections. How greatly all these evils are increased by the changes to which the workers are subject in consequence of fluctuations in trade, want of work, and the scanty wages in time of crisis, it is not necessary to dwell upon. Temporary want of sufficient food, to which almost every working-man is exposed at least once in the course of his life, only contributes to intensify the effect of his usually sufficient but bad diet.

Besides these, there are other influences which enfeeble the health of a great number of workers, intemperance most of all. All possible temptations, all allurements combine to bring the workers to drunkenness. Liquor is almost their only source of pleasure, and all things conspire to make it accessible to them. The working-man comes from his work tired, exhausted, finds his home comfortless, damp, dirty, repulsive; he has urgent need of recreation, he *must* have something to make work worth his trouble, to make the prospect of the next day endurable. Drunkenness has here ceased to be a vice, for which the vicious can be held responsible; it becomes a phenomenon, the necessary, inevitable effect of certain conditions upon an object possessed of no volition in relation to those conditions. They who have degraded the working-man to a mere object have the responsibility to bear.

Another source of physical mischief to the working-class lies in the impossibility of employing skilled physicians in cases of illness. English doctors charge high fees, and working-men are not in a position to pay them. They can therefore do nothing or are compelled to call in cheap charlatans, and use quack remedies, which do more harm than good. An immense number of such quacks thrive in every English town, securing their *clientèle* among the poor by means of advertisements, posters, and other such devices. Besides these, vast quantities of patent medicines are sold, for all conceivable ailments: Morrison's Pills, Parr's Life Pills, Dr Mainwaring's Pills, and a thousand other pills, essences, and balsams, all of which have the property of curing all the ills that flesh is heir to. It is by no means unusual for the manufacturer of Parr's Life Pills to sell twenty to twenty-five thousand boxes of these salutary pills in a week, and they are taken for constipation by this one, for diarrhoea by that one, for fever, weakness, and all possible ailments. As our German peasants are cupped or bled at certain seasons, so do the English working-people now consume patent medicines to their own injury and the great profit of the manufacturer. One of the most injurious of these patent medicines is a drink prepared with opiates, chiefly laudanum, under the name Godfrey's Cordial. Women who work at home, and have their own and other people's children to take care of, give them this drink to keep them quiet, and, as many believe, to strengthen them. They often begin to give this medicine to newly-born children, and continue, without knowing the effects of this 'heart's-ease', until the children die. The less susceptible the child's system to the action of the opium, the greater the quantities administered. When the cordial ceases to act, laudanum alone is given, often to the extent of fifteen to twenty drops at a dose. The Coroner of Nottingham testified before a Parliamentary Commission that one apothecary had, according to his own statement, used thirteen hundred-weight of laudanum in one year in the preparation of Godfrey's Cordial. The effects upon the children so treated may be readily imagined. They are pale, feeble, wilted, and usually die before completing the second year. The use of this cordial is very extensive in all great towns and industrial districts in the kingdom.

The result of all these influences is a general enfeeblement of the frame in the working-class. They are almost all weakly, of angular but not powerful build, lean, pale, and of relaxed fibre, with the exception of the muscles especially exercised in their work. Nearly all suffer from indigestion, and consequently from a more or less hypochondriac, melancholy, irritable, nervous condition. Their enfeebled constitutions are unable to resist disease, and are therefore seized by it on every occasion. Hence they age prematurely, and die early. On this point the mortality statistics supply unquestionable testimony.

According to the Report of Register-General Graham, the annual death-rate of all England and Wales is something less than $2\frac{1}{4}$ per cent. That is to say, out of forty-five persons, one dies every year. This was the average for the year 1839–40. In 1840–41 the mortality diminished somewhat, and the death-rate was but one in forty-six. But in the great cities the proportion is wholly different. I have before me official tables of mortality (*Manchester Guardian*, 31 July 1844), according to which the death-rate of several large towns is as follows: In Manchester, including Chorlton and Salford, 1 in 32.72; and excluding Chorlton and Salford, 1 in 30.75. In Liverpool, including West Derby (suburb), 31.90, and excluding West Derby, 29.00; while the average of all the districts of Cheshire, Lancashire, and Yorkshire cited, including a number of wholly or partially rural districts and many small towns, with a total population of 2,172,506 for the whole, is 1 death in 39.80 persons. How unfavourably the workers are placed in the great cities, the mortality for Prescott in Lancashire shows; a district inhabited by miners, and showing a lower sanitary condition than of the agricultural districts, mining being by no means a healthful occupation. But these miners live in the country, and the death-rate among them is but 1 in 47.54, or nearly $2\frac{1}{2}$ per cent, better than that for all England. All these statements are based upon the mortality tables for 1843. Still higher is the death-rate in the Scotch cities; in Edinburgh, in 1838–39, 1 in 29; in 1831, in the Old Town alone, 1 in 22. In Glasgow, according to Dr Cowen, the average has been, since 1830, 1 in 30; and in single years, 1 in 22 to 24. That this enormous shortening of life falls chiefly upon the working-class, that the general average is improved by the smaller mortality of the upper and middle-classes, is attested upon all sides. One of the most recent depositions is that of a physician, Dr P. H. Holland, in Manchester, who investigated Chorlton-on-Medlock, a suburb of Manchester, under official commission. He divided the houses and streets into three classes each, and ascertained the following variations in the death-rate:

| First class of Streets. Houses | I. class. Mortality 1 in 51 |
|---|---|
| „ „ „ | II. „ „ „ 41 |
| „ „ „ | III. „ „ „ 36 |
| Second „ „ | I. „ „ „ 55 |
| „ „ „ | II. „ „ „ 38 |
| „ „ „ | III. „ „ „ 35 |
| Third „ „ | I. „ Wanting – – |
| „ „ „ | II. „ Mortality „ 35 |
| „ „ „ | III. „ „ „ 25 |

It is clear from other tables given by Holland that the mortality in the *streets* of the second class is 18 per cent greater, and in the streets of the third class 68 per cent greater than in those of the first class; that the mortality in the *houses* of the second class is 31 per cent greater, and in the third class 78 per cent greater than in those of the first class; that the mortality in those bad streets which were improved, decreased 25 per cent. He closes with the remark, very frank for an English bourgeois:[1]

> When we find the rate of mortality four times as high in some streets as in others, and twice as high in whole classes of streets as in other classes, and further find it is all but invariably high in those streets which are in bad condition, and almost invariably low in those whose condition is good, we cannot resist the conclusion that multitudes of our fellow-creatures, *hundreds of our immediate neighbours*, are annually destroyed for want of the most evident precautions.

The death-rate is kept so high chiefly by the heavy mortality among young children in the working-class. The tender frame of a child is least able to withstand the unfavourable influences of an inferior lot in life; the neglect to which they are often subjected, when both parents work or one is dead, avenges itself promptly, and no one need wonder that in Manchester more than 57 per cent of the children of the working-class perish before the fifth year, while but 20 per cent of the children of the higher classes, and not quite 32 per cent of the children of all classes in the country die under five years of age.

Apart from the diverse diseases which are the necessary consequence of the present neglect and oppression of the poorer classes, there are other influences which contribute to increase the mortality among small children. In many families the wife, like the husband, has to work away from home, and the consequence is the total neglect of the children, who are either locked up or given out to be taken care of. It is, therefore, not to be wondered at if hundreds of them perish through all manner of accidents. Nowhere are so many children run over, nowhere are so many killed by falling, drowning, or burning, as in the great cities and towns of England. Deaths from burns and scalds are especially frequent, such a case occurring nearly every week during the winter months in Manchester, and very frequently in London, though little mention is made of them in the papers. I have at hand a copy of the *Weekly Dispatch* of 15 December 1844, according to which, in the week from 1 December to 7 December inclusive, *six* such cases occurred. These unhappy children, perishing in this terrible way, are victims of our social disorder, and of the property-holding classes interested in maintaining and prolonging this disorder. Yet one is left in doubt whether even this terribly torturing death is not a blessing for the children in rescuing them from a long life of toil and wretchedness, rich in suffering and poor in enjoyment. So far has it gone in England; and the bourgeoisie reads these things every day in the newspapers and takes no further trouble in the matter. But it cannot complain if, after the official and non-official testimony here cited which must be known to it, I broadly accuse it of social murder.

## Reference

1. Report of Commission of Inquiry into the State of Large Towns and Populous Districts, First Report, 1844. Appendix.

Frederick Engels, son of a German textile manufacturer, came to Manchester in 1842 to work in his father's factory. In 1845, aged 25, he published *The Condition of the Working Class in England* in Leipzig. The first British edition did not appear until 1892. The extract reproduced here is drawn from the translation of the full work by the Institute of Marxism–Leninism, Moscow, published by Panther Books, London, 1969.

# 22
# Inequalities in health: ten years and little further on

## J. N. MORRIS

On Aug 29, 1980, at the start of the summer bank holiday, the Department of Health and Social Security released the report of its Research Working Group on Inequalities in Health (of which I was a member), in minimal form and number, without any publicity, and prefaced by a summary rejection of its recommendations by the Secretary of State.[1] The media immediately spotted this unusual procedure and an impromptu press conference called by the group itself at the Royal College of Physicians attracted wide coverage. The issues raised in the 'Black report'[2,3] have continued to hold the interest of the public and have stimulated much critical examination and research in the UK and elsewhere.

The Black report dealt essentially with the official statistics of England and Wales, focusing on the steep gradient of mortality and life expectancy in 1970–72, from 'professional' social class I through to 'part-skilled' class IV and 'unskilled' class V. The gap between these occupational/social classes – the inequality in death rates – was of course long established but, apparently, was widening. After 30 years of the National Health Service and welfare state this was a grievous disappointment, provoking fundamental questions on health and social policy.

The working group considered several possible, plausible, explanations and concluded that material conditions of life, income, housing, and the working and general environments – with which education levels are closely associated – were the main factors. Class differences in these 'life chances' were largely responsible for their differences in health. It followed that poverty and deprivation were principal causes of the premature death and lesser life expectancy of the lowest classes, IV and V. This last and anything-but-new conclusion proved the most upsetting to received opinion.

### Research 1980–90

The 'longitudinal study'[4] of the Office of Population Censuses and Surveys, following a cohort identified in the 1971 census, used the same information on occupation/

social class throughout. The main technical flaw of previous analyses was thus overcome. In terms of social class they found the distribution as before. At the same time there was no support for the notion that 'slippage' because of ill-health was a major factor in social stratification. Moreover, the additional information now available[5] on such matters as housing tenure, car ownership, and education level allowed for more realistic allocations than occupational 'skill' and 'general standing in the community' alone. Findings were similar. The Whitehall study,[6] a quite independent body of data, with its detailed picture of four grades of civil servants, from the top administrative to men in support and unskilled services, showed even wider contrasts between these grades than the national figures. 'Ecological' studies, in another tradition, have compared *death* rates of small residential areas according to their *social conditions*, including levels of unemployment.[7,8] Close matching has been found and correspondence also to rates by conventional social class. Another, revitalised, approach[9] is the study of adult mortality in relation to social circumstances, favourable and adverse, at the beginning of life: powerful associations have emerged. The notion of an underclass, recently imported from [the] USA, seems merely to be another name for the 'undeserving poor' (because much their own fault, and so on). As educational failure is one of its main constituents this is scarcely a helpful formulation.[10,11]

### Lifestyles
Lifestyles have claimed the greatest attention in recent years because of their manifest importance and because of the access they offer to health education. *Cigarette smoking* became class-bound soon after the Royal College of Physicians' first report of 1962,[12] and manual workers have subsequently shown the least reduction in their smoking rates.[13] *Exercise* habits again differ in the familiar direction,[13] though adequate data on health-related exercise[14] must wait on the current National Fitness Survey.[15] The available data, 1977–86, show reductions in sex and age differentials as more women, and more older people, have participated, but there has been no narrowing of the gap between the classes. *Dietary* differences between income groups have been evident for many years – e.g., in fruit consumption and in vitamin C.[16] More encouraging, and worth greater study in so bleak a general scene, *all* income groups have latterly been improving their patterns of fat intake and showing increasing preference for brown/wholemeal bread. Be all this as it may, these behaviours plainly are embedded in the social structure. When questions are asked not merely how people behave but why they behave as they do, 'lifestyles' provide no release from the need to confront that structure – which also has so many other effects on health.

### Agenda
There has been little work on psychosocial aspects[17] or on inequalities away from poverty and deprivation – e.g., the superiority in health of social class I over II and of II over III non-manual.[12,18] And there has been disappointingly little advance in understanding of social-biological interactions.[19] Experimental approaches, for instance, with mothers and under-5s in inner cities, are notably few. Morbidity data confirm the general picture but are much scarcer than mortality data.[13]

## A disheartening decade

Mortality data for the 1980s are limited but discouraging. Official figures for 1979–83 suggested some increase in the class gradient since 1970–72.[20] The longitudinal study made similar observations to 1985, extending also to death rates among the elderly and the unemployed.[5,21]

The data on *income* are more disturbing.[22] The average rise of real incomes over 1979–87 was 23.1 per cent. But the rise in the bottom ten percent of the population was 0.1 per cent, in the next ten percent 2.4 per cent, and in the next, 2.8 per cent. During those years the proportion of children living on less than half average income, the nearest there is to an official (and European Community) poverty line, increased from 12 per cent to 26 per cent – now 3.1 million children. Large numbers of unmarried, divorced and separated 'single' mothers (the new major element), of the seriously disabled, of elderly persons without occupational or private pensions, and of the chronic unemployed also feature prominently in these statistics. Market forces, it is apparent, have not provided a solution; too little has trickled down.

The prospect has to be faced that inequalities in mortality, with unacceptably high rates among the poor, will continue, and it must be doubted that Britain will meet the WHO target (to which it is a signatory) and reduce inequalities by 25 per cent during the 1990s.[23]

## Contribution of medicine?

The first response to this situation must be public education. More directly *health education* has to be intensified, focusing on the disadvantaged. 'Look After Your Heart', the official campaign against coronary heart disease, now has more substantial funds, and its effectiveness in attacking the excess death rates among men in social classes IV and V will be critical. Discrimination of health service facilities in favour of the disadvantaged, as recommended in the original report, is a natural response, but with the NHS under siege it is too much to hope for a great effort in the foreseeable future.[24]

Has medicine a role beyond the treatment of these symptoms and end-stages of social failure? Can it respond to the poverty and deprivation which, to the best of our understanding, are the basis and a large part of the aetiology of one of our most persistent and serious national health problems? The mitigation of this poverty and deprivation, it is generally agreed, is the precondition of a solution. And evidently it cannot merely be left to others. This is to enter the central arena of politics – beyond the comparatively acceptable fields of smoking, alcohol, and so on – and such is the depth of ideological divide on questions of equality in Britain today that the dangers of any such intervention must be recognised. If, nevertheless, medicine, collectively, does decide to intervene, it is prudent to ask what would be the most 'medical' initiatives – and the least likely to provoke hostile criticism and be self-defeating?

Two fields may be mentioned which command much cross-party and non-party support and are unlikely to arouse contention on 'dependency culture' and the like. The classic public health concern for decent housing would make it natural to support Shelter, the national housing campaign; rising concern with homelessness highlights a continuing, too slowly reducing, national problem of inadequate housing.[25] Officially, in excess of 130,000 families are homeless (the figure has more than doubled in the

1980s) and even greater numbers of single persons and childless families are excluded from these statistics. The other campaigning area where support of medicine could be appropriate and likely to be effective is child poverty. Child benefit has been frozen for 3 years and the outlook for next year is dim. The Child Poverty Action Group has a scholarly record, one of seriously and responsibly keeping the needs before the public, and again it could claim our support. The British Medical Association has shown impressive political skills and its response to these issues would be welcome.

Alternatively, or perhaps in a complementary approach, our new public health medicine[26] and its Faculty, returning to its roots, could speak and act collectively on behalf of all.

## References

1. Department of Health and Social Security, *Inequalities in Health: Report of a Research Working Group* (D. Black (Chairman); J. N. Morris; P. Townsend; C. S. Smith), DHSS, London (1980).
2. Townsend, P. and Davidson, N. *Inequalities in Health: The Black Report*, Penguin, Harmondsworth (1988).
3. Whitehead, M. *The Health Divide*, Health Education Council, London (1987) and Penguin, Harmondsworth (1988).
4. Goldblatt, P. 'Mortality by social class, 1971–85', *Popular Trends*, **56**, 6–15 (1989).
5. Goldblatt, P. In: Goldblatt P. (ed.) *Longitudinal Study: Mortality and Social Organisation*, HM Stationery Office, London 163–92 (1990).
6. Marmot, M. G., Shipley, M. J., and Rose, G. 'Inequalities in death, specific explanations of a general pattern?', *Lancet*, i, 1003–1006 (1984).
7. Townsend, P., Phillimore, P., and Beattie, A. *Inequalities in Health in the Northern Region*, Northern RHA and University of Bristol, Newcastle and Bristol (1986).
8. Carstairs, V. and Morris, R. 'Deprivation and mortality, an alternative to social class?', *Community Medicine*, **11**, 210–19. *With erratum*, **11**, no. 3 (1989).
9. Barker, D. J. P., Winter, P. D., Osmond, C., Margetts, B., and Simmonds, S. J. 'Weight in infancy and death from ischaemic heart disease', *Lancet*, ii, 577–80 (1989).
10. Murray, C. *Losing Ground: American Social Policy, 1950–1980*, Basic Books, New York (1984).
11. Editorial. 'The underclass', *Lancet*, **335**, 1312–13 (1990).
12. Morris, J. N. 'Social inequalities undiminished', *Lancet*, i, 87–90 (1979).
13. Office of Population Surveys and Censuses, *General Household Survey*, HM Stationery Office, London (annual publication).
14. Morris, J. N., Clayton, D. G., Everitt, M. G., Semmence, A. M., and Burgess, E. H. 'Exercise in leisure-time, coronary attack and death rates', *British Heart Journal*, **63**, 325–34 (1990).
15. Fitness and Health Advisory Group of the Health Education Authority and the Sports Council, *Activity and Health 2000: Prospectus of the National Fitness Survey*, HEA, London (1988).
16. *Household Food Consumption and Expenditure*, HM Stationery Office, London (annual publication).
17. Jenkins, C. D. 'Behavioural perspectives on health risks among the disadvantaged'. In: Parron, D. L., Solomon, F., and Jenkins C. D. (eds) *Behaviour, Health Risks and Social Disadvantage*, National Academy Press, Washington, 3–12 (1982).
18. Morris, J. N. 'Inequality, poverty, and health', *Lancet*, ii, 632–33 (1986).
19. Markowe, H. L. J., Marmot, M. G., Shipley, M. J. *et al.* 'Fibrinogen, a possible link between social class and coronary heart disease', *British Medical Journal*, **291**, 1312–14 (1985).

20. Government Statistical Service, *Households Below Average Income: a Statistical Analysis 1981–1987*, HM Stationery Office, London (1990).
21. Office of Population Censuses and Surveys, *Occupational Mortality, Decennial Supplement 1979–1980, 1982–83*, HM Stationery Office, London (1986).
22. Moser, K., Goldblatt, P., Fox, J., and Jones, D. 'Unemployment and mortality'. In: Goldblatt, P. (ed.) *Longitudinal Study: Mortality and Social Organisation*, HM Stationery Office, London, 81–97 (1980).
23. World Health Organisation European Region, *Targets for Health for All – 2000*, WHO, Copenhagen (1985).
24. Delamothe, T. 'Deprived area payments', *British Medical Journal*, **300**, 1609–10 (1990).
25. Dean, M. 'Homelessness, a housing or health problem?', *Lancet*, **335**, 715–16 (1990).
26. Committee of Inquiry into the Future Development of the Public Health Function in England and Wales (*The Acheson Report*), HM Stationery Office, London (1988).

Professor J. N. Morris is in the Department of Public Health and Policy at the London School of Hygiene and Tropical Medicine, London. This article, reproduced here in full, was originally published in the *Lancet*, **336**, 491–493 (1990).

# 23
# Depression: a sociological view

## GEORGE W. BROWN

I have been asked for a personal statement about depression. Of all psychiatric conditions depression is perhaps the most fitting for a sociologist to study. It is an affliction of a person's sense of values; and an exploration of the way people give meaning to their world can be expected to throw some light on a condition whose central feature is a feeling that there is no meaning in the world, that the future is hopeless, and the self worthless. Around this three-fold sense of futility cluster different psychological and somatic symptoms none of which on their own are either sufficient or necessary for the diagnosis. But I will leave this aside and start at the heart of the matter – with aetiology.

I believe that depression is essentially a social phenomenon. (If this were not a personal statement I would say that present evidence does not make it unreasonable to hold this view.) I would not make the same claim for schizophrenia, though its onset and course are also greatly influenced by social factors. Society and depression are more fundamentally linked. I can envisage societies where depression is absent and others where the majority suffer from depression. While this is social science fiction something not too unlike it has been documented. At least a quarter of working-class women with children living in London suffer from a depressive disorder which, if they were to present themselves at an out-patient clinic, psychiatrists would accept as clinical depression; while women with children living in crofting households in the Outer Hebrides are practically free of depression no matter what their social class. (They do experience more anxiety conditions, but I believe that this is another story.) Moreover, I know of no compelling reason to believe that the many bodily correlates of depression such as those revealed by work on bioamines are any more than the *result* of social and psychological factors. This is not to deny the possible aetiological implications of recent biochemical research, nor the possible aetiological role of genetic and constitutional factors. But taking account of the need to explain differences in the rate of depression in whole populations, I do not think that there is likely to be any more than a very modest primary aetiological influence from biochemical processes, that is, from such processes alone. The evidence for such a primary role for psychological and social factors is certainly far more convincing.

Like most doing research in the field of depression I am firmly convinced of a multifactorial view: that factors at many levels can play a role in aetiology. But this perspective should not disguise the need to establish the *relative* contribution of the various levels. Lip-service tends to be given to a multifactorial view but often in practice, in teaching, in research, and in clinical work only a single class of factor is seriously considered. Ritual obeisance to many variables allows pursuit of one. A psychiatrist in 1967 who asserted that a woman attending his clinic could not be clinically depressed as her condition was clearly related to her bad housing was perhaps expressing in a somewhat unsophisticated way the same views as many of his colleagues. Clinicians understandably desire research that will justify intervention in clinical settings. They also want theories that would be both intellectually challenging and serve as a basis for their claims to professional expertise within medicine. The failure of sociological ideas and methods to make much of an impact on psychiatric teaching has meant that most psychiatrists see little intellectual challenge in a socio-logical approach concentrating on the current environment. This also means that many have remained tied to a narrow view of science in which only experimentation is given full honours.

Of course, during the last two decades there have been important changes not least due to the lead of Sir Aubrey Lewis. But social psychiatry still needs to devote more of its time to the heady and dangerous job of causal analysis in natural settings; only in this way is it likely to get the necessary challenge and impetus to develop measures and methods that will have the authority to influence psychiatry as a whole.

During the last eight years my colleagues and I have done our best to follow such a path: our ideas about depression cannot be said to diverge all that much from ideas expressed *somewhere* in the psychiatric literature. (Has any other discipline specu-lated quite so much?) Any claim to originality probably mainly rests on the way factors have been brought together on a causal model; and any claims to attention on the consideration we have given to methodological problems. Indeed the model is sufficiently well based for some interest to be shown in the theory that we have linked to it. But in what follows, model and theory should be kept distinct; claims made for our causal model cannot be made for our more speculative theory.

The job of creating such a model involves developing measures and research design so that a claim can be made that the factors, following the temporal order set out in the model (Figure 23.1), are in *some way* involved in bringing about depression. Obvious biases must be ruled out and objections that would trivialize the model must be met. (For example, while life-events do play a causal role they merely bring about a depressive disorder that would have occurred before long in any case without any pre-event occurring.) We have made some progress; certain kinds of severe life-events and difficulties do appear to bring about the majority of depressive disorders – both among women treated by psychiatrists and among women found to be depressed after being selected at random from the general population (see Table 23.1). The kind of depression does not matter: these *provoking agents* are as strongly associated with the onset of psychotic as neurotic depressive conditions. Perhaps the most challenging claim of the model is that provoking agents (i.e. events and difficulties) are rarely sufficient to bring about depression – although they do determine *when* the disorders occur.

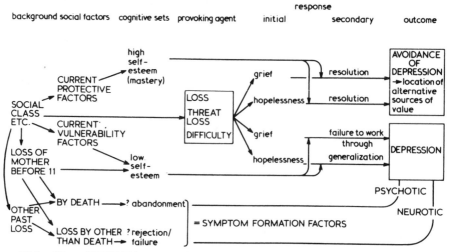

**Figure 23.1**  (Key: CAPITALS = Causal model)

**Table 23.1**  Proportion with at least one severely threatening event or at least one major difficulty in the period before onset for patients and onset cases or interviews for 'normal' and 'borderline' women

|  | patients (N = 114) % | onset cases (N = 37) % | 'normal' and 'borderline' women (N = 382) % |
|---|---|---|---|
| 1. severe event alone | 30 ⎫ | 41 ⎫ | 13 ⎫ |
| 2. severe event and major difficulty | 31 ⎬ 75 | 24 ⎬ 89 | 6 ⎬ 30 |
| 3. major difficulty | 14 ⎭ | 24 ⎭ | 11 ⎭ |
| 4. no severe event or major difficulty | 25 | 11 | 70 |

This is best illustrated by the way depression is linked to social class. Working-class women in London are not only far more likely to suffer from depression, they are also far more likely to develop a clear depressive disorder in the presence of a major life-event or difficulty (see Table 23.2). Something other than the provoking agent is at work.

There is in fact a second set of factors. If a woman does not have an intimate relationship with a husband or boyfriend – one in which she feels she can confide and trust – she is much more likely to break down in the presence of a major life-event or difficulty. Similarly she is also at greater risk if she has three or more children under fifteen at home, if she is unemployed, and if she lost her mother (but not father) before the age of eleven. We call these *vulnerability factors* – although more optimistically they can be seen in a reverse way and called protective factors. None are capable of producing depression on their own, but they greatly increase chances of breakdown in the presence of a provoking agent (Table 23.3). Some of the social class difference is explained by the fact that working-class women in London experience

**Table 23.2** Percentage of women developing a psychiatric disorder (i.e. caseness) in year by life-stage, social class, and whether preceded by a severe event or major difficulty (chronic cases excluded)

| | severe event/<br>major difficulty<br>% | no<br>severe event/<br>major difficulty<br>% |
|---|---|---|
| *women without child at home* | | |
| middle class | 22 (7/32) | 0 (0/62) |
| working class | 10 (3/30) | 2 (1/44) |
| *women with child at home* | | |
| middle class | 8 (3/36) | 1 (1/80) |
| working class | 31 (21/67) | 1 (1/68) |
| *all women* | | |
| middle class | 15 (10/68) | 1 (1/142) |
| working class | 25 (24/97) | 3 (2/112) |

**Table 23.3** Proportion of women developing psychiatric disorder in the year among women who experienced a severe event or major difficulty by vulnerability factors (intimacy, employment status, early loss of mother and 3 + children under 15 at home)

| | | *with event or<br>difficulty* | | *without event<br>or difficulty* | |
|---|---|---|---|---|---|
| 'a'* intimacy relationship regardless | employed | (4/53) 9% | } (9/88) 10% | (1/117) 1% | } (2/193) 1% |
| | not employed | (5/45) 11% | | (1/76) 1% | |
| non-'a'* intimacy relationship excluding early loss of mother or 3 + children under 15 living at home | employed | (6/39) 15% | | (0/34) 0% | |
| | not employed | (7/23) 30% | | (2/19) 11% | |
| non-'a'* intimacy relationship with early loss of mother or 3 + children under 15 living at home | employed | (5/8) 63% | | (0/7) 0% | |
| | not employed | (6/6) 100% | | (0/2) 0% | |
| | | (33/164) 20% | | (4/255) 2% | |

* Essentially an 'a' intimacy relationship is one where the respondent reports a confiding relationship (where both partners can talk to each other about any personal matter) and this person is either a man or a member of the respondent's household.

more untoward life-events and difficulties – in this sense their lives are much tougher. But most of the class difference is due to their excess of vulnerability factors which put working-class women at risk for depression at the time of a major life-event or difficulty. The low rate of depression in the Outer Hebrides is probably due to the much greater degree of protection their culture and society gives these women – but this has still to be documented in detail.

Recently a third factor has been added to this model. While only loss of a mother before eleven increases the risk of a woman developing depression, other past losses of close relatives, largely in childhood and adolescence, influence the type and severity of depression. We call these *symptom formation* factors. Loss by *death* is strongly associated with psychotic-like depressive symptoms and their severity and *loss by other means* (e.g. parents separating) to neurotic-like depressive symptoms (and their severity). Only loss of mother before eleven plays two roles – as a vulnerability factor increasing risk of depression and as a symptom formation factor. Otherwise past loss merely determines the form and severity of a depressive disorder once it has occurred.

This is a rough outline of the model – stated without necessary caveats. But what does it all mean? What about theory? Consider employment and its protective role for women. Is it because it improves her economic circumstances, alleviates her boredom, keeps her occupied, brings her a greater variety of social contacts, or enhances her sense of personal worth? And just why should any of these aspects play a protective role? A causal model is not enough: theory is needed to explain what is happening. Theory unfortunately takes longer than a causal model to develop and to test. Any theory concerning the aetiology of depression has to deal with two crucial 'facts' provided by our model. First, that on the whole provoking life-events mainly involve major losses (if this term is allowed a certain licence to include events such as learning of a husband's infidelity); major difficulties and threats of loss can also at times bring about a depressive disorder. Something more than loss must be involved. Second, in the absence of a vulnerability factor such provoking agents rarely bring about depression. In other words, no matter how catastrophic a loss depression will not follow without the presence of at least one vulnerability factor.

We have speculated that low self-esteem is the common feature behind all four vulnerability factors and it is this that makes sense of the results. It is not loss itself that is important but the capacity of a woman to hope for better things once an event or difficulty has occurred. In response to a provoking agent relatively specific feelings of hopelessness are likely to occur: the person has usually lost an important source of value – something that may have been derived from a person, a role, or an idea. If this develops into a *general* feeling of hopelessness it may form the central feature of the depressive disorder itself; and Beck's triad of cognitions accompanies the well known affective and somatic symptoms of depression. Essential in any such generalization of hopelessness is a woman's ongoing self-esteem, her sense of her ability to control her world, and her confidence that alternative sources of value will be available. If the woman's self-esteem is low *before* the onset of any depression she will be less likely to be able to see herself as emerging from her privation. And, of course, once depression has occurred feelings of confidence and self-worth can sink even lower.

It must not be overlooked that an appraisal of general hopelessness may be entirely realistic: the future for many women *is* bleak. But given an event or difficulty, low self-esteem will increase the chances of such an interpretation of hopelessness. Here inner and outer worlds meet, and internal and external resources come together. And from there the sociologist must go on to build links with the wider cultural, economic, and political systems. Psychiatry cannot rest in the consulting room or even within the confines of a person's immediate social circle. Study of self-esteem cannot stop at the borders of a woman's personal world. For instance, may not feelings of low self-worth have something to do with the fact women are not paid for what many see as their central tasks? Do we take work seriously if it is not paid? The bitterness created by the recent attempts at wage control in all strata of male society suggest that more than economic considerations are involved in payment for work in our society.

While I have emphasized the role of the current environment our own results make it clear that this should not be taken too far – it is intended as a corrective. We carry with us our pasts. But I would again emphasize cognitive factors in explaining the effect of past loss. Loss of a mother before eleven, for instance, can be linked to the learning of uncontrollability, and through this low self-esteem. Martin Seligman's concept of learned helplessness has got a good deal in common with the way we have interpreted the role of vulnerability and protective factors. But unlike him I see no reason to restrict our model to so-called 'reactive' or 'neurotic' depressive conditions. The various vulnerability factors increase the risk of all types of depression; for example, among our patients those with neurotic-like depressive symptoms were no more likely to have more vulnerability factors or provoking agents than those with psychotic symptoms; we also have seen that past loss in childhood and adolescence can greatly influence the much later expression of psychotic or neurotic symptoms.

Here again I would emphasize a cognitive interpretation – in this instance, concerning long held perceptions of abandonment for psychotic as against rejection and failure for neurotic depressive symptoms.

But this is particularly speculative and I have at this point pursued our theoretical ideas enough. I will just finally add that we have also argued for a second, but less important, aetiological mechanism in which self-esteem is again implicated. Low self-esteem can inhibit a woman carrying out the necessary grief work after a major loss – and complications leading to depression are then likely to arise. This would also make it more difficult for her to take advantage of alternative sources of value that might be available.

It is probably unnecessary to make the obvious point that these processes will have biological correlates. It is possible that certain occurrences (e.g. early loss of mother, a depressive illness) may lead to more or less irreversible biochemical changes in the brain, thereby perhaps changing the mechanism of reward for the individual.

I am conscious of many gaps. I would have liked to explore the convergence of ideas about depression. There is, for instance, clearly a parallel between our sources of positive value and the psychologist's 'reinforcers', the psychoanalyst's 'narcissistic supplies', and the social scientist's concern with 'meaning'. I am also aware of my failure to deal with the perennial issue of diagnosis. Some psychiatrists may wish to dispute the label of depressive psychiatric disorder we have given to women in the community – very few of whom were receiving psychiatric help. I would point out that this is likely to place psychiatry in a perplexing intellectual and ethical dilemma. The women do not appear to differ in any essential way from many seen and treated in out-patient clinics. Is a psychiatric label to be restricted to those who manage to present themselves in such clinics? Fresh ideas and new research are required to clarify this issue. Another topic which needs much more exploration is the boundary between normal grief and depression.

But most of all I am conscious of my failure to convey in human terms what I believe to be involved in depression and in avoiding depression. I comfort myself that the reader of the *Bethlem and Maudsley Gazette* least requires such an account. But, if my talk of value resources, provoking agents, vulnerability factors, and protective factors has not lost you, Shakespeare may be able to illustrate our theory and to suggest the power of alternative sources of value to rescue a person from the onset of depression.

> 'When in disgrace with Fortune and men's eyes
> I all alone beweep my outcast state,
> And trouble deaf heaven with my bootless cries,
> And look upon myself, and curse my fate,
> Wishing me like to one more rich in hope,
> Featur'd like him, like him with friends possess'd,
> Desiring this man's art, and that man's scope.
> With what I most enjoy contented least;
> Yet in these thoughts myself despising,
> Haply I think on thee,—and then my state,
> Like to the lark at break of day arising
> From sullen earth, sings hymns at heaven's gate;
>   For thy sweet love remember'd such wealth brings
>   That then I scorn to change my state with kings.'
>                                   (Sonnet XXIX)

George W. Brown is a Medical Research Council External Staff Member and Honorary Professor of Sociology at Bedford College, London. 'Depression' was first published in the *Bethlem and Maudsley Gazette*, Summer 1977, pp. 9–12. It was republished in *Basic Readings in Medical Sociology*, Tuckett, D. and Kaufert, J. M. (eds), Tavistock, London (1978).

# 24
# Entitlement and deprivation

## JEAN DRÈZE AND AMARTYA K. SEN

### Deprivation and the law

In a private ownership economy, command over food can be established by either growing food oneself and having property rights over what is grown, or selling other commodities and buying food with the proceeds. There is no guarantee that either process would yield enough for the survival of any particular person or a family in a particular social and economic situation. The third alternative, other than relying on private charity, is to receive free food or supplementary income from the state. These transfers are, as things stand now, rather rare and limited.

For a large part of humanity, about the only substantial asset that a person owns is his or her ability to work, i.e. labour power. If a person fails to secure employment, then that means of acquiring food (e.g. by getting a job, earning a wage, and having food with this income) fails. If, in addition to that, the laws of the land do not provide any social security arrangements, e.g. unemployment insurance, the person will, under these circumstances, fail to secure the means of subsistence. And that can result in serious deprivation – possibly even starvation and death.

It should also be added that even a person who is engaged in growing food and who succeeds in growing more (even, much more) than enough food for survival may not necessarily survive on this basis, and may not even have the legal right to do so. In many famines the majority of the victims come from the class of agricultural labourers. They are often primarily engaged in growing food. However, the legal nature of their contract, which is often informal, basically involves a wage payment in exchange for employment. The contract typically includes no right to the output grown by the person's own labour – no entitlement to the food output which could be the basis of survival for that person and his or her dependants.

Even if a person is lucky enough to find employment and is paid a certain sum of money for it as a wage, he or she has to convert that into food by purchase in the market. How much that wage commands would, of course, depend on the price of food. If food prices rise very rapidly, without money wages rising correspondingly, the labourers who have grown the food themselves may fail to acquire the food they need to survive. The food grown belongs to the employer (typically the owner of the land), and the wage payment is the end of the grower's right to the produce, even if that wage does not yield enough to survive.

Similarly, a person who acquires food by producing some other commodity and selling it in the market has to depend on the actual ability to sell that product and also on the relative price of that product *vis-à-vis* food. If either the sale fails to materialise, or the relative price of that product falls sharply *vis-à-vis* food, the person may again have no option but to starve.

It is also important to realise that uncertainty and vulnerability can be features of subsistence production (involving 'exchange with nature') as well as of market exchange. This precariousness is particularly visible in African famines, where a substantial proportion of the victims often come from the ranks of small farmers who are hit *inter alia* [among other things] by a collapse of their 'direct entitlement' to the food they normally grow. It would be a misleading simplification to regard self-provisioning as synonymous with security. The peasant farmer, like the landless labourer, has no guaranteed entitlement to the necessities of life.

### Entitlement failures and economic analysis

If a group of people fail to establish their entitlement over an adequate amount of food, they have to go hungry. If that deprivation is large enough, the resulting starvation can lead to death. There is nothing particularly novel in the recognition that starvation is best seen as a result of 'entitlement failure'. Since the aggregate food supply is not divided among the population through some distributive formula (such as equal division), each family has to establish command over its own food. Even though this fact is elementary enough, it is remarkable that food analysis is often conducted just in terms of production and total availability rather than taking note of the processes through which people establish their entitlements to food.

Entitlement analysis has been used in recent years to study various famines, e.g. the Bengal famine of 1943, the Malawi (in fact, Nyasaland, as it was then called) famine of 1949–50, the Sahel famines of the 1970s, the Bangladesh famine of 1974, the Ethiopian famines of 1973–85, and also a number of historical and recent cases of widespread starvation.

Just as there have been major famines in private ownership economies without state guarantee of basic subsistence rights, there have also been famines in socialist countries with their own systems of legality (e.g. in Ukraine in the early 1930s, in China during 1958–61, in Kampuchea in the late 1970s). The entitlements guaranteed by the law have, on those occasions, failed to provide the means of survival and subsistence to a great many people. In some cases, e.g. in the Ukrainian famines, state policy was in fact positively geared to undermining the entitlements of a large section of the population.

In analysing the causation of famines and in seeking social changes that eliminate them, the nature of entitlement systems and their workings have to be understood and assessed. The same applies to the problem of regular hunger and endemic under-nourishment. If people go hungry on a regular basis all the time, or seasonally, the explanations of that have to be sought in the way the entitlement system in operation fails to give the persons involved adequate means of securing enough food. Seeing hunger as entitlement failure points to possible remedies as well as helping us to understand the forces that generate hunger and sustain it. In particular, this approach compels us to take a broad view of the ways in which access to food can be protected or promoted, including reforms of the legal framework within which economic relations take place.

Since food problems have often been discussed in terms of the availability of food without going into the question of entitlement (there is a substantial tradition of concentrating only on food output per head, going back at least to Malthus's famous *Essay On the Principle of Population* of 1798), it is particularly important to understand the relevance of seeing hunger as entitlement failures. Such failures can occur even when food availability is not reduced, and even when the ratio of food to population (on which Malthus concentrated) goes up rather than down. Indeed, the relentless persistence of famines and the enormous reach of world hunger, despite the steady and substantial increase in food availability per head, makes it particularly imperative for us to reorientate our approach away from food availability to entitlements.

This can be done without losing sight of the elementary fact that food availability must be *among* the factors that determine the entitlements of different groups of people, and that food production is one of the important determinants of entitlements.

## Availability, command and occupations

The links between food availability and entitlements are indeed numerous and often important. First, for some people, the output of food grown by themselves is also their basic entitlement to food. For example, for peasants engaged mainly in growing food crops, the output, availability, and entitlement of food for the family can be much the same. This is a matter of what may be called 'direct entitlement'. Second, one of the major influences on the ability of anyone to purchase food is clearly the price of food, and that price is, of course, influenced by the production and availability of food in the economy. Third, food production can also be a major source of employment, and a reduction in food production (due to, say, a drought or a flood) would reduce employment and wage income through the same process that leads to a decline in the output and availability of food. Fourth, if and when a famine develops, having a stock of food available in the public distribution system is clearly a major instrument in the hands of the authorities to combat starvation. This can be done either by distributing food directly (in cooked or uncooked form), or by adding to the supply of food in the market, thereby exerting a downward pressure or a moderating influence on possibly rocketing prices. For these and other reasons, food entitlements have close links with food availability and output. It would be amazing if such links were absent, since the physical presence of food cannot but be an influence on the possibility of acquiring food through direct ownership or exchange.

However, as was discussed earlier, the actual command over food that different sections of the population can exercise depends on a set of legal and economic factors, including those governing ownership, production, and exchange. The overall availability of food is thus a very poor guide to the fortunes of different socio-economic groups.

The inadequacy of the availability view is particularly important to note in the context of the making of economic policy. Indeed, an undue reliance – often implicit – on the availability view has frequently contributed to the development or continuation of a famine, by making the relevant authorities smug about the food situation. For instance, there have been famines, e.g. in Bengal in 1943 and in Ethiopia in 1973, when the absence of a substantial food availability decline has contributed to official smugness.

The possibly contrary nature of the availability view and the entitlement view can be illustrated by considering the food availability picture during the Bangladesh famine of 1974. The availability in 1974 – the year of the famine – was higher than in any other year during 1971–6. And yet the famine hit Bangladesh exactly in that year of peak food availability! The families of rural labourers and other occupation groups who died because of their inability to command food were affected by a variety of influences (including loss of employment, the rise in food prices etc.), and this occurred despite the fact that the actual availability of food in the economy of Bangladesh was at a peak.

The failure of the availability view of famine can be further brought out by comparing different districts of Bangladesh in terms of their food availability in 1974 vis-à-vis their experience of famine.

It turns out that among the nineteen districts of Bangladesh, one of the famine districts (Dinajpur) had the *highest* availability of food in the entire country, and indeed all four of the famine districts were among the top five in terms of food availability per head. Even in terms of change in food availability per head over the preceding year, *all* the famine districts without exception had a substantial increase, and three of the four were among the top six in terms of food availability increase among all the nineteen districts.

The entitlement failure of the famine victims in Bangladesh related to a variety of factors, over and above output and availability of food. The floods that afflicted Bangladesh (particularly the famine districts) caused some havoc during June to August of 1974. The availability of food in the economy, however, remained high since the primary crop of Bangladesh (the *aman* crop, which tended to contribute substantially more than·half of the total food output of the country) is harvested during November to January, and this had been high in the *preceding* year (i.e. harvested in November 1973 to January 1974). The floods that hit Bangladesh did, of course, reduce the harvest in late 1974, including the primary *aman* crop. The famine, however, developed and peaked much before those reduced harvests arrived, and indeed by the time the primary crop (*aman*) was harvested, the famine was over and gone. During the famine months, the physical availability of food per head in Bangladesh thus remained high. And this was especially so for the famine districts, since they happened to have had rather good crops earlier, boosting the 1974 availability, even though the floods would eventually affect the availability of food in these districts in the *following* year (1975).

Among the influences that led to the collapse of entitlements of a large section of the population of Bangladesh in 1974 was the loss of employment as a result of the floods, which affected the planting and particularly the transplanting of rice, traditionally carried out in the period following the one in which the floods occurred. This would reduce the food output later, but its impact on employment was immediate and vicious.

The disruption of the economy of Bangladesh as a result of the floods was not, however, confined only to the decline of employment. The effect of the floods on the future output and availability of food and therefore on the expectation of food prices also played a major part. The poor and chaotic functioning of rice markets, fed by alarmist anticipations, led to price explosions following the flood, resulting in a collapse of food entitlements for those who found the already low purchasing power of their earnings further undermined.

The failure of the government to institute a suitable stabilising response also contributed to the unstable behaviour of the rice market. Rural labourers found a sharply diminished ratio of food command per unit of employment, and on top of that many had, in fact, lost employment as a result of floods, especially in the famine districts.

There is, therefore, no paradox in the fact that the Bangladesh famine of 1974 occurred at a time when the physical availability of food in the economy was at a local peak. It is the failure of large sections of the population, particularly of the labouring families, to command food in the market that has to be examined in order to understand the causation of that major catastrophe.

The terrible story of the Bangladesh famine of 1974 brings out the folly of concentrating only on the physical availability of food in the economy, and points to the necessity of investigating the movements of food entitlements of the vulnerable occupation groups and the causal influences (including market operations) that affect these movements. Similar lessons can be drawn from other famines as well.

### The 'food crisis' in sub-Saharan Africa

Alarm has often been expressed at the possibility of a decline in the amount of food available per person in the modern world. Indeed, there is a good deal of discussion centring on prospects of disaster, based on modern variants of Malthusian fears. As a matter of fact, however, there has not been any declining trend in food availability per head for the world as a whole in recent decades (nor, of course, any such trend since Malthus's own days). Obviously, any such future gazing is hard to do, but it seems unlikely that the real dangers in the near future can lie in the prospect of food output falling short of the growth of population.

Table 24.1 presents the trends in food output per head over the last half decade and the last decade (i.e. from 1981–3 to 1986–8, and from 1976–8 to 1986–8) for some of the major regions in the world.

The fact that the trend of food output per head is so sharply upward for developing economies in particular is, naturally a source of comfort. But it could be false comfort. In fact, different developing economies have done very differently over the last few decades. Specifically, Africa has been plagued by production problems – in addition to other problems – over nearly two decades now. The aggregate picture for the developing economies put together is thus, quite misleading.

This having been said, we must, however, resist the oversimplified suggestion that Africa's recent problems of hunger arise simply from declines in food output and supply. While food production and availability are undoubtedly among the more important influences in the determination of food entitlements, the connections are complex and there are also other matters involved (such as the performance of industries and non-food agriculture, and the general role of employment and economic participation).

Table 24.1   World trends in food output per head

| Region | The last half decade: 1986–8 average over 1981–3 average | The last decade: 1986–8 average over 1976–8 average |
|---|---|---|
| All developed economies | up 2% | up 3% |
| All developing economies | up 5% | up 11% |
| Europe | up 5% | up 13% |
| USA | down 7% | up 7% |
| Africa | down 2% | down 8% |
| South America | unchanged | up 2% |
| Asia | up 8% | up 17% |

*Source*: Calculated from data obtained from *FAO Production Yearbook 1988*, Table 4 and *FAO Quarterly Bulletin of Statistics*, vol. i, pt 4, 1988.

It must be borne in mind that food production is not only a source of food supply, it is also a major source of income and livelihood for vast sections of the African population. As a result, any reduction in food output per head in Africa also tends to be associated with a reduction in overall income for many occupation groups. However, the observed decline in food output per head in Africa need not have resulted in a collapse of food entitlements, if that decline had been compensated by an expansion of alternative incomes usable to acquire food from other sources, e.g. through imports from abroad.

Several economies elsewhere have experienced comparable or even greater declines in food output per head (in some cases as large as 30 or 40 per cent), without having any problems of the kind which have afflicted these African countries. This is so both because food production is a less important source of income and entitlement in these other economies, and also because they have achieved a more than compensating expansion of *non-food* production with favourable effects on incomes and entitlements. What may superficially appear to be a problem of food production and supply in Africa has to be seen in the more general terms of entitlement determination.

One important implication of this perspective is that even though current problems of hunger and famines in sub-Saharan Africa are undoubtedly connected *inter alia* with the decline of food production, remedial action need not necessarily take the form of attempting to reverse that historical trend. Other avenues of action, such as the diversification of economic activities and the expansion of public support, deserve attention as well.

Amartya K. Sen is Lamont University Professor of Economics and Philosophy at Harvard University and Jean Drèze is a freelance development economist. This article is an edited and amended extract from Chapter 3 of their book, *Hunger and Public Action*, Clarendon Press, Oxford, 1989.

# 25
# Deaths under 50

## MEDICAL SERVICES STUDY GROUP OF THE ROYAL COLLEGE OF PHYSICIANS OF LONDON

### Summary and conclusions

The Medical Services Study Group has started a collaborative study in the Mersey, West Midlands, and Grampian regions to examine the causes of death among medical inpatients aged 1 to 50. The cause of death was determined from the case notes and the consultant's opinion. The rate of ascertainment of cases was initially low, though it is increasing; despite this limitation an analysis of the first 250 cases showed one important finding. No fewer than 98 patients contributed to their own deaths through overeating, drinking, smoking, or not complying with treatment.

### Introduction

The consultants in hospitals in the Merseyside and West Midlands regions were visited and told about the study. The project put forward was a broad one – namely, to look in detail at the causes and circumstances of all deaths of patients aged 1 to 50 years in medical wards. For this the information contained in the case notes and the consultant's opinion on the patient were needed.

After it had started the physicians in the Grampian Region asked to participate.

### Ascertainment

The total population of the three regions under investigation is around 8 million – that is, about a sixth of the population of England and Wales. We would expect about 1,000 sets of case notes on medical patients dying in hospital each year.

From October 1977 to September 1978 over 400 were submitted. At present the rate of ascertainment is therefore about 50 per cent though there has been great variation between hospitals that promised support, some sending us all their deaths and some very few or none.

## Results of analysis

Table 25.1 shows the causes of death in the first 250 patients. Through studying the case notes in detail we have been able to assess the background to each case; in no fewer than 98 cases the patients contributed in large measure to their own deaths.

### The 98 cases of 'self-destruction'

Eight patients died from deliberate self-poisoning. In one there was no evidence of any previous psychiatric illness, but of the other seven, one had schizophrenia, one had a psychopathic personality, one was hopelessly dependent on alcohol, and the other four were depressives. Fashions in suicidal agents change and three used paraquat to kill themselves. One who died from barbiturate poisoning had had every conceivable treatment for schizophrenic depression: had been admitted for self-poisoning on three previous occasions; had slashed her wrists in an attempt to kill herself; and in her final illness had spent ten days in an intensive care unit. During her time in the intensive care unit she underwent 94 laboratory tests and 8 radiographic examinations – a sad example of the frequent inescapable commitment of skills and resources to patients beyond hope of being saved or restored to any worthwhile life.

Six of the 98 died from alcoholic cirrhosis of the liver, and another, whose liver disease was not primarily alcoholic in origin, accelerated his death by a high intake of alcohol. Though this group is small they exemplify the difficulty of helping alcoholics and the enormous demand they make on the health and social services. One 24-year-old man, who suffered cardiac arrest and irretrievable brain damage during acute alcoholic intoxication, occupied a bed in a teaching hospital for four months before he died, though it was clear from the outset that no recovery was possible.

Thirteen patients who died from carcinoma of the bronchus were strongly addicted to cigarettes, some smoking as many as 60 a day. Three other heavy cigarette smokers died from chronic airway obstruction and one from bronchopneumonia.

Among those whose death was attributable to myocardial infarction there were 25 with one or more causal factors within their own control. Twelve were grossly overweight; 22 smoked large numbers of cigarettes; two diabetics and two hypertensives did not comply with their treatment; and three others had had symptoms for a long time before they consulted a doctor.

Nine of the 98 patients delayed in seeking medical advice and in four this probably cost them their lives, for two died from gastroenteritis, one from meningococcal infection, and one from myxoedema. The patient with myxoedema had been ill for many years but had refused to see a doctor. Two of the other five might have survived and the remaining three lived longer had they sought help earlier.

Thirty-seven of the 98 patients refused admission to hospital, were unwilling to submit to investigation, discharged themselves from hospital, defaulted from diabetic clinics, or did not co-operate in taking medication. These attitudes were often encouraged by their spouses. It is impossible to quantify this factor, but certainly in many cases it was to some extent responsible for the fatal issue, while in others it hastened death. An anxious and nervous temperament was responsible in many instances but

**Table 25.1**  Summary of cause of death in the 250 patients surveyed

| Causes of death | | No. of cases |
|---|---|---|
| Malignancies: | | 47 |
|   Carcinomas (primary site): | | |
|     Ampulla of Vater | 1 | |
|     Breast | 5 | |
|     Bronchus | 14 | |
|     Colon | 2 | |
|     Stomach | 3 | |
|     Undetermined | 2 | |
|   Sarcomas | 2 | |
|   Gliomas | 4 | |
|   Myelomatosis | 3 | |
|   Leukaemias | 7 | |
|   Lymphomas | 4 | |
| Haematological conditions | | 7 |
| Cardiovascular conditions | | 96 |
|   Myocardial infarction | 31 | |
|   Cerebrovascular accidents | 51 | |
|   Thromboembolic disease | 7 | |
|   Miscellaneous | 7 | |
| Respiratory conditions | | 14 |
|   Asthma | 6 | |
|   Respiratory failure | 8 | |
| Alimentary conditions | | 7 |
|   Crohn's disease | 2 | |
|   Small intestine gangrene | 4 | |
|   Oesophageal perforation | 1 | |
| Neurological conditions: | | 4 |
|   Multiple sclerosis | 3 | |
|   Muscular dystrophy | 1 | |
| Infections: | | 25 |
|   Pneumonia | 6 | |
|   Acute laryngoepiglottitis | 3 | |
|   Encephalitis | 6 | |
|   Meningitis | 5 | |
|   Bacterial endocarditis | 2 | |
|   Gastroenteritis | 3 | |
| Hepatic failure: | | 12 |
|   Cirrhosis | 10 | |
|   Acute hepatic necrosis | 2 | |
| Renal failure | | 11 |
|   Chronic | 8 | |
|   Acute | 3 | |
| Diabetes | | 2 |
| Congenital abnormalities, brain damage at birth, etc. | | 10 |
| Self-poisoning (1 accidental) | | 9 |
| Others | | 6 |
| Total | | 250 |

in others lack of co-operation seemed to stem from fecklessness or a psychopathic attitude to life and to doctors in particular. There was little to indicate that lack of intelligence played any significant part.

## Discussion

Our initial finding will come as no surprise to the profession. Doctors have been saying for years that the causes of many of the killing diseases of middle life are not mysteries, but are contributed to by overeating, excess alcohol, and tobacco. Doctors' pronouncements tend not to be popular – some are contradictory and some are frankly disbelieved, and the disbelief is reinforced by the fact that the 'patient' often feels quite well. Health education is often derided ('It won't happen to me'), but there is an astonishing statistic which can stand much repetition. In 1930–32 the standard mortality ratio for ischaemic heart disease in social class I was 237 (normal 100). Over the next four decades it gradually fell to 88, but from 1951 to 1971 the crude mortality rate from ischaemic heart disease in all males almost doubled. Much the most likely explanation for this is that people in social class I do heed such advice whereas other groups do not.

The 'deaths under 50' project may be criticised on statistical grounds, but any bias in ascertaining the cases of 'self-destruction' is probably in the direction of under-reporting. The study's great merit lies in the fact that the information on causes of death is obtained from case notes and the clinicians' expert opinions, whereas in many surveys where the rate of ascertainment is better this information comes from death certificates.

'Deaths under 50' forms part of a report prepared by the Medical Services Study Group of the Royal College of Physicians of London. The report was compiled by Sir Cyril Clarke, director of the study group, and Dr George Whitfield, assistant director. A number of clinicians participated in the study. The full article was published in the *British Medical Journal*, **2**, 1061–1062 (1978).

# 26
# Malingering

## RICHARD ASHER

I define malingering as the imitation, production or encouragement of illness for a deliberate end. The patient is quite conscious of what he is doing and quite cognisant of why he is doing it. With that definition, pure malingering – the planned fraudulent faking of illness – is, in my experience, a very rare condition. Either that, or else I am a very gullible physician. I know I have been mistaken before now and it is possible that many malingerers have deceived me without being suspected.

True malingering is best classified by motives rather than by techniques – the principal prime movers being Fear, Desire and Escape.

*Fear*: fear of call-up, fear of overseas duty, fear of warfare.

*Desire*: desire for compensation, desire for a comfortable pension, desire for revenge against a surgeon for some (usually imagined) wrong. Desire for the comforts of hospital life. Desire to stay in the ward longer because one has fallen in love with the staff nurse.

*Escape*: escape from a prisoner-of-war camp by incurable disability, escape from prison by transfer to hospital, escape from an impending court case, escape from battle.

Malingering by prisoners of war has evolved a variety of ingenious techniques, even to the extent of passing borrowed albuminuric urine, secreted in a false bladder and passed in the presence of a suspicious German doctor, through a hand-carved and hand-painted penis of life-like verisimilitude.

It is well known that opposing forces try to weaken the enemy's army by dropping pamphlets persuading them to malinger. A particular pamphlet dropped in large numbers early in 1945 on English troops in Italy is worthy of your attention. Neatly produced in book-match form (to make it easy to hide), it opens with Three Golden Rules for Malingering which I do not think could be beaten:

1. You must make the impression you hate to be ill.
2. Make up your mind for one disease and stick to it.
3. Don't tell the doctor too much.

There is only time to give details about one of those. Here is how to have tuberculosis – according to the instruction book:

'First you must smoke excessively to acquire a cough. Then tell the doctor that you have lost weight, you do not feel well and that you cough a great deal. Say that sometimes you cough up streaks of blood. Sometimes you wake drenched with sweat. Stick to those symptoms, do not invent any new ones.'

Mental as well as physical disease can be simulated. Those with little experience of mental disease may learn with surprise that it is very hard to pretend to be mad. For instance, the peculiar distorted thinking of the schizophrenic is something a sane person cannot manage. An experiment was done in which twenty normal people were asked to feign insanity; they, and twenty genuinely psychotic patients, were interviewed by psychiatrists (who had no other means of telling which was which). The psychiatrists were able to pick out the malingerers in nearly 90 per cent of the cases.

I now pass to those cases of illness which, though self-produced or prolonged, do not constitute malingering. They do not have so definite a purpose. I have grouped them together as The Borderland of Malingering.

### The Borderland of Malingering

A. Illness as a comfort
   (a) Hysteria.
   (b) The Proud Lonely Person (Lucy's disease).

B. Illness as a hobby
   (a) The Grand Tour Type (rich hypochondriac).
   (b) The Chronic Out-Patient (poor hypochondriac).
   (c) The Eccentric Hypochondriac (faddist).
   (d) The Chronic Convalescent (daren't recover).

C. Illness as a profession
   (a) Anorexia Nervosa.
   (b) The Chronic Artefactualists.
   (c) Munchausen's Syndrome.

Hysterics differ from malingerers because, although they may produce illness and enjoy it, they are unaware of what they are doing. They possess a capacity for self-deception; they can wall off part of their mind so that it is impervious to self-scrutiny. This process, dignified by psychiatrists with the term 'dissociation', is colloquially called 'kidding yourself'. Some cases of hysteria are very close to malingering. Others start as malingerers, and as they become better at kidding others, they finally succeed in kidding themselves, and become hysterics.

I have seen very little proven hysteria and I diagnose the condition only with diffidence. A fair proportion of 'hysterics' turn out to have organic disease, as many of us know to our cost.

Notice that among illness as a comfort I have put the proud, lonely person. Allow me to explain this. This pathetic type of case usually occurs in later life when praise and companionship are hard to come by. To lonely people a medical consultation may represent an event of great importance. It supplies that need to be noticed that exists in all human beings. A visit from the doctor allows them the illusion of seeking medical advice rather than companionship. A patient may be too proud to complain of loneliness, but there is no loss of pride in complaining of symptoms. Lonely people miss, not only companionship, but also the advice and criticism that go with it.

Turning to the hypochondriacs, first we have the rich hypochondriac. I call this one The Grand Tour Type, because she spends much of her time touring the larger cities in Europe visiting consultants. She always carries a large dossier, opinions from consultants, X-rays and laboratory reports; and usually a list of her own symptoms which she has carefully written out. During her tour she may have persuaded surgeons to remove some of her less essential organs. She has usually had her gall bladder and a quota of her pelvic organs removed by the time she reaches one's consulting room. To the consultant in private practice they are a familiar, tedious and lucrative burden.

The poor hypochondriac (or perpetual out-patient). Every hospital has a number of out-patients who have attended for many years. Whenever they are discharged from one department they turn up in another, thus acquiring a very large collection of documents, rivalling that of the rich hypochondriac although written on less luxurious writing paper and penned by less illustrious names. Though some have genuine chronic illness, many of them attend because they like the companionship of hospital; instead of going to the local public house for a glass of beer and a chat with the landlord, they go to the local hospital for a bottle of medicine and a chat with the other patients. One enlightened doctor tried the experiment of arranging out-patient sessions where the patients did not see the doctor at all unless they asked for him. It was a great success.

The eccentric hypochondriacs. These people like peculiar or unorthodox treatments. They believe with apostolic fervour in nature cures, osteopaths, astrologers and herbalists. Their preoccupation is more with treatment than with illness and they are harmless and often entertaining.

The chronic convalescent. When a patient has had longstanding organic disease for many years it becomes so familiar to him that it is almost a friend. If the illness is suddenly cured, he may feel deserted and friendless. He misses the familiar pain, the sympathetic enquiries of his friends and the security of his medical routine. He does not really want to get well; he has become a hypochondriac.

Now the last group: Illness as a profession. First, I consider anorexia nervosa. The reason why these people go to such lengths to avoid eating is rarely clear. They will resort to a variety of artifices to avoid food. They will hide food in their bed lockers, pour milk into their hot-water bottles and insist on starving in the midst of plenty.

The next group is that of the chronic artefactualists, who may spend years in self-mutilation or the production of spurious fevers. Skin diseases are most favoured by the sufferers from chronic autogenous disease, but various other forms of self-damage are reported.

Lastly, Munchausen's syndrome. This is the strangest and rarest form of chronic autogenous disease. The patient with this syndrome is nearly always brought into hospital by police or bystanders, having collapsed in the street or on a bus with an apparently acute illness, supported by a plausible and yet dramatic history. Though his history seems most convincing at first, later his story is found to be largely false, and his symptoms and signs mostly spurious. He is discovered to have attended and deceived an astounding number of other hospitals. At several of them he may have been operated upon, and a large number of abdominal scars is often found. So skilfully do these people imitate acute illness that the diagnosis may be quite unsuspected until a passing doctor, ward sister or hospital porter says 'I know that man – we had him in St Quinidines last September. He says he's an ex-fighter pilot shot in the chest, in the last War, and he coughs up blood; or sometimes he's been shot through the head in the last war and has fits.'

Common varieties are:

(a) The abdominal type: laparotomophilia migrans.
(b) The bleeding type: haemorrhagica histrionica, colloquially called haematemesis merchants, haemoptysis merchants, and so on.
(c) The type specialising in faints, fits, convulsions and paralysis (neurologica diabolica).

These people differ from other chronic artefactualists in their constant progression from one hospital to another, often under a variety of false names, but nearly always telling the same false story, faking the same fictitious symptoms and submitting to innumerable operations and investigations. It seems that nothing can be done to prevent their continuing clinical depredations. Most doctors are so pleased if they succeed with detection and ejection they never think about protection. Though serious psychiatric studies of these people have been made, nobody can yet answer the two fundamental questions:

(a) Why do they do it?
(b) How can we stop them doing it?

All that can be said about them, and indeed about the whole subject of malingering, are these words of Robert Burns:

But human bodies are such fools
For all their colleges and schools
That when no real ills do perplex them
They make enough themselves to vex them.

The best explanation for all this self-manufactured disease is simply this: That human beings are such fools.

Richard Asher was a leading British physician who worked both in public health and hospital medicine from 1934 to 1963. This article is an extract from the book *Talking Sense*, a collection of his papers edited by Sir Francis Avery Jones, published by Pitman Medical (1972).

# 27
# Why must I be a teenager at all?

## BARRY BOGIN

What biological characteristics set us apart from other animals? The answer seems easy enough. To start with, we have a large brain, or more precisely, a large cerebral cortex. Then comes bipedality, a complex material culture and our decidedly peculiar reproductive biology (where else in nature do you find permanent breasts, concealed ovulation, a conspicuous penis and continuous sexual receptivity in both sexes?). Those in the know might add to this list our unique combination of large molar and small incisor and canine teeth. Yet the chances are that few biologists and anthropologists would mention the adolescent growth spurt.

This is an odd omission. For no other mammals, primates included, experience the equivalent period of growth, and at no other time in our lives do our physical and social attributes change quite so dramatically. Indeed, the uniqueness of our adolescent dash for maturity makes for some challenging puzzles, not least concerning its evolutionary origins. Why did adolescence evolve only in humans and not other primates? What, if any, advantage did it offer our ancestors?

We must first be clear about what adolescence is and where it falls within the human life cycle. Infancy starts at birth and ends when the child is weaned, which in pre-industrial societies occurs most often at 18 to 24 months. Childhood is defined as the period following weaning, when the youngster still depends on older people for feeding and protection. It usually spans the ages of two to eight years, whereupon the child becomes a juvenile. In girls, the juvenile period ends at about the age of 10, two years before it usually ends in boys; the difference reflects the earlier onset of puberty in girls. The adolescent stage begins with puberty, marked by some visible sign of sexual maturation such as pubic hair. Adolescence ends with the attainment of adult stature, which occurs at about age 17 in girls and 21 in boys.

The clearest evidence for these developmental stages comes from studies of human growth rates. During infancy growth rate plummets, to be followed by a period of slower decline during childhood and the juvenile stage. The onset of adolescence is marked by a sudden and rapid increase in growth rate, which peaks at a level unequalled since early infancy.

Most other mammals progress from infancy to adulthood seamlessly, experiencing no childhood and no adolescent growth spurt. Indeed, animals such as mice, guinea pigs, rabbits and cattle all reach sexual maturity with their growth rates in decline: puberty follows hard on the heels of weaning. This trend is broken only by the most social mammals – primates, wolves, elephants and so on – which follow infancy with a period of juvenile growth and behaviour, when they no longer need parental care but are not yet sexually mature. But in these animals, too, puberty occurs while the rate of growth is still decelerating and there is no detectable growth spurt.

That this is true even in our closest living relatives, the apes, makes the evolutionary origins of adolescence all the more puzzling. Why did our ancestors evolve the growth spurt? The conventional theory rests on the observation that humans alone require prolonged stages of infant, childhood and juvenile growth to learn the complex technical and social skills that make up human culture. The growth spurt, so the theory goes, evolved because at the end of this period our ancestors were left with proportionately less time for procreation than most mammals, and therefore needed to attain sexual maturity quickly. In an age when life was 'brutish and short', young-sters who matured and reached adult size quickly would have produced more offspring than their more sluggish cousins.

So genetic traits encouraging an adolescent growth spurt emerged in humans not because of any intrinsic value but to compensate for time 'lost' to learning in early life. In a sense, childhood begot adolescence: that, at least, is the idea.

### Growing up ain't easy

But surely this cannot be the whole story. For one thing, the argument that adolescence evolved to compensate for a prolonged childhood does not explain its timing. Girls experience the growth spurt before becoming fertile, but for boys the reverse is true. Why the difference? More fundamentally, the conventional theory assumes a simple, cosy relationship between adult stature and fertility, and between fertility and reproductive success. The reality is more complex: there is much more to raising a child than fertilising an egg, and body size is not linked in a simple way to sexual development.

The complexity of the links between adolescence, fertility and body size suggests that the human growth spurt has its own intrinsic value, and is not just a by-product of slow pre-pubertal development. In short, it evolved because it somehow made our ancestors better equipped to reproduce.

Human beings are a reproductive success story. Even people lacking the benefits of modern medicine raise half their infants to adulthood (chimpanzees manage to rear less than 36 per cent of their offspring to adulthood). The physical roots of this reproductive prowess undoubtedly lie in our capacity for learning complex behaviours and survival skills – language, cooperation, hunting, tool making and so on. And these, in turn, depend in part on the dramatic growth of the brain early in life. Yet the question remains: when and how do young people learn all those exclusively adult behaviours related to sex and child rearing?

As children and juveniles, perhaps. The problem here is that pre-pubescent boys and girls look very similar in terms of size and the amount of muscle and fat that they carry. Not looking like reproductive beings, they are unlikely to be treated as such by adults. Moreover, pre-pubescents have very low levels of testosterone and oestrogens – hormones thought to play an essential part in priming a young person's interest in adult sexual and social behaviour. Pre-pubescents are ill-placed to learn from adults the social behaviours that underpin reproductive success.

Even with the onset of puberty, when girls and boys become hormonally and physically attuned to sexual behaviour, the road to reproductive maturity is long and winding. In girls, the first outward sign of puberty is the development of the breast buds and wisps of pubic hair. This is followed by the laying down of fat on the hips, buttocks and thighs, the growth of more body hair, the adolescent growth spurt and, finally, menarche – the onset of menstruation. Menarche is usually followed by a period of one to three years of adolescent sterility, in which menstrual cycles occur but without ovulation. So it is often not until a young woman is 14 or more years old that she becomes fertile.

Fertility, however, does not necessarily imply reproductive maturity. Becoming pregnant is only a part of the business of reproduction. Maintaining the pregnancy to term and raising offspring to adulthood are equally important. In Western countries today, the risk of spontaneous abortions and complications of pregnancy for girls under 15-years-old is more than twice as high as that for women of 20 to 24 years. Babies born to American mothers under 15 years of age are more than twice as likely to be of 'low birth weight' than infants born to women aged 25 to 29.

A mother's age, of course, is not the only factor affecting her baby's survival prospects: low socioeconomic status, smoking, a failure to put on weight during pregnancy and ethnic origins are important, too. However, holding all these other factors constant still leaves the teenage mother and her infant at risk.

Why? Part of the answer lies with basic biology. A decade ago Marquisa LaVelle, a physical anthropologist now at the University of Rhode Island, uncovered evidence of a physical reason for the high percentage of small babies born to teenage mothers. Examining pelvic X-rays from a group of healthy girls, LaVelle noticed that their pelvic inlets – the bony opening of the birth canal – reached adult size only when the girls were 17 or 18-years-old, four or five years after menarche. The implication was as unexpected as it was profound. The adolescent growth spurt does not influence the size of the girl's pelvis. Rather, the pelvis has its own slow pattern of growth which continues for several years after a girl has reached adult stature.

The fact that women must wait up to a decade from the time of menarche to reach full reproductive maturity suddenly begins to make sense. So, too, does the observation that the average ages at which women in cultures as diverse as the Kikuyu tribe of Kenya and urban North America marry and have their first child all tend to cluster around 19 years. Yet the slow development of the female pelvis raises questions as well as answering them. Why should evolution have selected a developmental trait that hinders successful childbirth for teenage girls?

The answer may lie with the need to learn social skills. A mother-to-be must acquire information about pregnancy and experience in adult sociosexual relations and child care. And this, in my view, is where adolescence comes into play.

The dramatic physical changes that girls experience during adolescence serve as efficient advertisements for their sexual and social maturation – so efficient that they stimulate adults to include adolescent girls in their social circles and encourage the girls themselves to practise adult social interactions: male–female bonding, 'aunt-like' caring for children and so on. As anthropological research shows, girls in every human culture, on reaching adolescence, display a surge of interest in the sexual behaviour of adult women.

In our female ancestors, then, adolescence evolved because it enabled girls to learn how to be more reproductively successful as young women. But is there any direct evidence for this? Some support comes from the fact that first-born infants of monkeys and apes are more likely to die than those of humans. Studies of yellow baboons, toque macaques and chimpanzees show that between 50 and 60 per cent of their first-born offspring die in infancy. By contrast, in hunter-gatherer human societies, such as the !Kung of southern Africa, only about 44 per cent of first-born children die in infancy.

## Life-saving experience

Furthermore, studies of wild baboons by Jeanne Altmann of the University of Chicago show that although the rate of infant mortality for the first-born is as high as 50 per cent, it drops to 38 per cent for the second infant, and 25 per cent for the third and fourth infants. This improvement in infant survival is in part due to the experience the mother gains with each birth – experience girls accumulate during adolescence. The initial human advantage may seem small, but it means about 16 more people than baboons or chimpanzees survive out of every 100 first-born infants – more than enough over the vast course of evolutionary time to make human adolescence an overwhelmingly beneficial adaptation.

A further evolutionary advantage may accrue from female adolescence. By priming girls to help their older siblings rear children, adolescence enables women to give birth to more infants than primates can. The primatologist Jane Goodall finds that female chimpanzees have their first baby at about 13 years and must wait an average of 5.6 years between successful births, because each infant is totally dependent on its mother. As a result, few chimpanzee females produce more than three offspring. In traditional human societies, by contrast, women usually have their first baby at 19 and then go on to produce an infant every two to four years. This means they can easily have six or more children.

So much for adolescence in girls; what of boys? Boys become fertile well before they assume adult size and the physical characteristics of men. The little fertility research done on boys suggests that they begin producing sperm at an average age of 14.5 years. Yet the cross-cultural evidence is that few boys successfully father children before their late teenage years. When Carol Worthman, now at Emory University in Atlanta, Georgia, lived with the Kikuyu tribe in Kenya, she found that it is customary for the men to defer marriage and fatherhood until the age of about 25, though they become sexually active following their circumcision rite at around 18. The National Center for Health Statistics in the US reports that only four per cent of all births in the US are fathered by men under 20-years-old.

Why the lag between sperm production and fatherhood? One explanation may be that the sperm of younger adolescents do not swim well enough to reach an egg cell in the woman's fallopian tubes. But it could be that the average boy of 14.5-years-old is only beginning his adolescent growth spurt. In terms of physical appearance, physiological status and psychosocial development, he is still more a child than an adult. Young men display the opposite developmental trend to that of girls in that they experience a delay between reaching reproductive maturity and *later* advertising this maturity with an increase in physical size, body hair, muscularity and other secondary sexual characteristics.

To trace the evolutionary advantage of this delay, one must turn to the subtle psychological effects of testosterone and the other androgen hormones released from the male gonads during early adolescence. In effect, these hormones 'prime' boys to be receptive to their future roles as men. Over the past three decades, studies on a cross-section of youths in Europe, North America and Japan have established that as blood levels of testosterone begin to increase, but before the growth spurt reaches its peak, there is an increase in psychosexual activity. Nocturnal emissions begin and masturbation, dating and infatuation all intensify, as do feelings of guilt, anxiety, pleasure and pride. At the same time boys become more interested in adult activities, adjust their attitude to parental figures, and think and act more independently. In short, they begin to behave like men.

However – and this is where I believe the survival advantage lies – they still look like boys. Because their adolescent growth spurt occurs late in sexual development, young males can practise behaving like adults before they are actually perceived as adults. The socio-sexual antics of young adolescent males enable boys to fine-tune their sexual and social roles before either their lives, or those of their offspring, depend on them. In many traditional societies, for example, competition among males for women can be fierce, even fatal, and older men usually come off best. In such circumstances, the 'cute', childlike appearance of an adolescent male may be life-saving.

My argument, then, is this. Girls best learn their adult social roles while they are infertile but perceived by adults as mature; boys best learn their adult social roles while they are fertile but not yet perceived as such by adults. Without the adolescent growth spurt this unique style of social and cultural learning could not occur. And this is why adolescence deserves to stand alongside our large cerebral cortex, bipedality and unique sexual behaviour as a factor defining us as human. Indeed, all these characteristics stem from the same underlying biological trait: our uniquely human pattern of growth.

Barry Bogin is Professor of Anthropology at the University of Michigan, USA. He is the author of, amongst other things, *Patterns of Human Growth* (Cambridge University Press, 1988) and 'The evolution of human childhood' (*BioScience*, January, 1991). This article is an edited extract from a longer text, which was first published in *New Scientist*, 6 March (1993) pp. 34–38.

# 28

# A new division of the life course

## PETER LASLETT

Dividing life experience into numbered stages is as old as the study of age and ageing, and the various usages are often to be met with in our literature. William Shakespeare, for example, was following a commonplace, a threadbare literary tradition when he put the speech about the seven ages of man into the mouth of Jaques in *As You Like It*. Large numbers of titles and principles of division have been suggested; some of them have been used, a few have been very widely used and survive into our own generation. The phrase which has been the most recent to arrive is the *Third Age*. The *Third Age* has not as yet been employed at all systematically, as far as I know, that is in relation to a First Age, a Second Age and perhaps a Fourth Age or even higher number of ages. Here however it will be taken as belonging to a numerical order of the whole life course, and the quadripartite division can be justified as follows.

First comes an era of dependence, socialization, immaturity and education; second an era of independence, maturity and responsibility, of earning and of saving; third an era of personal fulfilment; and fourth an era of final dependence, decrepitude and death. Such a fourfold numbered system has many precedents and many rivals. The present scheme differs from its predecessors in several ways, one of them quite radical.

In this analysis of life experience the divisions between the four ages do not come at birthdays, nor do they even lie within clusters of years surrounding birthdays. Moreover the life career which is divided into these four modules has its culmination in the Third Age, the age of personal achievement and fulfilment, not in the Second Age and emphatically not in the Fourth. It follows logically enough that the ages should not be looked upon exclusively as stretches of years, and the possibility has to be contemplated that the Third Age could be lived simultaneously with the Second Age, or even with the First. Since the Third Age is identified here as that during which the apogee of personal life is achieved, anyone who reaches the goal at the same time as money is being earned and accumulated, a family founded and sustained, a successful career brought to a pitch of attainment, could be said to live the Third Age alongside the Second. No passage from one to the other need occur, for an individual with these characteristics is doing his/her own thing from maturity until the final end. Artists, the consummate artists, are the best examples. An athlete, on the other hand, usually has to attain his peak during the First Age, and so live part of the Third Age then.

The ageing both of populations and of societies can be effectively analysed in this way, with some inconsistencies which have yet to be resolved. It does provide, however, clear and definite ideas for individuals thinking about their own ages, those of their spouses, children and friends.

There can be no doubt whatever that dependence and decrepitude have always been inseparably associated with becoming old, however active, useful and healthy many people have been at the high, higher, and even highest calendar ages. Such an association can never have been more than partially justified as a general description of a particular calendar age. The effect of failing to make the distinction implied in the phrase the Third Age, therefore, must have fastened upon the senior members of all societies, past and present, inappropriate and damaging descriptions of their physical and mental state. This obstinate unwillingness to see the Third Age apart from the Fourth has sanctioned their exclusion from activities, especially earning activities, for which nearly all of them have been perfectly well suited, has debased their status in the eyes of their juniors, and above all has devalued them in their own estimation of themselves. To live as you wish to live after your sixty-fifth, seventieth and especially your eightieth birthday, you still have to have something of the quality ascribed to Shakespeare by Matthew Arnold.

### Self-school'd, self-scanned, self-honour'd, self-secure
Now that a fifth and more of the whole of our population is classed as retired, the results of this seemingly deliberate mass depreciation scarcely bear contemplation. The waste of talent and experience is incalculable. The fact that those who write off the elderly are also writing off themselves, as they will be in a decade or two's time, defies understanding. The only explanation offered here calls upon the somewhat unsatisfactory terms of cultural lag, even of false-consciousness.

The physical dependence of failing individuals in their final years, and sometimes their mental depreciation too; the dilemma of younger persons obliged to look after them, and frequently to look after other dependants as well; the burdens on the social services; the difficulties of the social workers; the poverty of the working class elderly and the intensification of social divisions which come with age; the problems presented by residential homes for the great and growing numbers of those in the Fourth Age and their horrendous cost – all these are extremely serious issues and they are pre-eminently issues of our time. So is the question of how British society will be able to meet the costs of supporting the elderly and of providing ever more expensive medical care. It is easy to see why nearly all the writings about ageing are about need and dependence, and it is understandable, if deplorable, that an effect of this preponderance is to intensify the conviction that the older population is a problem.

Rearranging these facts by redividing the life course and giving its most important component, from the elderly point of view, a somewhat novel name, may not go very far. But something can be done in this way to make it clear that the challenges are interesting as well as difficult, in human as well as intellectual terms. It is indeed, as I believe, an entirely new world which has opened up and beckoned us within.

If it is necessary to be clear and careful about the terms which have to be used for whole divisions of the course of life, it is also necessary to keep watch on the rest of the language which is used in reference to ageing, even down to the similes and metaphors which have worked themselves into the language. For the subject of this essay, growing old, teems with tired metaphors, unthinkingly applied.

These figures of speech derived by analogy from many of the characteristics of the natural world, and the implied comparison of the time of day and the season of the year with the stages of life are prominent amongst them. Such analogies were natural enough in a traditional society, close to the land and the vicissitudes of the seasons. But they still pervade the jocularity, the sentimentality, the sententiousness which are so often found in discussions of later life, devices no doubt to try to ensure that the more menacing themes shall be kept in the wings. Being old is not in fact at all like evening or like winter, for the good reason that the day and the year are not at all like human life itself. Whiteness, snowy whiteness, no more justifies the vaguely comforting description of being old as the winter of life, than the colour of the light from the declining sun justifies the excruciating description 'golden oldies'. Thinking by analogy and relying upon metaphor makes for muddle: a consistent, realistic vocabulary is imperative if we are to get the fact and circumstance of ageing clear.

Even the word *age* itself has a range of meanings. We shall distinguish five separate senses for the age of a person: calendar age will be seen to differ from biological age, from social age, from personal age and from subjective age. You may think yourself to be young, or old, in any of these senses, and others may judge you in a similar way. But there can be ambiguities. Consider for a moment what may be meant by the remark, 'she is young for her age'.

Someone in the Third Age is here addressing not first and foremost his own coevals, though they are clearly caught up in the discussion at every point, but the middle-aged, and especially middle-aged women themselves soon to join the ranks of those already in the Third Age. It is natural that he should see things from the senior point of view and defend what he sees to be the interests of the elderly, as they now are and as they will inevitably be. It has not been often that the older part of society has spoken in its own voice in such a way: championship has usually come from younger sympathizers.

Nevertheless, I should not wish it to be thought that I myself had a previously fixed opinion on the gravest of all the questions raised by the subject of ageing, the most demanding and the most intriguing to the intellectual enquirer. This is the issue of justice between age groups, both contemporary age groups, those living alongside each other, and those now separated by death, inter-generational equity as it is coming to be called.

[There is a] suspicion that those about to succeed to the status of the Third Age have been privileged by time, enriched in comparative terms to an extent never attained by their predecessors and not being accorded to those who will be their successors. If such can be demonstrated, we are faced with the first recognized and defined opportunity for providing against victimization by lottery of the date of birth. Since they are the only age group in society who can be identified as trustees for the future, those in the Third Age must do all they can to elaborate the principles of inter-generational equity, and make whatever provision is open to them to see that justice will be done, even if this is to some extent at their own expense. This is not the only challenge which arises out of taking account of the need to be our age.

Peter Laslett is a social historian and Fellow of Trinity College, Cambridge. This article is an edited version of Chapter 1 of his book *A Fresh Map of Life: The Emergence of the Third Age*, published in 1989 by Weidenfeld and Nicolson, London.

# 29
# Prevention is better. . . .

## HELEN ROBERTS, SUSAN SMITH AND CAROL BRYCE

The publication in July 1992 of the government White Paper *The Health of the Nation*[1] heralds a new dawn for health promotion. This document makes much of the importance of both education and information in reducing ill health. But as strategies for reducing health problems, what do we know about their effectiveness? We need to know two things about which little has been published. Do education and information affect behaviour, and does behaviour affect health status? A consequence of the White Paper is likely to be an increase in preventive work. This paper seeks to challenge this approach to preventive work in the child accident field (one of the areas targeted in the White Paper) by drawing on examples of prevention in practice in a recent Scottish study. This work illustrates fundamental differences in approach between citizens and professionals in prioritising preventive measures, and suggests that careful needs assessment in this area is needed to ensure that any investment in health promotion in this area is effective.

### Accidents: the potential for prevention

As the leading cause of death to children after the age of one in the United Kingdom and elsewhere in the developed world, child accidents are a legitimate focus of preventive activity. In the UK for instance, the majority of deaths to the under-fives are the result of an accident in the home, and to older children the result of a road traffic accident.

The main thrust of accident prevention directed towards children and their parents continues to make heavy use of advice, safety campaigns and competitions for children to design posters, all punctuated with reminders to mothers that the main responsibility is theirs.

Health education programmes in child safety which have been evaluated have been disappointing, or have concentrated on inappropriate outcome measures. There is little point in knowing that every health visitor working in a certain area has put a leaflet into the hand of every mother of an under-five, and given personalised advice, if we do not know whether the accident rate is reduced, increased or unchanged by these measures. And we cannot take it for granted that health education messages have no adverse effects. The generation of anxiety in otherwise healthy populations, in the absence of any measurable health gain may be an undesirable consequence of vigorous and enthusiastic health education.

## The Corkerhill study

In what follows, we describe some findings from a study set in a Glasgow housing estate and designed to identify factors predisposing children to be at risk of, and protected from, accidents. Fieldwork comprised group interviews with four 'citizens' groups and one group of 'professionals', a household survey and a series of case studies of successful and unsuccessful accident prevention strategies identified during the survey. For the purposes of this paper, we describe some differences in professional and parental perspectives on accidents and their preventability which became evident during the group interviews. These are supplemented by data from our case studies based on both 'real' accidents and near-misses.

### The 'citizens' groups
Two groups of parents and one teenage group were recruited and interviewed on three occasions each. A further smaller group of parents was interviewed twice.

### The 'professionals' group
The 'professionals' group comprised seven individuals, most but not all of whom had a degree of occupational responsibility relating specifically to Corkerhill. The group comprised a health visitor, two health promotion officers, a police sergeant, a representative of the housing department, a fire prevention officer and a road safety officer.

### The case studies
In the course of the household survey, we sought to identify all accidents in the previous year to a child of 14 or under resulting in hospital admission, a trip to the Accident and Emergency (A&E) department, a visit to the GP or dentist, or treatment at home. We also sought details of near-misses and averted accidents.

The findings discussed below are those which compare and contrast key elements of parents' and professionals' accounts of accident risks in the community and their rather different preventive strategies and describe some of the parents' views collected in the course of the case studies.

### The community
Corkerhill is a post-war housing scheme of 580 dwellings in Glasgow. It has a chip shop, a newsagent, a pub, and as community premises, a community 'shop' (in effect, a meeting room) and a tenants' hall. The estate is bounded to the north by a railway line and railway yard, to the south by a river, and to the west by a busy trunk road with a dual carriageway. In contrast, there is an area of parkland immediately to the east of Corkerhill. The single environmental asset in Corkerhill is shortly to be cut

off from the community by a major new road. This is unlikely to be of major benefit to Corkerhill where almost 60 per cent of households do not have access to a car or a van. Well over a third of the families in Corkerhill are headed by a lone parent, and most of the families live in conditions of considerable hardship.

**What is an accident?**

We found little support for the existence of a fatalistic view of accidents, although conceptually, there are clear differences between the views of the parent and professional groups on what comprised an accident. The parents see accidents as just one element of insecurity and one further hazard for people living in damp, cold houses. Thus in discussing risk factors for accidents, parents relate their children's asthma and other respiratory problems to damp housing and chemicals used to treat the mould associated with the damp. 'Your house is damp . . . Your house isn't safe . . .' (Group interview). 'I had to go to my mother's house [because of damp] and every time we came back, my wee boy had diarrhoea and the inspector told me not to cover the dampness' (Case study).

This broad view of what accidents are underpins a related conviction that many events labelled accidents are not accidents at all. Parents felt that many risks in their environment render accidents foreseeable, and with known causes. In what sense, argued the parents, are incidents arising from known hazard accidents? The fact that many of the tenements have balconies with a gap at crawler's eye level just wide enough for a small child to creep through was identified by parents not so much as an accident risk as a frank disregard for child safety on the part of planners, builders and architects. Similar views were expressed about kitchen design; the lack of adequate play facilities; the fact that the housing scheme with its low car ownership was designated a free car parking area for other people's cars; the electrical wiring system in the houses (many plugs were of the old fashioned three holes in the wall type with no switch) and the old fashioned immersion heaters where it was difficult to adjust the heat of bath water at source. It was suggested to us in all the parents' groups that factors such as these do not lead to 'accidents'. It can be foreseen that they will lead to injury, so that the risks that they entail are not accidental at all: 'They're no designed with safety in mind at all, and yet they call them family houses . . .' (Group interview). 'These windows, the weans can open them no bother . . .', 'Then they say [dampness is caused by] lack of ventilation so you go around opening all your windows, and it is freezing' (Case studies).

Professionals had a rather narrower conception of accidents. Not surprisingly, they (like us) did not refer to asthma or respiratory ailments in their discussion of accidents, and kept rather closer to conventional definitions of what an accident is. In discussing accidents in general, they drew on their professional knowledge. Reference was made to the work of a local senior registrar in public health medicine whom some of the group had heard describe the epidemiology of accidents in Glasgow: 'For pre-fives, the incidence of home accidents was much higher . . . But even within the home, I think the main one, the main category, was burns and scalds . . .' Accidents were thus described in terms of the injuries which were caused rather than risks or hazards which led to them, and in terms of the patterns which had become clear to them as health workers, police officers or road safety officers. In this sense, the professionals were far more likely to conceptualise accidents in terms of their sequelae (injury or damage) than in terms of their antecedents.

## What are the risk factors for child accidents in Corkerhill?

Parents and teenagers apparently carry clear mental maps of risk factors and risky areas. Road works, pavements dug up, and building works were identified as evident hazards: '... they dug up a bit of pavement and just went away home and left it like that ... and if you didn't have somebody with you and you had a pram, you couldn't get across because you needed someone to help you over' (Group interview). The playpark was identified as unsafe by the teenagers: 'There was four swings between about all the kids.... The grass is a mess, it's just all broken glass and things like that.' Broken glass was a recurring theme: 'When the glaziers come to replace the windows, they smash out the old window into the garden' (Case study). Some of the parents meanwhile identified nearby playing fields as a no-go area as children had to cross a fast main road in order to get there: 'Some wee weans are banned from Nethercraigs [the play area] because they have tae cross the road, and the parents havnae always got the time to go with them and wait with them until they come back' (Group interview). An unmanned railway station adjacent to Corkerhill was identified as a danger: 'There's a hole in the fence roon the side and it wis seen being done and it wis actually the workmen who were clearing up the railway taking a short cut to the chippie. That's the kind of thing that the kids would get blamed for ...' (Group interview).

The professional group saw risk in terms of the characteristics of the children: 'for that age group, 0–4, the main risks are in the home ...' Only the health visitor made a comment on two specific risk factors in Corkerhill. The first was related to burns: 'There's no heating in some of the houses so a lot of the parents use electric fires so you get a lot of accidents with the smaller kids from the electric fires.' The second related to needlestick injuries: '... drug abusers with needles, kids picking up needles in the streets and the closes ...' When the group was pressed by the interviewer on other specific hazards and risks, none were offered and the discussion was moved on by a participant referring to work in another part of the city associating chip pan fires with drunkenness.

Some risks which parents had raised were downplayed by the professionals: '... there is a general perception that the cars are travelling faster than they actually are ...' and 'if you look at the roads and the amount they get used, and the complexity of them, they're not really that dangerous.' The theme of popular perceptions of external risk being mistaken was taken up by another group member who suggested a sign saying: ' "You are now entering the most dangerous place in the world – your home". And that's about the size of it. I mean we've got a saying in the Fire Brigade that there's only three causes of fires and generally it's men, women and children, and that's the sad fact of it ...'

## Responsibility for safety

Both the 'citizens' and the 'professional' groups were exercised by the question of responsibility for accidents. All of the groups agreed that the maintenance of safety is a parental (or more usually maternal) responsibility. The parents described their commitment to the positive exercise of individual and collective responsibility: 'You've got to watch them constantly and make sure they don't dae anything . . . you've got tae think about things . . . you're constantly on the alert . . . you're constantly mcving things'. There was a recognition that mistakes were made: 'I am fairly safety conscious. It is quite difficult in this kind of house . . . your safety awareness comes by things which nearly happen, just managing to avert them . . . Unfortunately, sometimes they do happen' (Case study). A small percentage of families was viewed as irresponsible: 'One per cent unsocial tenants in this scheme. It's probably a wee bit mair than that now, but they're the people you hear about all the time. You don't hear about the folk who look after their kids' (Group interview).

This view was acknowledged by the professionals who agreed that the community is a good one. Where the parents' and professional groups diverge is in their views on the responsibility which people or institutions *other* than parents have for safety. The parents, while recognising their pivotal place in the maintenance of child safety expressed the view that the regional council, the roads department, the local housing office, workmen coming into the area and British Rail, among others, have a responsibility for child safety in Corkerhill. 'With the amount of scaffolding that is in the scheme, you would think they would have a watchman of some description.' 'It was the company [repairing the pavements], and especially it wasn't just a couple of men doing the job. It was about three dozen of them, and to me, they could have done it bit by bit. Sometimes they would go away on a Friday and come back on a Monday, and the pavements would be left just as they were' (Case studies). An ability to identify the hazards and risks which led to accidents by no means meant that parents absolved themselves from blame: 'I am going to murder the person who left that [socket] cover off, and it was probably me . . . because I am usually the last person using it.' 'I blame myself, I should have been more careful,' 'You feel it is your fault' (Case studies).

The professional group, which recognising a *generalised* social responsibility for accidents was less inclined to link specific problems for specific hazards with specific bodies whose responsibility it is, or should be, to reduce those hazards. As one of the professional group bluntly put it: 'The house is there and there's no money to change [in] terms of safety. We couldn't look at that at all. We look at family composition in terms of nuisance and everything else, but we don't look at the insides because there just isn't the money'.

### How can accidents be prevented in Corkerhill?

The final week of the 'citizen' interviews, and the final part of the interview with professionals specifically addressed the preventability of accidents, asking the groups what might be done with low funds, no funds or more substantial funds. In other words, what their priorities were for preventive measures given different levels of resources. Parents were also asked in the case studies about accident prevention and accident avoidance.

There was virtual unanimity among the parents' groups that housing was the place to start. 'Raze them to the ground, and make wee front and back doors' '. . . Upstairs, downstairs, back and front garden . . .' 'Aye, that's everybody's ideal isn't it?'

'Window frames, insulation, oh there must be aboot a hundred things you should do in the house – get started with a wee drawing...' 'Outside the house: I'd start with a play area, and a one way street.' 'And sleeping policemen in the street.' 'And limited times when they're allowed to come in 'cause it's a play area 'cause there's so many kids.'

With less money to spend, priorities would include re-wiring (many electric sockets in Corkerhill have no on/off switches), a high cupboard in the kitchen, smoke alarms and funds for the sort of community business which would tackle safety issues. Also suggested were thermostats on the water tanks, and gas fires provided with guards ready fixed rather than as an optional extra. The teenagers group would improve the play area.

Among the 'no cost' preventive measures were a 10mph speed limit within the housing scheme, shared childcare, passing on equipment, changing routines for the bin men (who at the time came to the housing scheme as children were leaving for school, with the consequence that pavements piled high with black bags were impassable).

The professionals were more modest in their preventive ambitions and focussed solidly on education. 'Even if we had the money to put all these things right, education needs to be done as well,' and 'it's a bit more than making sure equipment is available' were remarks received with nods and murmurs of agreement. There was no such thing as a no cost solution for the professionals. They rightly pointed out that: '...if you're going to try and change what people do at home, then that's going to cost something.' But low cost solutions included advice on the use of chip pans, and 'just basic things like that and things like when you're running a bath, don't run scalding water first.' Another possibility was 'Having ongoing videos and displays [in mother toddler groups].' Higher cost solutions were also educational. 'There's one or two teaching packages being taken up at the moment' and if only one or two things were possible: 'educating the parents, obviously, with a lot of reinforcement'... 'a scheme of paid instructors for training child pedestrian skills...' Although the interviewers suggested moving on to specific features within the home which might be changed, the message from the professionals was much the same: 'we have to educate them that the home is really the most unsafe place you can be.'

## Discussion

The educational approach to accident prevention invokes a deficit model of parents, so that for instance a number of RoSPA posters work on the exhortation principle. Posters on sale in the current catalogue include: (showing two mothers outside a school) 'Meet them: Don't let them die on the roads.' This is in spite of evidence that *more* children are met by their parents from school now than was the case twenty years ago, and that ironically, since some of these children are brought to school by cars this may pose an additional risk to children arriving on foot. An educational approach of this kind flies in the face of the study reported in this paper. In a low income, high risk council estate, we found little evidence from the group interviews, the household survey or the case studies that knowledge and awareness were lacking.[2] With the exception of a good knowledge of first aid, general knowledge about accidents is high in the community, and specific knowledge about local hazards and risks is quite considerably more detailed among the citizens than among the professionals.

It was clear from the group interviews that parents already exercise a wide range of preventive activities. In relation to building works in the street, one mother said: 'I went away in and I kicked up merry hell aboot the fact that there wasnae a board or anything put over it and it ended up two workmen came oot and lifted the pram over the hole and then left somebody there on guard . . . By the time I got back, they had a workman standing on it, they had boards across it, and by the next morning it was all cemented. So I think part of the thing that we have tae dae is to be more voluble – is to shout and to say, "C' mon, get the finger oot, it's time something was done."' Plans were made for an equipment loan scheme (which failed as the local health promotion department was unable to provide any support, offering instead a specially commissioned – and thus not inexpensive – poster). Meanwhile old cots were cut down to make safety gates or playpens. In brief, parents were using the resources they had to hand to try and create a safer environment.

Much health promotion appears to ignore this kind of achievement, and to under-estimate the difficulties associated with 'standard solutions' such as the purchase of safety goods. A number of the mothers we spoke to therefore experienced health promotion messages about constant vigilance and the importance of having a variety of safety goods as itself anxiety-provoking (and in that sense, a health hazard). 'You can get really depressed and think about the things your children should have – things that you're told all the time, all this equipment you should have and it can end up, "I'm no bringing my child up properly. I don't have this and I don't have that" and add that to all the other stresses you've got – living in bad housing or poverty and you can get depressed and distracted and that's when accidents are more likely to happen – when you're under stress' (Group interviews).

## Conclusion

Currently, education is the cornerstone of accident prevention policy. However, while education is one of the less costly options in the reduction of accidents, there is little evidence that it results in a decrease in injury. This work indicates that parents have a good understanding of the causes of accidents in general, clear views on hazards and risks in their own environments, and that they are effective most of the time in keeping children safe in unsafe conditions. However cheap it may be when compared with other public health measures, to 'educate' parents and children, if it is not effective, then it cannot be cost effective.

Just as the introduction of child resistant containers for medicine has been associated with a steep drop in childhood poisonings, our work indicates a number of areas where preventive efforts based on environmental rather than (though in association with) behavioural change might usefully focus.

Further, our view is that to base preventive work on injury and death data is misconceived. A focus on risks and hazards may be more productive, since these provide the context in which parents negotiate their everyday safe keeping behaviour.

Outcome studies of preventive work tend to be poorly conceived, concentrating on delivery or reception of the health message rather than health gain. It is unclear what part, if any, educational health promotion messages have played in the reduction of accidents. Our study suggests one reason for this is the markedly different views held by professionals and 'their' public on the character of accident and accident risk, and the nature of safekeeping. A first step for the Department of Health should be to explore whether, in spending public funds on education and information, they will be getting good value for money. A pre-requisite for doing this is to consult those whose day to day lives are a reservoir of effective safekeeping strategies.

## References

1. HMSO. *The Health of the Nation*, London (1992).
2. Roberts, H., Smith, S. J. and Bryce, C. *Safety as a Social Value*, Final report to the Scottish Office Home and Health Department, Public Health Research Unit, University of Glasgow (1993).

Helen Roberts and Carol Bryce were employed at the Public Health Research Unit of the University of Glasgow, and Susan Smith was at the University of Edinburgh when the fieldwork for this research was carried out. Helen Roberts is currently Co-ordinator, Research and Development, in the Policy and Development Unit of the children's charity Barnardo's, London. The article, an edited extract of which appears here, was originally published in *Sociology of Health and Illness*, **15**, 447–463 (1993).

# Part 4
## The role of medicine

## INTRODUCTION

In the first half of the nineteenth century, the effectiveness and humanity of medicine came under systematic and vehement criticism from both within and without the medical profession. This was the first era of 'therapeutic nihilism'. After that period, with the growth of a more scientific medicine, the prestige of the profession rose to previously unattained heights. But over the past forty years, the role of medicine has once again been questioned. The critics have included epidemiologists and economists, feminists and sociologists, doctors and moral philosophers, social historians and theologians. They have focused on two particular issues – the effectiveness of medicine and the wider role of doctors in society.

Assessment of the effectiveness of medicine has taken two main forms – historical analysis and evaluation of contemporary practice. The leading exponent of the former has been Thomas McKeown, a British doctor and demographer, who has argued that medicine played only a minor role in the dramatic decline in infectious diseases and in the growth of population in the United Kingdom since the seventeenth century. For McKeown, these changes resulted instead largely from improvements in nutrition and other social conditions. 'The medical contribution' summarizes his evidence and conclusions.

McKeown's views have been so immensely influential that they have almost become a new orthodoxy. Simon Szreter, a medical historian, does not dispute McKeown's core argument that medicine played a very limited role in the decline of mortality. But he does take issue with McKeown's conclusion that the decline in mortality can be attributed instead to nutritional improvements and rising living standards. In 'The importance of social intervention in Britain's mortality decline c. 1850–1914: a re-interpretation of the role of public health', he bases his case on a close reading of the same evidence used by McKeown. Szreter argues that McKeown was methodologically suspect, and also misinterpreted the evidence on the contribution of different diseases to declining mortality, and on the chronology of the decline. Medicine's role may have been small, concludes Szreter, but the contribution of public health measures in improving the urban environment have been underestimated.

Scepticism about the value of *contemporary* medical practice gained widespread attention, at least in the United Kingdom, with the publication in 1972 of a book entitled *Effectiveness and Efficiency*, written by the epidemiologist and doctor Archie Cochrane; an extract is included in this part of the book. His work was strongly influenced by his experiences in the Second World War, when he was captured and put in charge of medical care for his fellow prisoners. He had almost no medicines and yet, to his surprise, most of his patients made a full recovery. In his later work he went on to explore the dangers of simply assuming that medicine was necessarily effective in combating illness, and argued strongly for the systematic collection and review of evidence on effectiveness, particularly by means of randomized controlled trials. One legacy of his work has been the development, during the 1990s, of a worldwide Cochrane Collaboration, aiming to perform systematic reviews of existing evidence on health interventions.

Randomized controlled trials, for all their virtues, are not without problems. Some of the ethical and indeed practical issues they raise are illustrated by the collection of articles, editorials and letters entitled 'Ethical dilemmas in evaluation – a correspondence', concerning trials to investigate the effect of vitamin supplements in preventing the occurrence of neural tube defects (such as spina bifida). Initial evidence of such an effect was questioned and a trial proposed, but a trial was itself considered either impractical or unethical by many. In the event, as the final contributions to this collection show, a randomized controlled trial was eventually performed and cleared many if not all uncertainties.

The issue of randomized controlled trials also arises in 'Assessment of screening for cancer', by Carlo La Vecchia and colleagues. The authors are entirely in favour of screening as a technology, and marshall evidence that it can be very effective in the early detection of specific cancers, with consequent potential for a reduction in mortality. But they also emphasize the complexity of screening programmes, and the immense difficulties in evaluating them, especially by means of randomized controlled trials of screening. Effectiveness is easier to assess in some areas than others.

Marc Strassburg takes as his subject a health programme of absolute effectiveness, 'The global eradication of smallpox'. As a result of the intervention which Strassburg describes, smallpox was eradicated from Europe and North America by the 1970s, but a number of major reservoirs of the virus still existed. By 1980 the World Health Organization declared the world to be free of smallpox, a feat that had been achieved through the application of medical knowledge and technology by a global organization, based on elaborate economic, political and social coordination. If smallpox can be eradicated, will a future world be free of other major infectious diseases? The answer is probably no. Smallpox was a prime candidate because much was known of the process and progress of the disease, and a vaccine was available. A similar programme to eliminate malaria has not been successful, largely because of the existence of a reservoir of the malaria parasite in mosquitoes.

Many of the assessments of the effectiveness of medicine considered so far have given little formal consideration to the role of doctors *per se*. But some critiques of the role of medicine have started from the power relationship between doctors and the laity which, it is argued, has enabled them to perpetuate a hierarchy of advantaged and disadvantaged in society. At their most extreme, these critiques have argued that doctors not only perpetuate existing structures, but actually cause harm (iatrogenesis, or doctor-made disease). Probably the best known example of such an analysis is the work of Ivan Illich, an Austrian theologian who has lived in Mexico since 1960. In 'The epidemics of modern medicine', Illich argues that the ills of society result from individuals' loss of self-reliance, which in turn is a consequence of industrialization. Thus, just as education becomes the province of the teacher, so, equally undesirably, health has become the responsibility of doctors who now tyrannize the laity, causing more harm than good.

While Illich sees the basic struggle as one in which individuals must 'regain' their self-reliance and liberty from the oppressive nature of industrialization, Vicente Navarro views it as a struggle against a particular mode of industrial society – capitalism. Navarro, an American doctor originally from Spain, is one of the leading Marxist critics of modern medical care. In 'The mode of state intervention in the health sector' he argues that doctors aid the capitalist process by promoting the view that illness results from decisions made by individuals. This, he argues, is far from the reality of most people's lives, in which the opportunities to exercise free choice are severely circumscribed. In this situation, doctors are seen as an integral support for capitalism and therefore for the health-damaging nature of such an economic and social system. In this extract from his book, *Medicine under Capitalism*, Navarro argues that increasing State intervention in health care is made necessary by the damage done to people's health by a capitalist system that produces great social inequalities.

Finally, Alan Williams, a leading British health economist, adopts a position which concerns the effectiveness of modern medicine, but also has implications for the wider role of doctors in society. Williams shares many suspicions concerning the effectiveness of modern medicine and, like Cochrane, believes that the appropriate response to this uncertainty is to subject all health interventions to scientific appraisal. But to Williams, this means evidence about costs as well as effectiveness. He adheres to the view that, in a world in which health care possibilities invariably exceed the available resources, it is necessary to have a coherent framework for establishing priorities. To do this, health gains need first to be measured (for example by means of the Euroqol© system of rating health states, which he illustrates), and then costed. As for the role of doctors, they have failed in the past to obtain good value for money, and cannot be expected to do so unaided in the future: 'Priority setting in the NHS', Williams concludes, is 'too big and important a task to be left to the experts'.

# 30
# The medical contribution

## THOMAS McKEOWN

Until recently it was accepted, almost without question, that the increase of population in the eighteenth century, and by inference later, was due to a decline of mortality brought about by medical advances. This conclusion was suggested by Talbot Griffith, who was impressed by developments in medicine in the eighteenth century. They included expansion of hospital, dispensary and midwifery services; notable changes in medical education; advances in understanding of physiology and anatomy; and introduction of a specific protective measure, inoculation against smallpox. Taken together these developments seemed impressive, and it is scarcely surprising that Griffith, like most others who considered the matter, should have concluded that they contributed substantially to health. This conclusion, however, results from failure to distinguish clearly between the interests of the doctor and the interests of the patient, a common error in the interpretation of medical history. From the point of view of a student or practitioner of medicine, increased knowledge of anatomy, physiology and morbid anatomy are naturally regarded as important professional advances. But from the point of view of the patient, none of these changes has any practical significance until such time as it contributes to preservation of health or recovery from illness. It is because there is often a considerable interval between acquisition of new knowledge and any demonstrable benefit to the patient, that we cannot accept changes in medical education and institutions as evidence of the immediate effectiveness of medical measures. To arrive at a reliable opinion we must look critically at the work of doctors, and enquire whether in the light of present-day knowledge it is likely to have contributed significantly to the health of their patients.

The obvious way to do this is to assess the contribution which immunization and therapy have made to the control of the infectious diseases associated with the decline of mortality. Since this can be done reliably only from the time when cause of death was certified, I shall examine the influence of medical measures in the post-registration period.

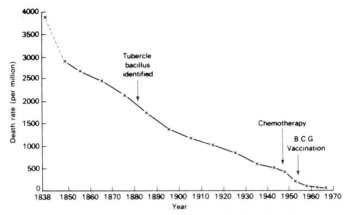

**Figure 30.1**   Respiratory tuberculosis: death rates, England and Wales

## Airborne diseases

### Tuberculosis
Figure 30.1 shows the trend of mortality from respiratory tuberculosis in England and Wales since 1838. This is the disease which, if any, was critical for the fall of the death rate. It was much the largest single cause of death in the mid-nineteenth century, and it was associated with nearly a fifth of the total reduction of mortality since then.

The time when effective medical measures became available is not in doubt. The tubercle bacillus was identified by Koch in 1882, but none of the treatments in use in the nineteenth or early twentieth century had a significant influence on the course of the disease. The many chemotherapeutic agents that were tried are now known to have been ineffective, as was also the collapse therapy practised from about 1920. Effective treatment began with the introduction of streptomycin in 1947, and immunization (BCG vaccination) was used in England and Wales on a substantial scale from 1954. By these dates mortality from tuberculosis had fallen to a small fraction of its level in 1848–54; indeed most of the decline (57 per cent) had taken place before the beginning of the present century. Nevertheless, there is no doubt about the contribution of chemotherapy, which was largely responsible for the rapid fall of mortality from the disease since 1950. Without this intervention the death rate would have continued to fall, but at a much slower rate.

### Whooping cough
The trend of mortality from whooping cough is shown in Figure 30.2, based on mean annual death rates of children under 15 in England and Wales. Mortality began to decline from the seventh decade of the nineteenth century, and the disease contributed 2.6 per cent to the reduction of the death rate from all causes.

Treatment by sulphonamides and, later, antibiotics was not available before 1938 and even now their effect on the course of the disease is questionable. Immunization was used widely after 1952; the protective effect is variable, and has been estimated to be between less than 20 and over 80 per cent. Clearly almost the whole of the decline of mortality from whooping cough occurred before the introduction of an effective medical measure.

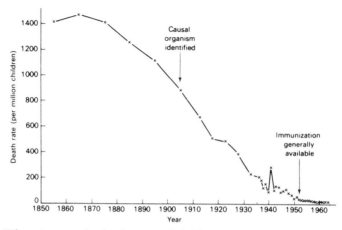

**Figure 30.2**   Whooping cough: death rates of children under 15, England and Wales

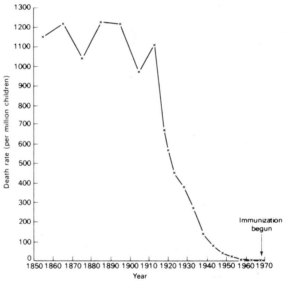

**Figure 30.3**   Measles: death rates of children under 15, England and Wales

*Measles*
Again Figure 30.3 is based on deaths of children under 15 in England and Wales. The picture is among the most remarkable for any infectious disease. Mortality fell rapidly and continuously from about 1915. Effective specific measures have only recently become available in the form of immunization, and they can have had no significant effect on the death rate. However, mortality from measles is due largely to invasion by secondary organisms, which have been treated by chemotherapy since 1935. Eighty-two per cent of the decrease of deaths from the disease occurred before this time.

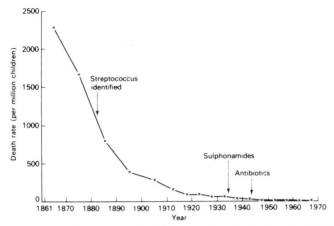

**Figure 30.4**    Scarlet fever: death rates of children under 15, England and Wales

*Scarlet fever*
Because scarlet fever was grouped with diphtheria in the early years after registration of cause of death, the trend of mortality from the disease in children under 15 is shown from the seventh decade in Figure 30.4. There was no effective treatment before the use of prontosil in 1935. But even by the beginning of the century mortality from scarlet fever had fallen to a relatively low level, and between 1901 and 1971 it was associated with only 1.2 per cent of the total reduction of the death rate from all causes. Approximately 90 per cent of this improvement occurred before the use of the sulphonamides.

*Diphtheria*
Figure 30.5 is based on the mean annual death rate of children under 15, from the eighth decade of the nineteenth century. It is perhaps the infectious disease in which it is most difficult to assess precisely the time and influence of therapeutic measures. Antitoxin was used first in the late nineteenth century and has been the accepted form of treatment since then. It is believed to have reduced the case fatality rate, which fell from 8.2 per 100 notifications in 1916–25 to 5.4 in 1933–42, while notifications remained at an average level of about 50,000 per year. The mortality rate increased at the beginning of the last war but fell rapidly at about the time when national immunization began.

It is tempting to attribute much of the decline of diphtheria mortality between 1900 and 1931 to treatment by antitoxin and the rapid fall since 1941 to immunization. Nothing in British experience is seriously inconsistent with this interpretation. However, experience in some other countries is not so impressive; for example there are American States where the reduction of mortality in the 1940s did not coincide with the immunization programme. Moreover, several other infections, particularly those that are airborne, declined in the same period in the absence of effective prophylaxis or treatment. While therefore it is usual, and probably reasonable, to attribute the fall of mortality from diphtheria in this century largely to medical measures, we cannot exclude the possibility that other influences also contributed, perhaps substantially.

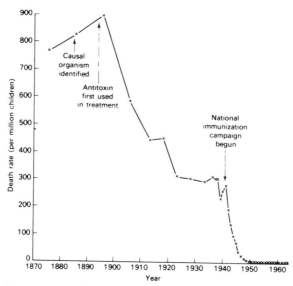

**Figure 30.5**   Diphtheria: death rates of children under 15, England and Wales

*Smallpox*

The death rate from smallpox in the mid-nineteenth century was a good deal smaller than that of the infections already discussed, and the somewhat erratic trend of mortality since then is shown in Figure 30.6. Vaccination of infants was made compulsory in 1854 but the law was not enforced until 1871. From that time until 1898, when the conscientious objector's clause was introduced, almost all children were vaccinated. Most epidemiologists are agreed that we owe the decline of mortality from smallpox mainly to vaccination. Since the mid-nineteenth century the decrease has been associated with only 1.6 per cent of the reduction of the death rate from all causes.

*Infections of ear, pharynx and larynx*

Together these diseases also were associated with only a small part (0.8 per cent) of the decrease of deaths. The main therapeutic influences have been chemotherapy and, in some ear infections, surgery. It is difficult to give a time from which surgical intervention can be said to have been beneficial, but in view of the small contribution made by these diseases it is perhaps not very important to assess it more precisely than by saying that one-third of the decline (0.3 per cent of mortality from all causes in this century) occurred before the use of sulphonamides in 1935.

In summary, the airborne diseases accounted for two-fifths of the reduction of mortality from all causes from the mid-nineteenth century to 1971. Vaccination against smallpox was the only medical measure which contributed to the fall of deaths before 1900, and this disease was associated with only a small part (1.6 per cent) of the decrease of the death rate from all causes. In this century antitoxin probably lowered mortality from diphtheria, and surgery may have reduced deaths from ear infections, but together these influences had little effect on total deaths. With these exceptions, effective medical intervention began with the chemotherapeutic agents which became

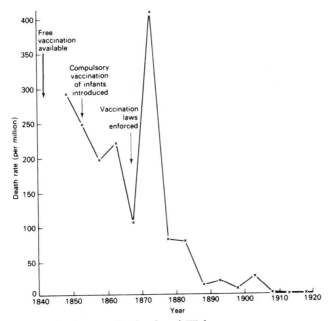

**Figure 30.6**   Smallpox: death rates, England and Wales

available after 1935, particularly the sulphonamides and antibiotics. By this time mortality from airborne infections had fallen to a small fraction of its level in the mid-nineteenth century; and even after the introduction of chemotherapy, with the important exception of tuberculosis, it is probably safe to conclude that immunization and therapy were not the main influences on the further decline of the death rate.

## Water- and food-borne diseases

### Cholera, diarrhoea and dysentery
In the mid-nineteenth century cholera was grouped with other diarrhoea diseases in the Registrar General's classification; however, the last epidemic in Britain was in 1865, so from that time the contribution of cholera was negligible. Mortality from the diarrhoeal diseases fell in the late nineteenth century; it increased between 1901 and 1911 but then decreased rapidly.

It is unlikely that treatment had any appreciable effect on the outcome of the diseases before the use of intravenous therapy in the nineteen thirties, by which time 95 per cent of the improvement had occurred. For the main explanation of the decline of mortality we must turn to the hygienic measures which reduced exposure.

### Non-respiratory tuberculosis
Non-respiratory tuberculosis was an important cause of death in the nineteenth century. Although mortality fell quite rapidly after 1901, there was still a considerable number of deaths in England and Wales (197) in 1971.

Interpretation of this trend is complicated by the fact that non-respiratory tuber-culosis is due to both human and bovine infections; the abdominal cases are pre-dominantly of bovine origin, whereas those involving other organs such as bones are often caused by the human organism. The human types can be interpreted in the same terms as the pulmonary disease, but a different explanation must be sought for the bovine infection. It is unlikely that treatment contributed significantly to the fall of mortality, since the level was already low when streptomycin – the first effective measure – was introduced in 1947.

### Typhoid and typhus

Mortality from typhus fell rapidly in the late nineteenth century and there have been few deaths in the twentieth. It can be said without hesitation that specific medical measures had no influence on this decline.

The decline of the enteric fevers was also rapid, and began before the turn of the century, somewhat earlier than the fall of deaths from diarrhoea and dysentery. Effective treatment by chloramphenicol was not available until 1950, but by that time mortality from enteric fever was almost eliminated from England and Wales. Al-though immunization was used widely in the armed services during the war, its effectiveness is doubtful and it can have had little influence on the number of deaths.

In summary, the rapid decline of mortality from the diseases spread by water and food since the late nineteenth century owed little to medical measures. Immunization is relatively ineffective even today, and therapy of some value was not employed until about 1950, by which time the number of deaths had fallen to a very low level.

## Other diseases due to micro-organisms

### Convulsions and teething

Most of the deaths included under these unsatisfactory terms were due to infectious diseases of childhood, for example to whooping cough, measles, otitis media, men-ingitis and gastro-enteritis. These infections are mainly airborne, and the general conclusions concerning the time and influence of immunization and therapy on air-borne diseases may be accepted for them. That is to say, it is unlikely that medical measures had any significant effect on the frequency of death before the introduction of sulphonamides and antibiotics, and even after that time they were probably less important than other influences.

### Syphilis

Although syphilis was associated with only 0.3 per cent of the reduction of mortality from the mid-nineteenth century to 1971, it remained an important cause of sickness and death until about 1916, when salvarsan was made available free of charge to medical practitioners. From this time the number of deaths fell, and it was quite low in 1945 when penicillin largely replaced the arsenical preparations.

The decline of syphilis since its introduction to Europe in the fifteenth century was not due mainly to therapy, for after several centuries of exposure of the population the disease had changed to a milder form. Nevertheless it seems reasonable to attribute the reduction of mortality since 1901 essentially to treatment. It should of course be recognized that effective treatment, as in the case of tuberculosis, not only benefits those affected by the disease, but also reduces the number of persons who spread the infection. It seems right to regard this secondary effect as a further contribution of medical measures.

## Appendicitis, peritonitis
Mortality from these causes increased slightly during the nineteenth and early twentieth centuries – probably because of more accurate certification of cause of death – but declined after 1921. This improvement, which accounted for 0.4 per cent of the fall of death rate from all causes, can be attributed to treatment.

## Puerperal fever
The death rate from puerperal fever declined from the beginning of this century, but more rapidly after the introduction of the sulphonamides (1935) and, later, penicillin. It seems probable that the initial fall was due mainly to reduced exposure to infection, as the teaching of Semmelweis in the previous century began to improve the practice of the developing midwifery services; but from 1935 these services were greatly reinforced by chemotherapy. Both influences can be credited to medical interventions.

## Other infections
The 'other conditions' are a miscellaneous group, including some well recognized infectious diseases which caused few deaths, either because they were uncommon in this period (as in the case of malaria, tetanus, poliomyelitis and encephalitis) or because although common they were not often lethal (as in the case of mumps, chicken pox and rubella). They also include some relatively uncommon certified causes of death which are ill defined, such as abscess, phlegmon and pyaemia. In addition, there is a very small number of deaths due to worm parasites which, strictly, do not belong among conditions due to micro-organisms.

These infections were associated with 3.5 per cent of the fall of mortality between the mid-nineteenth century and 1971. In view of their varied aetiology it is not possible to assess accurately the major influences, but it is unlikely that therapy made much contribution before 1935. More than half of the reduction of deaths occurred before this time.

To summarize: except in the case of vaccination against smallpox (which was associated with 1.6 per cent of the decline of the death rate from 1848–54 to 1971), it is unlikely that immunization or therapy had a significant effect on mortality from infectious diseases before the twentieth century. Between 1900 and 1935 these measures contributed in some diseases: antitoxin in treatment of diphtheria; surgery in treatment of appendicitis, peritonitis and ear infections; salvarsan in treatment of syphilis; intravenous therapy in treatment of diarrhoeal diseases; passive immunization against tetanus; and improved obstetric care resulting in prevention of puerperal fever. But even if these measures were responsible for the whole decline of mortality from these conditions after 1900 – which clearly they were not – they would account for only a very small part of the decrease of deaths which occurred before 1935. From that time the first powerful chemotherapeutic agents – sulphonamides and, later, antibiotics – came into use, and they were supplemented by improved vaccines. However, they were certainly not the only influences which led to the continued fall of mortality. I conclude that immunization and treatment contributed little to the reduction of deaths from infectious diseases before 1935, and over the whole period since cause of death was first registered (in 1838) they were much less important than other influences.

Thomas McKeown was Professor of Social Medicine at the University of Birmingham from 1945 to 1977. This article is taken from Chapter 5 of his book *The Modern Rise of Population*, published by Edward Arnold, London (1976).

# 31

# The importance of social intervention in Britain's mortality decline *c.* 1850–1914: a re-interpretation of the role of public health

SIMON SZRETER

## Introduction

As most undergraduates today in medicine or modern history will know, it is now widely considered that the belief that directed human agency informed by medical and sanitary science was the principal source of improvement in the nation's health, has been apparently conclusively deflated and debunked by the historical epidemiological research project of Professor Thomas McKeown and associates.

The main purpose of this article will be to argue that McKeown's analysis of the empirical data has been misleading. It will be urged that the public health movement working through local government, rather than nutritional improvements through rising living standards, should be seen as the true moving force behind the decline of mortality in this period.

Professor Thomas McKeown's book, *The Modern Rise of Population*, was published in 1976 as an accessible summary of over two decades of painstaking empirical work. It effectively demonstrated that those advances in the science of medicine which form the basis of today's conventional clinical and hospital teaching and practice, in particular the immuno- and chemo-therapies, played only a very minor role in accounting for the historic decline in mortality levels. McKeown simply and conclusively showed that many of the most important diseases involved had already all but disappeared in England and Wales before the earliest date at which the relevant scientific medical innovations occurred.

However, in addition to this *negative* finding that the forward march of modern 'scientific medicine' cannot be given the credit for the historical fall in mortality, McKeown also propounded a *positive* explanatory thesis. He claimed that his analysis of the epidemiological evidence showed that the major factor responsible was 'a rising standard of living, of which the most significant feature was improved diet'.

McKeown believed that his empirical work on the nineteenth-century evidence had conclusively established this in two ways. First, that part of the mortality decline supposedly attributable exclusively to increased nutrition was claimed to have occurred earliest, whereas public health measures came along relatively late in the day, when the momentum of declining mortality was already established. Secondly, that on etiological[1] grounds, according to the available epidemiological records tracking changes in the incidence of different causes of death, sanitary measures could only have had at the maximum the potential to eliminate roughly a quarter of all deaths, whereas rising nutritional standards had probably been responsible for about twice that proportion. Thus, nutritional improvements were unequivocally presented as the prime moving and primary sustaining forces in accounting for the Victorian mortality decline. However, it is shown below that neither of these arguments can be sustained on a careful re-examination of the historical evidence.

**The 'McKeown thesis'**

The analysis of death-rates in nineteenth- and twentieth-century Britain which was presented by McKeown *et al.* is based on a uniquely detailed historical source material. These are the returns of deaths classified by age and certified cause of death which are available for the entire population of Britain, excluding Scotland, from July 1837 onwards. Details about the numbers dying from each disease by age and sex were combined with comparable information regarding the total population alive at each of the national censuses taken every ten years to produce a series of age-specific, cause-specific death-rates, published decennially by the Registrar-General in a special supplement.

McKeown grouped the individual diseases into four broad etiological categories, according to what modern medical science understands to be the main pathways of transmission involved in the spread of each particular disease. Three of McKeown's four categories relate to diseases which are due to the invasion of the human host by a micro-organism, meaning usually bacteria or a virus. First, there is the airborne category of diseases, where the microbes in question can simply float about in suspension in the air usually associated with tiny droplets of water vapour or saliva spray from the exhalations of infected victims or carriers. Secondly, there are the diseases caused by water- and food-borne microbes. Thirdly, there is a small residual category of other diseases also attributable to micro-organisms, where the vector of transmission is neither air- nor food- nor water-borne. These include strictly contagious diseases, that is, those passed by direct contact between animals and humans (e.g. plague, typhus) or just between humans (e.g. sexually transmitted diseases). Finally, there is the category of afflictions which are not micro-biotically caused, such as

---

1. Often spelt 'aetiological' in English texts; aetiology (or etiology) is the study of the causes of disease.

congenital defects and the degenerative diseases which are associated with the normal processes of ageing (subject, of course, to modification by lifestyle, diet, and overall environment). These include cancers and coronary heart diseases as the most significant examples.

With this simple but very useful classification system established, McKeown went on to argue that any observed fall in the incidence of a disease must be due to one of the following causes:

(i)   an autonomous decline in the virulence of the micro-organism itself;
(ii)  an improvement in the overall environment so as to reduce the chances of initial exposure to potentially harmful organisms. This could either be:
  (a)  as a result of scientific advances in immunisation techniques;
  (b)  through a public health policy designed to sanitise the urban environment – McKeown calls this 'municipal sanitation' or 'hygiene improvements';
(iii) an improvement in the human victims' defensive resources *after* initial exposure to hostile organisms. This could occur either:
  (a)  through the development of effective scientific methods of treating symptoms;
  (b)  via an increase in the level and quality of the exposed population's average nutritional intake, that is better and more abundant food, thereby improving the individual's own natural defences.

McKeown's strategy in presenting his argument was to assess each of these candidate 'causes' of mortality decline in turn, regarding their possible proportionate contributions to the overall observed fall in mortality levels.

First, he dealt with (i) the possibility that there might have been a spontaneous change in the virulence of some of the infective micro-organisms. McKeown was willing to allow that two of the airborne diseases, scarlet fever and influenza, probably declined spontaneously in this manner. However, the impression was given, by taking a wider sweeping perspective including the eighteenth and twentieth centuries as well, that this factor was relatively insignificant and could be more or less ruled out as a significant component of the mortality decline.

McKeown next dealt with what was called the medical contribution (iia and iiia), by which was meant, first, scientific advances in protective immunisation and, secondly, scientific advances in chemotherapy and hospitalised treatment of sufferers. Hospitals were dismissed outright.

He then proceeded to demonstrate for each of the major diseases in turn that, with the exception of smallpox and diphtheria, the dates at which either effective immunisation procedures or scientific medical treatments first became available were often far too late in time to be able to account for all but the last few percentage points of the overall decline of the disease. This was certainly true of respiratory tuberculosis, measles, and scarlet fever, and broadly true for whooping cough and the bronchitis, pneumonia, and influenza group.

Having eliminated in this fashion both aspects of advances in medical science, McKeown was now left with just two possible causal factors out of the original list, to account between them for the lion's share of the decline in mortality.

The argument presented was as follows. It can only have been the water- and food-borne diseases which could have been controlled by (iib) municipal sanitation and similar preventive public health measures in the nineteenth and early twentieth centuries. Airborne diseases by contrast could not be prevented in this way from spreading or from occurring. It was admitted that isolation of individuals with symptoms might have some net effect, but then the efficacy of the hospitals had already been roundly dismissed, whilst it was pointed out that many airborne diseases could be carried and spread by persons not even manifesting symptoms. McKeown argued, therefore, that any real decline in the incidence of mortality from the airborne category of diseases could *only* be the result of (iiib) improvements in the potential victim's resistance to the disease by virtue of an improved nutritional and dietary status, since the chances of initial exposure to the disease could not be affected by public health preventive measures.

Using this *a priori* argument, McKeown's data apparently showed that the airborne category of diseases was responsible for about twice the percentage share of the total reduction in death-rates in both periods, before and after 1901. Accordingly, this constituted irrefutable evidence that above all else it has been improvements in nutritional intake brought about by rising living standards, rather than any other factor – including public health measures – which has been the most important cause of the decline in mortality in Britain.

### Critique of McKeown's interpretation

First, as has been pointed out by many others, the weight of presumption in favour of improvements in nutrition as the primary causal factor in the registered mortality decline emerged merely by default, as a result of the sceptical devaluation of other factors including medical intervention, rather than because of any convincing positive evidence in its favour.

Secondly, and related to this, the argument by exclusion is only legitimate if *all* the suspects have been correctly identified and are separately examined. But here 'the standard of living' acts very much as a conceptual, residual catch-all, simply subsuming by fiat a variety of other possible factors, which are, therefore, not explicitly addressed in the analysis.

One might at least have expected in a study coming out so strongly in favour of nutrition as the major factor that there would at the very least have been some detailed consideration given to the history of food adulteration and the battle for its regulation and control. But all this is blandly subsumed under the economistic term, 'standard of living'. McKeown's interpretation of the epidemiological evidence has, therefore, been crucially misleading in suggesting that these social, cultural, and political dimensions can quite properly be conceived merely as the automatic corollary of changes in a country's per capita real income.

In his interpretation of the data, McKeown was particularly impressed with the importance of the overall long-run decline of the single airborne disease, respiratory tuberculosis (TB). In 1848–54 this had been the most lethal single cause of death, accounting for 13.3 per cent of all deaths occurring at that time. However, if attention is concentrated more closely on the nineteenth century, McKeown's own evidence provides far from unequivocal support either for the contention that a fall in airborne disease is the leading epidemiological feature of the period, or for the derivative conclusion that this could *only* be primarily the reflection of general improvement in dietary standards and nutritional levels.

Apart from respiratory TB, there were two other airborne diseases which declined very significantly in the nineteenth century, scarlet fever and smallpox. However, neither of these can be used to support the nutrition hypothesis, although they are within the airborne category. It has long been recognised that human intervention, in the form of inoculation starting in the eighteenth century and then vaccination, quarantining, and isolation procedures in the nineteenth century, must be granted the major role in the case of smallpox. As for scarlet fever, McKeown is prepared to acknowledge that the epidemiological evidence strongly suggests that this was in all probability a disease which burned itself out spontaneously. But most disconcerting of all for McKeown's general interpretation, is the behaviour of the composite airborne category, 'bronchitis, pneumonia and influenza', which has so far been omitted from the discussion. This was the second most important cause of death in 1848–54, accounting for 10.25 per cent of all deaths. It actually registered a very considerable *absolute increase* in mortality of well over 20 per cent down to 1901. By the turn of the century this category was clearly the most important single killer, contributing over 16 per cent of all deaths, a greater proportion of the total than respiratory TB had represented in the mid-nineteenth century.

Thus, McKeown would have us treat the airborne diseases as a single unitary group, which between them accounted for about half of the decline in mortality before 1901 and would have us believe that nutritional improvements, made possible by a rising standard of living, can alone be considered responsible for the large-scale reduction of the group as a whole. Yet, on closer examination, we find that this completely ignores the important contrary trend exhibited by one of the two most lethal disease categories in the group. Furthermore, we find that the nutrition argument applies almost exclusively to only *one* of the several diseases within the group, respiratory TB.

But how strong is McKeown's case that even this one disease's reduction was due to rising living standards and food consumption *alone*? First, contrary to McKeown's sweeping assertion, it should be pointed out that overall exposure of the population to airborne diseases would have been affected by the general level of crowding and ventilation in domestic or working environments. Thus incidence of airborne diseases probably was influenced by certain public health and preventive measures.

Secondly, the etiology of respiratory TB is a highly complex one, which is far from completely understood. Although it is probable that absence of malnutrition in a population is a necessary condition for the elimination of tuberculosis mortality altogether, it is equally probable that danger is decreased if other risk factors are reduced; particularly, frequency of incidence of other infectious diseases; but also overcrowding, lack of sunlight, air ventilation, and various occupational hazards.

It would certainly seem presumptuous, therefore, to attribute a long-term reduction in TB mortality to one single factor, such as improving nutritional standards. What, then, were McKeown's grounds for this bold assertion? The critical factor was the apparent empirical finding that respiratory TB was already declining from the late 1830s and 1840s, before any other major disease had begun to fall (apart from smallpox which had probably been on the wane since the latter part of the eighteenth century). An examination of the evidence originally adduced by McKeown to demonstrate the early decline of TB is, in fact, far from convincing.

There is, in fact, no good evidence for TB's chronological priority in the mortality decline. And in any case, there had always been the claim of the much earlier, medically induced decline in smallpox, the quantitative importance of which McKeown failed to acknowledge. Although smallpox did not appear to be a predominant factor in the civil registration returns which McKeown analysed, this was precisely because it had already been beaten back considerably by the 1830s. All the evidence of medical testimony in the eighteenth and early nineteenth centuries suggest that it had been a major scourge, especially of childhood.

Finally, there still remains to be taken into account the strong counter-trend, already remarked upon, which the increasingly lethal bronchitis group of airborne respiratory diseases exhibited throughout the rest of the nineteenth century. This constitutes the most awkward and serious general caveat on the validity of McKeown's airborne 'nutritional determinism' interpretation, however it is explained.

With the anomalous rise in bronchitis-group fatalities properly acknowledged, the classic sanitation diseases come to the fore in quantitative terms. These two water/food-borne categories would between them be responsible for at least 8 per cent and perhaps 10 per cent of the overall mortality decline. That is one-third part of the nineteenth-century reduction, or over half as much again as that attributable to the airborne combination of TB and the bronchitis group.

Improvement in respiratory TB would, then, no longer appear to have been either chronologically prior or the quantitatively predominant feature of the nineteenth-century mortality decline in England and Wales. According to the logic of McKeown's own arguments, the foregoing would indicate a primary role for sanitary reform and public health measures, rather than rising nutritional levels or living standards. The changing incidence of mortality from respiratory TB in Victorian Britain, rather than being cast in the role of a leading and determining influence can be seen as a dependent function of the general intensity and frequency of *other* debilitating diseases.

### An alternative interpretation: urban congestion remedied by social intervention

Between 1801 and 1871 the rate of urban growth in Britain was quite unprecedented, both in the provinces and the metropolis. At the commencement of the nineteenth century no provincial town contained as many as 100,000 inhabitants. By 1871 there were seventeen cities over this size on mainland Britain, apart from London.

National aggregate mortality patterns only indirectly reflect the full impact of this period of intensive but chaotic and disorganised urban expansion on the nation's health. According to the best single summary measure currently available, Wrigley and Schofield's series for the expectation of life at birth, average life expectancy at birth rose from around 30 years to about 40 years, then slowed to a halt at the end of the first quarter of the nineteenth century. For about half a century, from the 1820s until the 1870s, there was virtually no perceptible further improvement. Thereafter, a gradual rise to about 47–8 years by the end of the century, followed by a somewhat faster rise, to just over 60 years by 1931. Paradoxically – for McKeown's thesis – it had been almost exactly at this same point in time, when the long eighteenth-century rise in life expectancy had stalled to a halt, that a concomitant eighteenth-century *fall* (or at best stagnation) in national aggregate real wages was reversed and there had begun a trend of continual, although not continuous, improvements in average real wages throughout the rest of the nineteenth century.

The explanation of the inverse relationship is not, however, difficult if it is simply accepted that the relative state of insalubrity in the expanding urban environments, rather than improvements in average real wages or the food supply, must have been the more predominant factor influencing national mortality trends in the nineteenth century. It is simply two sides of the same coin that this process could simultaneously engender higher wage-rates for the industrial workers and their families congregating at places where new enterprises were emerging, yet also simultaneously exert a negative influence on their average life expectancy because of the crowded and chaotic living conditions prevalent in the mushrooming towns and cities created by the rapidly expanding employment opportunities.

Whilst increasingly huge populations continued to concentrate ever more intensively in townships growing into cities but lacking the appropriate social overhead capital to preserve – let alone promote – health, then morbidity and mortality risks inevitably proliferated. Equally inevitably, these multiplying and compounding health hazards could only be alleviated through the appropriate social and political responses; the technical development of, and proper deployment of, precisely that infrastructure which was previously largely unnecessary. For instance, despite its rapid growth and the unhealthy over-crowded conditions which this implied, a mains sewer system for London as a whole, which dumped the waste securely downstream of its population, was not completed until 1865 – the first such large-scale integrated system in the country.

On the assumption that it was the three middle decades of the nineteenth century when most progress was occurring in the field of public health, the lack of any obvious chronological fit between public health advances and the general fall in mortality from infectious and sanitary diseases, which did not occur until the last third of the century, has perhaps discouraged historians from assigning any particular significance to the expansion of preventive public health measures as the major influence on mortality patterns.

However, despite the slowing down in *central* government activity and the relative quiescence of sanitarians in and around Westminster and Whitehall, it was in fact the last 30 years of the nineteenth century when most of the significant improvements and works of construction and concrete applications of preventive health measures went forward and were actually occurring on the ground throughout the provincial cities and towns of Britain.

For instance, the 1872 Public Health Act obliged local authorities as one of their statutory duties to ensure a pure water supply. In turn, this led to pressure for the 1878 Public Health (Water) Act whereby municipal purchase of private waterworks was made truly financially feasible. Whereas in 1879 only 415 urban local authorities were in charge of their water supplies, by 1905 over two-thirds of the 1,138 urban sanitary authorities then in existence were running the local waterworks, so that the health of the populace was decreasingly left in the hands of the likes of the East London Waterworks Co. Another example is that of the increasingly close regulation of the quality of the urban food supply, which duly resulted from the attention which Medical Officers in the 1860s had begun to pay to adulterated and defective food-stuffs, particularly meat and milk, as a source of disease. The Adulteration of Foods Acts followed in the 1870s leading to the appointment of professional inspectors and public analysts by most local authorities in the 1880s; also Weights and Measures Acts in 1878 and 1889 and a final consolidating Sale of Food & Drugs Act 1899.

The last third of the century was the classic period in which all the hectic activity of the Public Health political and administrative pioneers finally began to bear fruit and to take concrete effect. Of course, all this was only achieved as a result of innumerable unsung local skirmishes between frequently underpaid health officials, often lacking security of tenure, and their local allies – other sanitary officials, the district registrars of births and deaths, perhaps the town's press and occasionally some members of the local councils themselves – as against the parsimonious representatives of the majority of ratepayers. It is precisely the importance and *necessity* of this slow dogged campaign of a million Minutes, fought out of town-halls and the local forums of debate all over the country over the last quarter of the nineteenth century which has been missing in our previous accounts of the mortality decline.

I would argue, therefore, that there is a sound *prima facie* case to be answered that the decline in mortality, which began to be noticeable in the national aggregate statistics in the 1870s, was due more to the eventual successes of the politically and ideologically negotiated movement for public health than to any other positively identifiable factor. The resulting implementation of preventive measures of municipal sanitation and regulation of the urban environment and food market actually arrived on the ground in the many new cities throughout the country during the last third of the nineteenth century and the first decade of the twentieth.

The all but complete eradication by the end of the century of typhoid, cholera, and smallpox each testify in different ways to the importance and effectiveness of various aspects of the large-scale strategic public health measures which were introduced during this period. Provision of a suffcently clean local water supply was essential in the cases of both typhoid and cholera. Due to their epidemic nature, elimination of cholera and smallpox additionally required a properly functioning national system of surveillance to identify and snuff out local outbreaks which could otherwise quickly become major incidents. Port sanitary authorities established by the 1872 Public Health Act, alongside the initiative of the General Register Office in establishing regular communications with foreign authorities so as to gain advance warning of any outbreaks abroad, helped to ensure – in the absence of an entirely secure national water supply – that Britain successfully evaded all three subsequent European visitations of Asiatic cholera in 1873, 1884–6 and 1892–3.

By contrast, the apparent rise in the bronchitis group of airborne respiratory diseases may well be evidence that in those areas of the urban and industrial environment where preventive legislation and action was *not* forthcoming, serious consequences followed. Clean air was one obvious omission from the late nineteenth-century sanitary reform arsenal and one need look no further than the appalling urban smogs to explain such anomalously high levels of respiratory disease in the Victorian period. For instance, male textile workers in the 1890s, a numerically large segment of the factory working class, had a two-and-a-half times higher death-rate from respiratory diseases than agricultural labourers, despite their considerably higher pay and better access to a varied diet – the main factors stressed by McKeown in accounting for secular falls in the incidence of airborne diseases.

Whereas the reduction in the mortality of elder children and younger adults throughout the last third of the nineteenth century reflected improvement of the urban environment at the strategic level outside the home, that of infants had to await the more probing and detailed regulations and the expansion of skeletal social services, which had only just begun by the turn of the twentieth century to penetrate into and improve the conditions existing in the infant's 'environment': the working-class domestic household itself.

## Conclusions

In the course of this most brilliant attack on the historical claims of his main target, 'scientific medicine', McKeown's detailed historical research work led him to produce an ambitious general interpretation of the causes of mortality decline, which minimalised the role of directed human agency in general, not just that which could be identified as the precursor of modern hospital and clinical practice.

It has been argued here that the historical epidemiological evidence presented by McKeown *et al.* does not in fact offer the conclusive and exclusive support, which it has long been assumed to do, for the contention that rising living standards and associated nutritional improvements have been the predominant source of mortality decline in Victorian and Edwardian Britain.

The revised account indicates a primary role for those public health measures which combated the early nineteenth-century upsurge of diseases directly resulting from the defective and insanitary urban and domestic environments created in the course of industrialisation. The 'invisible hand' of rising living standards, conceived as an impersonal and ultimately inevitable by-product of general economic growth, no longer takes the leading role as historical guarantor of the nation's mortality decline. Indeed, economic growth in itself, even with rising real wages, seems just as likely to harm as to benefit the nation's health, witness the urban experience of the first two-thirds of the last century.

It seems, then, that it all depended on how the fruits of that growth were deployed. This, in turn, depended on the cumulative net outcome of a rich history of political, ideological, scientific, and legal conflicts and battles at both national and local levels throughout the period under review. Fallible, blundering, but purposive human agency is returned to centre stage in this account of the mortality decline.

Simon Szreter is a demographer and social historian working at Gonville and Caius College, Cambridge. This article is an edited and amended extract from a very much longer article first published by *The Society for the Social History of Medicine*, pp. 1–37 (1988).

# 32
# Effectiveness and efficiency

## A. L. COCHRANE

The critical step forward which brought an experimental approach into clinical medicine can be variously dated. At any rate there is no doubt that the credit belongs to Sir Austin Bradford Hill. His ideas have only penetrated a small way into medicine, and they still have to revolutionize sociology, education, and penology. Each generation will, I hope, respect him more.

The basic idea, like most good things, is very simple. The randomized controlled trial (RCT) approaches the problem of the comparability of two groups the other way round. The idea is not to worry about the characteristics of the patients, but to be sure that the division of the patients into two groups is done by some method independent of human choice, i.e. by allocating according to some simple numerical device such as the order in which the patients come under treatment, or, more safely, by the use of random numbers. In this way the characteristics of the patients are randomized between the two groups, and it is possible to test the hypothesis that one treatment is better than another and express the results in the form of the probability of the differences found being due to chance or not.

The RCT is a very beautiful technique, of wide applicability, but as with everything else there are snags. When humans have to make observations there is always a possibility of bias. To reduce this possibility a modification has been introduced: the 'double-blind' randomized trial. In this neither the doctor nor the patients know which of the two treatments is being given. This eliminates the possibility of a great deal of bias, but one still has to be on one's guard.

There are other snags: first a purely statistical one. Many research units carry out hundreds of these so-called tests of significance in a year and it is often difficult to remember that, according to the level of significance chosen, 1 in 20 or 1 in 100 will be misleading. Another snag has been introduced by the current tendency to put too much emphasis on tests of significance. The results of such tests are very dependent on the number in the groups. With small numbers it is very easy to give the impression that a treatment is no more effective than a placebo, whereas in reality it is very difficult indeed to exclude the possibility of a small effect. Alternatively, with large numbers it is often possible to achieve a result that is statistically significant but may be clinically unimportant. All results must be examined very critically to avoid all the snags.

Another snag is that the technique is not always applicable for ethical reasons. There is, of course, no absolute medical ethic but the examples I quote here represent the majority of medical opinion at present, though I do not necessarily agree with them myself. They are: surgery for carcinoma of the lung, cytological tests for the prevention of cervical carcinoma, and dietetic therapy for phenylketonuria. No RCTs have ever been carried out to test the value of these standard therapies and tests. In the first two cases the RCT technique was not available when the surgical and medical innovations were made for carcinoma of the lung and cervix. By the time such RCTs were considered by medical scientists the one-time 'innovations' were embedded in clinical practice. Such trials would necessarily involve denying the routine procedure to half a group of patients and at this stage are nearly always termed unethical. It can be argued that it is ethically questionable to use on patients a procedure whose value is unknown, but the answer is that it is unethical not to do so if the patient will otherwise die or suffer severe disability and there is no alternative therapy. Such trials, it must be accepted, cannot be done in areas where the consensus of medical opinion is against them. This means, on the one hand, that patients' interests are very well protected and on the other that there are sections of medicine whose effectiveness cannot at present be measured and which, *in toto*, probably reduce the overall efficiency of the NHS.

There are other limitations on the general applicability of the RCT. One important area is the group of diseases where improvement or deterioration has to be measured subjectively. It was hoped that the double-blind modification would avoid this trouble, but it has not been very successful in, say, psychiatry. Similarly the assessment of the 'quality of life' in such trials has proved very difficult. A good example is the various forms of treatment attempted for recurrences after operation for carcinoma of the breast. We have so far failed to develop any satisfactory way of measuring quality.

Another very different reason for the relatively slow use of the RCT in measuring effectiveness is illustrated by its geographical distribution. If some such index as the number of RCTs per 1,000 doctors per year for all countries were worked out and a map of the world shaded according to the level of the index (black being the highest), one would see the UK in black, and scattered black patches in Scandinavia, the USA, and a few other countries; the rest would be nearly white. It appears in general it is Catholicism, Communism, and underdevelopment that appear to be against RCTs. In underdeveloped countries this can be understood, but what have Communism and Catholicism against RCTs? Is authoritarianism the common link, or is Communism a Catholic heresy? Whatever the cause this limitation to small areas of the world has certainly slowed down progress in two ways. There are too few doctors doing the work and the load on the few is becoming too great. An RCT is great fun for the co-ordinator but can be very boring for the scattered physicians filling in the forms.

In writing this section in praise of the RCT I do not want to give the impression that it is the only technique of any value in medical research. This would, of course, be entirely untrue. I believe, however, that the problem of evaluation is the first priority of the NHS and that for this purpose the RCT is much the most satisfactory in spite of its snags. The main job of medical administrators is to make choices between alternatives. To enable them to make the correct choices they must have accurate comparable data about the benefit and cost of the alternatives. These can really only be obtained by an adequately costed RCT.

If anyone had any doubts about the need for doing RCTs to evaluate therapy, recent publications using this technique have given ample warning of how dangerous it is to assume that well-established therapies which have not been tested are always effective. Possibly the most striking result is Dr Mather's RCT in Bristol[1] in which hospital treatment (including a variable time in a coronary care unit) was compared with treatment at home for acute ischaemic heart disease. The results do not suggest that there is any medical gain in admission to hospital with coronary care units compared with treatment at home. Equally striking are the results of the multi-centre American trial on the value of oral anti-diabetic therapy, insulin, and diet in the treatment of mature diabetics.[2,3] They suggest that giving tolbutamide and phenformin is definitely disadvantageous, and that there is no advantage in giving insulin compared with diet. Dr Elwood, in my unit, has demonstrated very beautifully how ill-founded was the general view of the value of iron in pregnant women with haemoglobin levels between 9 g and 12 g per 100 ml in curing the classical symptoms of anaemia.[4]

I have neither the ability, knowledge, time, nor space to classify all present-day therapies. All I feel capable of is a rough classification:

1. Those therapies, with no backing from RCTs, which are justified by their immediate and obvious effect, for example, insulin for acute juvenile diabetes, vitamin $B_{12}$ for pernicious anaemia, penicillin for certain infections, etc.
2. Those therapies backed by RCTs. The best example is the drug therapy of tuberculosis, but there are, of course, many others.
3. Those where there is good experimental evidence of some effect, but no evidence from RCTs, of doing more good than harm to the patient, particularly in the long-term. A good example, mentioned above, is the effect of iron on raising haemoglobin levels. This rise is very simply demonstrated, and there was a general belief that raising the haemoglobin level cured all the symptoms traditionally associated with low levels, until Dr Elwood published his results.
4. Those therapies which were well established before the advent of RCTs whose effectiveness cannot be assessed because of the ethical situation, but where there is some real doubt about the effectiveness, for example treatment for carcinoma of the bronchus and of the breast.
5. Those therapies where the evidence from RCTs is equivocal. The best example is tonsillectomy.
6. Those therapies under-investigated by RCT, although there are no ethical constraints, which are over-ripe for them. Psychotherapy and physiotherapy are probably the most important members of this group.

If effectiveness has been rather under-investigated, efficiency has hardly been investigated at all.

1. The most important type of inefficiency is really a combination of two separate groups, the use of ineffective therapies and the use of effective therapies at the wrong time. They are closely connected; for instance I should, without thinking, have classified tonics as ineffective but many of them contain medicaments which

could be effective in some circumstances. Iron and the vitamins, which are common ingredients of tonics, can, of course, on occasions be very effective. It is important to distinguish the very respectable, conscious use of placebos. The effect of placebos has been shown by RCTs to be very large. Their use in the correct place is to be encouraged. What is inefficient is the use of relatively expensive drugs as placebos.

At the other end of the scale are the therapies for which there is no evidence of effectiveness, but where something has to be done. Simply mastectomy is a case in point for carcinoma of the breast. This I do not consider inefficient, but on present evidence I would not classify the use of radical mastectomy as efficient.

2. The incorrect place of treatment. This is possibly the least-recognized type of inefficiency, but it seems probable that the increasing cost of hospitalization will force attention to it. There are in general five places where treatment can be given: at the GP's surgery, at home, at the out-patient department, in hospital, or more recently in a 'community' hospital. Traditions have grown up as to the correct place for treatment for particular diseases, and until very recently no one has treated these traditional decisions as hypotheses which should be tested. I have already mentioned Dr Mather's comparison of the treatment of acute ischaemic heart disease at home and in a hospital with a coronary care unit. Weddell has compared the treatment of varicose veins in hospital and in the out-patient department using the RCT technique.[5] No evidence was found of any advantage associated with hospitalization for those cases without skin damage. It is to be hoped that such demonstrations that RCTs are possible and ethical will encourage others to follow suit in this new sphere.

3. Incorrect length of stay in hospital. It is not surprising, given the economic and psychological facts of the NHS, that the average length of stay in hospital in this country is higher than in some other countries. In addition, evidence has been accumulating of large differences in length of stay between regions and between different consultants when treating the same disease. The most striking evidence (and the most accurate) comes from Heasman and Carstairs[6] from whose paper Figure 32.1 is taken. The extent of the differences is really surprising when hospitalization in a district general hospital is one of the costliest treatments that can be prescribed, and that the majority of patients wish to leave hospital as soon as possible. The only condition in which length of stay has been much investigated is hernia. One group were discharged on the first day post-operatively. [No] serious disadvantages of early discharge [were] noted, but early discharge of herniorrhaphies has hardly become routine. The mean length of stay for hernia in England and Wales in 1967 was 9.1 days for males.

Unfortunately this observational evidence does not take us very far. All the consultants cannot be right, but this does not help us to determine the optimum length of stay. This can again be best approached by RCTs, but it will not be easy. The main index will have to be the incidence of complications and as these will in general not be high, very large populations are required to establish an optimum.

I am conscious that I have only scratched the surface of inefficiency. I could have stressed the rising percentage of hospital admissions for iatrogenic diseases; I could have stirred the dirty waters of medical administration, but I think for my limited purposes I have done enough.

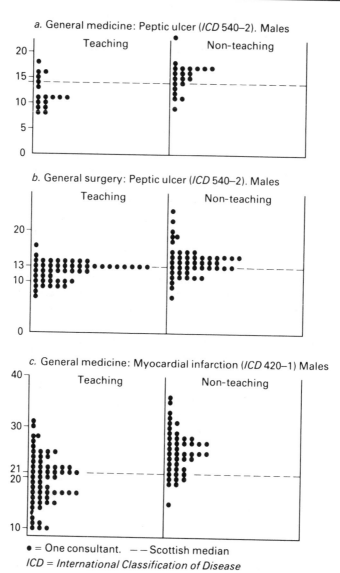

*a.* General medicine: Peptic ulcer (*ICD* 540–2). Males

*b.* General surgery: Peptic ulcer (*ICD* 540–2). Males

*c.* General medicine: Myocardial infarction (*ICD* 420–1) Males

● = One consultant.   — — Scottish median
*ICD = International Classification of Disease*

**Figure 32.1**  Median duration of stay in days for two diagnoses for individual consultants in Scotland (data for 1967), in teaching and non-teaching hospitals

## An illustrative example: pulmonary tuberculosis

The change in the tuberculosis world between 1944 when I was burying my POW tuberculosis patients in Germany and the present day when TB deaths are the subject of a special investigation, as in theory they should not happen, is one of the most cheering things I have experienced in my life. The way in which the new treatments and preventive measures were introduced can also serve as a model for the introduction of all new treatments in the future. RCTs were used from the very beginning, and

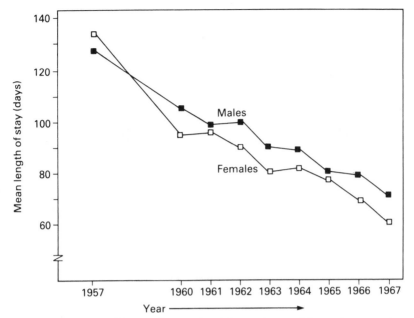

**Figure 32.2**   Mean length of hospital stay (days) for patients with respiratory tuberculosis (*ICD*, 7th revision, causes 001–008) in England and Wales, 1957–67

through this the correct dosages and combinations of drugs were quickly established; 'resistance to drugs' was quickly identified and means found of preventing it; each new drug was carefully assessed as it came on the market. The result is that there now are effective methods of treatment and prevention for TB. The speed of its development is very much to the credit of the MRC, WHO, and the British Tuberculosis Association, but it would have been impossible without the technique of the RCT.

On the efficiency side there is also a great deal to the credit of this branch of medicine. 'Place of treatment' was first investigated by an RCT when hospital and home care for the tuberculous were compared in Madras[7] and various studies in this country and the USA have confirmed the Madras finding that bed rest was unimportant.[8,9,10]

In spite of the striking evidence about the unimportance of bed rest, it is surprising to find how slowly the mean length of stay in hospitals in England and Wales is falling (Figure 32.2), and how much the variation in length of stay seems to depend on individual consultants (Figure 32.3). The real problem is how to ensure that patients take their chemotherapy after leaving hospital. Some doctors react by keeping their patients longer in hospital, others try biweekly supervised chemotherapy. The correct solution is still unknown, and until it is the treatment will not be completely efficient.

There are other details which need tidying up. There are remarkable differences for instance in radiographic routine. In an unpublished study of a twelve-month follow-up of all cases admitted during one year the type of case admitted to three hospitals were reasonably comparable, but in one hospital only 10 per cent, in another 52 per cent, and in the third, 85 per cent had at least one tomogram.

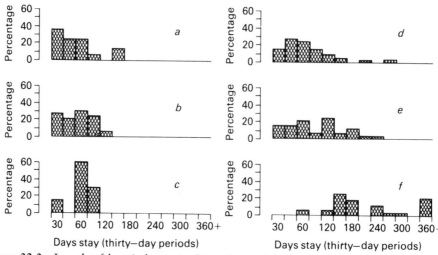

**Figure 32.3** Length of hospital stay in thirty-day periods for male patients with pulmonary tuberculosis (*ICD*, 8th revision, cause 011) before discharge home from six selected chest hospitals in 1969

Someone, rather sardonically asked me once how far I was prepared to take this 'randomizing game'. I answered, without thinking, 'You should randomize until it hurts (the clinicians).' In spite of my great admiration for the effective therapy and the efficiency with which it has been applied in this field I still think there is room for improvement. The TB world has not randomized until it hurts.

## References

1. Mather, H. G., Pearson, W. G., Read, K. L. Q., Shaw, D. B., Steed, G. R., Thorne, M. G., Jones, S., Guerrier, C. J., Eraut, C. D., McHugh, P. M., Chowdhury, N. R., Jafary, M. H., and Wallace, T. J. 'Acute myocardial infarction: Home and hospital treatment', *Br. Med. J.* 3, 334 (1971).
2. Universities Group Diabetes Program 'A study of the effects of hypoglycemic agents on vascular complications in patients with adult-onset diabetes. II, Mortality results', *Diabetes*, 19, suppl. 2 (1970).
3. Knatterud, G. L., Meinhert, C. L., Klimit, C. R., Osborne, R. K., and Martin, D. B. 'Effects of hypoglycemic agents on vascular complications in patients with adult onset diabetes', *J. Am. med. Ass.* 217, 6, 777 (1971).
4. Elwood, P. C., Waters, W. E., Green, W. J., and Wood, M. M. 'Evaluation of a screening survey for anaemia in adult non-pregnant women', *Br. med. J.* 4, 714 (1967).
5. Piachaud, D., and Weddell, J. M. 'The economics of treating varicose veins', *International J. Epid.* 1(3), 287–294 (1972).
6. Heasman, M. A., and Carstairs, V. 'Inpatient management variations in some aspects of practice in Scotland', ibid. 1, 495 (1971).
7. Dawson, J. J. Y., Devadatta, S., Fox, W., Radharkrishna, S., Ramakrishnan, C. V., Somasundarah, P. R., Stott, H., Tripathy, S. P., and Velu, S. Tuberculosis Chemotherapy Centre, Madras 'A five year study of patients with pulmonary tuberculosis – a current comparison of home and sanatorium treatment for 1 year with isoniazid plus P. A. S.', *Bull. Wld Hlth Org.* 34, 533 (1966).

8. Tuberculosis Society of Scotland 'The treatment of pulmonary tuberculosis at work: a controlled trial', *Tubercle. Lond.* **41**, 161 (1960).
9. Spriggs, E. A., Bruce, A. A., and Jones, M. 'Rest and exercise in pulmonary tuberculosis: A controlled study', ibid. **42**, 267 (1961).
10. Tyrell, W. F. 'Bed rest in the treatment of pulmonary tuberculosis', *Lancet*, i, 821 (1956).

A. L. (Archie) Cochrane was Director of the Medical Research Council's Epidemiology Unit in Cardiff before his retirement. These extracts are taken from his book, *Effectiveness and Efficiency; Random Reflections on Health Services*, produced for the 1971 Rock Carling Fellowship, published by Nuffield Provincial Hospital Trust.

# 33

# Ethical dilemmas in evaluation – a correspondence

The following (edited) article appeared in *The Lancet* on 16 February 1980.

## Possible prevention of neural-tube defects by periconceptional vitamin supplementation

R. W. Smithells, S. Sheppard, and C. J. Schorah
*Department of Paediatrics and Child Health, University of Leeds*

M. J. Seller
*Paediatric Research Unit, Guy's Hospital, London*

N. C. Nevin
*Department of Medical Genetics, Queen's University of Belfast*

R. Harris, and A. P. Read
*Department of Medical Genetics, University of Manchester*

D. W. Fielding
*Department of Paediatrics, Chester Hospitals*

### Summary

Women who had previously given birth to one or more infants with a neural-tube defect (NTD) were recruited into a trial of periconceptional multivitamin supplementation. One of 78 infants/fetuses of fully supplemented mothers (0.6 per cent) had an NTD, compared with 13 of 260 infants/fetuses of unsupplemented mothers (5.0 per cent).

## Introduction

The well-known social-class gradient in the incidence of neural-tube defects (NTD) suggests that nutritional factors might be involved in NTD aetiology. A possible link between folate deficiency and NTDs in man was first reported in 1965.[1] More recently, significant social-class differences in dietary intakes in the first trimester,[2] and in first-trimester values for red cell folate, leucocyte ascorbic acid, red-blood-cell riboflavin, and serum vitamin A have been reported,[3] dietary and biochemical values being higher in classes I and II than in classes III, IV, and V. Furthermore, seven mothers, of whom six subsequently gave birth to NTD infants and one to an infant with unexplained microcephaly, had first-trimester mean values for red cell folate and leucocyte ascorbic acid that were significantly lower than those of controls.

These observations are compatible with the hypothesis that subclinical deficiencies of one or more vitamins contribute to the causation of NTDs. We report preliminary results of an intervention study in which mothers at increased risk of having NTD infants were offered periconceptional multivitamin supplements.

## Patients and methods

Women who had one or more NTD infants, were planning a further pregnancy, but were not yet pregnant were admitted to the study. All women referred to the departments involved in the study and who met these criteria were invited to take part. Patients came from Northern Ireland, South-East England, Yorkshire, Lancashire, and Cheshire. One hundred and eighty-five women who received full vitamin supplementation (see below) became pregnant.

The control group comprised women who had had one or more previous NTD infants but were either pregnant when referred to the study centres or declined to take part in the study. Some centres were able to select a control for each supplemented mother, matched for the number of previous NTD births, the estimated date of conception, and, where possible, age. There were 264 control mothers. The numbers of fully supplemented (S) and control (C) mothers in each centre were as follows: Northern Ireland S 37, C 122; South-East England S 70, C 70; Yorkshire S 38, C 35; Lancashire S 31, C 27; Cheshire S 9, C 10.

All mothers in supplemented and control groups were offered amniocentesis. Six mothers in Northern Ireland (three supplemented; three controls) declined amniocentesis and their pregnancies continue. They are not included in the figures above or in the accompanying table. All mothers with raised amniotic-fluid alpha-fetoprotein (AFP) values (one supplemented, eleven controls) accepted termination of pregnancy.

Study mothers were given a multivitamin and iron preparation ('Pregnative Forte F' Bencard), one tablet three times a day for not less than twenty-eight days before conception and continuing at least until the date of the second missed period, i.e. until well after the time of neural-tube closure.

## Results

One hundred and eighty-seven control mothers have delivered 192 infants (including five twin pairs) without NTDs, and a further thirty-eight have normal amniotic-fluid

**Table 33.1** Outcome of pregnancy in fully supplemented and control mothers

|  | Fully supplemented | Controls |
|---|---|---|
| Infant/fetus with NTD | 1 | 12 |
| Infant without NTD | 140(3) | 192(5) |
| Subtotal (1) | 141(3) | 204(5) |
| Normal amniotic AFP | 26 | 38 |
| Subtotal (2) | 167(3) | 242(5) |
| Spontaneous abortions | | |
| Examined, NTD | 0 | 1 |
| Examined, no NTD | 11 | 17 |
| Subtotal (3) | 178(3) | 260(5) |
| Not examined | 10 | 9 |
| Total | 188(3) | 269(5) |

All numbers relate to infants/fetuses.
Figures in parentheses indicate numbers of twin pairs included.

AFP values (see Table 33.1). Thirteen mothers have been delivered of NTD infants/fetuses. Seventeen fetuses of a further twenty-six control mothers who aborted spontaneously were examined and had no NTD. The provisional recurrence-rate of NTDs is 5.0 per cent (13 in 260), consistent with those previously reported and widely adopted in genetic counselling.

One hundred and thirty-seven fully supplemented mothers have given birth to 140 babies (including three twin pairs) without NTD, twenty-six have normal amniotic-fluid AFP values and their pregnancies continue, and one has had a further affected infant. Eleven fetuses of twenty-one mothers who aborted spontaneously were examined; none had an NTD. The provisional recurrence-rate in the supplemented group is therefore 0.6 per cent (1 in 178).

Comparison of NTD frequencies in the supplemented and control groups by Fisher's exact test showed significant differences (p < 0.01) for subtotals (1), (2), and (3) (Table 33.1).

## Discussion

Despite problems with choosing controls, the control women in this study have shown recurrence-rates for NTDs entirely consistent with published data. By contrast the supplemented mothers had a significantly lower recurrence-rate. Possible interpretations of this observation include the following:

(1) *A group of women with a naturally low recurrence risk has unwittingly selected itself for supplementation.* Apart from geographic and secular variations there is no evidence to suggest that any particular sub-group within populations, whether by social class or any other division, has a higher or lower recurrence risk. In genetic counselling clinics it is customary to quote the same risk for all mothers after one

affected child. We cannot exclude the possibility that women who volunteered and cooperated in the trial might have had a reduced risk of recurrence of NTD.

(2) *Supplemented mothers aborted more NTD fetuses than did controls.* The proportion of pregnancies ending in spontaneous abortion is similar in the two groups (supplemented 11.4 per cent, control 9.6 per cent). If the supplemented mothers have aborted more NTD fetuses, they must have aborted fewer other fetuses or had a lower initial risk of abortion. Eleven of twenty-one abortuses of supplemented mothers have been examined and none had an NTD. Eighteen of twenty-seven had an NTD. An explanation based on selective abortion of fetuses with NTD seems improbable.

(3) *Something other than vitamin supplementation has reduced the incidence of NTDs in the treated group.* This is an almost untestable hypothesis, but if anything has reduced the incidence of NTDs it needs to be identified urgently.

(4) *Vitamin supplementation has prevented some NTD.* This is the most straightforward interpretation and is consistent with the circumstantial evidence linking nutrition with NTDs. If the vitamin tablets are directly responsible, we cannot tell from this study whether they operate via a nutritional or a placebo effect.

We hope that the data presented will encourage others to initiate similar and related studies.

## References

1. Hibbard, E. D. and Smithells, R. W. 'Folic acid metabolism and human embryopathy', *Lancet*, i, 1254–56 (1965).
2. Smithells, R. W., Ankers, C., Carver, M. E., Lennon, D., Schorah, C. J. and Sheppard, S. 'Maternal nutrition in early pregnancy', *Br. J. Nutr.* 38, 497–506 (1977).
3. Smithells, R. W., Sheppard, S. and Schorah, C. J. 'Vitamin deficiencies and neural tube defects', *Arch. Dis. Childh.* 51, 944–50 (1976).

The three following letters appeared in *The Lancet* on 22 March 1980.

## Possible prevention of neural-tube defects by periconceptional vitamin supplementation

Sir, Professor Smithells and others believe they have observed a preventive effect of periconceptional vitamin supplementation on the recurrence of neural-tube defect (NTD). Their conclusions are based on the observation that the incidence of NTD in 185 fully supplemented women was significantly lower than that in 264 unsupplemented or control women.

Such an interpretation of the data rests upon the assumption that both the supplemented and the control women were, initially, at equal risk of conceiving a further affected fetus. A geographical analysis of the total sample shows that this was probably not so. In the accompanying Table (Table 33.2) the study subjects are characterised as falling into one of two groups – a 'relatively high risk' group, residing in Northern Ireland, Lancashire, and Cheshire; and a 'relatively low risk' group residing in south-east England and Yorkshire. (The varying geographical risk of NTD is well established.) It is clear that the supplemented sample is as heavily biased towards

**Table 33.2**   Geographical distribution of supplemented and control mothers

| | Relatively high risk areas No. (%) | Relatively low risk areas No. (%) | Total No. (%) |
|---|---|---|---|
| Supplemented mothers | 77 (41.6) | 108 (58.4) | 185 (100) |
| Control mothers | 159 (60.2) | 105 (39.8) | 264 (100) |

'relatively low risk' areas as the control sample is towards 'relatively high risk' areas. The higher incidence of recurrent NTD in the control group is therefore hardly surprising.

Why, I wonder, did Professor Smithells and his co-workers not evaluate their interesting hypothesis by means of a randomised controlled trial, which would have been eminently practicable, would have minimised selection bias, and would have been more likely to convince the sceptics?

David H. Stone
University of Glasgow, Social Paediatric and Obstetric Research Unit, Glasgow

Sir, with the wisdom of hindsight, we should have stated in our preliminary communication that our original intention had been a double-blind controlled study for which placebo tablets had already been prepared, but that the protocol was rejected by three separate hospital research ethics committees, and we had to resort to a less satisfactory design.

The number of fully supplemented (S) and 'control' mothers (C) was almost identical in all centres except Northern Ireland which had an excess of controls (Northern Ireland S 37, C 122; S-E England S 70, C 70; Yorkshire S 38, C 35; Lancashire S 31, C 27; Cheshire S 9, C 10). The recurrence rate of NTDs in the controls was in keeping with earlier reports. The excess of controls in Northern Ireland does not alter the fact that there was only one recurrence among the progeny of 185 fully supplemented mothers.

The geographical variation in the *incidence* of NTD is well recognised. What is relevant to our study is geographical variation in *recurrence* rate, about which little is known.

Dr Stone makes reference to what we 'believe', to our 'conclusions', and to 'an interpretation'. In our paper we subscribe to no belief, reach no conclusions, and offer four possible interpretations, of which the first covers the point Dr Stone raises.

We are not trying 'to convince the sceptics', among whom we count ourselves. We present some observations (which will be fully detailed in a later paper) and would welcome further studies to assist in their interpretation.

R. W. Smithells, S. Sheppard

Sir, Professor Smithells and his colleagues have opened the next chapter in the saga of neural-tube defects. Since a deficiency of some nutrient has been proposed as the source of nearly every ailment since antiquity, why not propose another? An unfortunate effect of this form of communication is that women will be induced to self-administer large quantities of vitamins, some of which may be teratogenic. I hope that future studies will incorporate properly selected controls treated with placebos and that nutritional assessment of the mother, before and during therapy, will be done.

Paul M. Fernhoff

Department of Pediatrics, Emory University School of Medicine, Atlanta, Georgia

The following extract is from an editorial which appeared in *The Lancet* on 17 May 1980.

## Vitamins, neural-tube defects and ethics committees

Some years ago Renwick[1] suggested that a specific teratogen present in blighted potatoes might be the causal agent. The plausibility of Renwick's hypothesis did draw attention to the possibility of maternal nutritional factors in the aetiology of neural-tube defects. An investigation reported in *The Lancet* in February suggests that subclinical maternal vitamin deficiency may be one of these factors.

At a time when the reduction in birth incidence of neural-tube defects rests largely on alpha-fetoprotein screening and selective abortion, this is an exciting finding. However, the study by Smithells *et al.* depends critically on the assumption that the vitamin-supplemented group and their controls were equally at risk of conceiving a further affected fetus. On this point there must be some doubt.

The vitamin-supplemented group were recruited on the basis of their ability to adhere to a fairly stringent regimen of tablet-taking while the controls were those who could not or would not adhere to the required protocol. Thus, selection was based on self-motivation and self-discipline, and one suspects that such women will have better-than-average outcome of pregnancy. A randomised control trial would have been more appropriate. But, as Professor Smithells[2] explains, such a study was proposed by the investigators and rejected by three separate hospital research ethics committees. As a result a far less satisfactory design was chosen.

How much does this matter? The results achieved by Smithells *et al.* are so striking that they provide a strong argument for the immediate vitamin supplementation of all mothers who are at risk of bearing a child with a neural-tube defect. If vitamins were completely harmless one could perhaps extend this argument to all mothers. But already there is evidence that at least one of the components of the multivitamin preparation, vitamin A, is a teratogen in rodents.[3,4] Doctors are thus faced with a dilemma; if they ignore the results of the Smithells study they may be allowing the conception of infants with neural-tube defects whose malformations might have been prevented. If they advise vitamin supplementation to all would-be mothers they may be contributing to the induction of a different range of congenital abnormalities whose appearance may not be recognised for some time.

The problem would probably be best resolved by a large randomised controlled trial on a general population of mothers, with vitamins being administered to one group and placebos to the other. But if this design has already been rejected by an ethics committee, it is even less likely to be acceptable now that the results of the Smithells trial are known. This raises the question of accountability. Research workers are quite properly called upon to explain and justify any investigation involving patients, both directly to an ethics committee and indirectly in the publication of their results. Ethics committees are less subject to scrutiny. They may explain their decision to individual workers, but many researchers find these arbitrary and lacking the coherence necessary to stand up to public examination. Perhaps the time has come to devise a system for making those ubiquitous committees more accountable.

## References

1. Renwick, J. H. 'Anencephaly and spina bifida are usually preventable by avoidance of a specific unidentified substance present in certain potato tubers', *Br. J. Prev. Soc. Med.*, 26, 67–88 (1972).
2. Smithells, R. W. and Sheppard, S. 'Possible prevention of neural tube defects by periconceptional vitamin supplementation', *Lancet*, i, 647 (1980).
3. Seller, M. J., Embury, S., Polani, P. F. and Adinolphi, M. 'Neural tube defects in curly-tail mice. II Effect of maternal administration of vitamin', *Proc. Roy. Soc. Lond. B.*, 206, 95–107 (1979).
4. Nakamura, H. 'Digital anomalies in the embryonic mouse limb cultured in the presence of excess vitamin A', *Teratology*, 14, 195–202 (1977).

The following letter appeared in *The Lancet* on 14 June 1980.

## Vitamins, neural-tube defects, and ethics committees

Sir, As a result of the study by Professor Smithells and his colleagues there is now a suggestion that periconceptional multivitamin supplementation may reduce the incidence of fetal neural tube defect (NTD). This possibility is of great interest in Ireland where the incidence of NTD is high.

Some of the shortcomings of the research design used by Smithells *et al.* have been discussed in your editorial and in your correspondence columns. The essential problem is the lack of comparability of the supplemented and non-supplemented mothers: we do not know whether the favourable outcome in the fully supplemented mothers is greater than might be expected for such a highly selected group.

You emphasise, as do your correspondents, need for a randomised controlled trial but suggest that such a design is even less likely to be acceptable to research ethics committees now in the light of the Smithells study. If this is so, then it is a matter for concern. Perhaps the most serious consequence of not testing this hypothesis with the most appropriate research design is the possibility that millions of mothers-to-be may take multivitamin preparations around the time of conception in the as yet unproven belief that to do so significantly reduces the risk of having a baby with NTD. Furthermore there is the important question of possible teratogenic effects. How certain are we that the ingestion by mothers of considerable qualities of this multivitamin, iron, and calcium preparation ('Pregnative Forte F') during the period of most rapid fetal organogenesis is safe? By rejecting randomised controlled trials, ethics committees are sanctioning what amounts to a situation of uncontrolled experimentation on mothers and their babies. In so doing can they be said to be carrying out their function of protecting the welfare of patients?

The weight of medical scientific opinion is that only a large randomised controlled trial will permit us to say with confidence whether periconceptional multivitamin supplementation reduces the incidence of NTD, and whether such regimes are free from teratogenic effects. Our professional duty would seem to be clear – to conduct such a trial as soon as possible.

Peadar N. Kirke
Medico-Social Research Board, Dublin, Ireland

The following (edited) article appeared in the *British Medical Journal* on 9 May 1981.

# Double-blind randomised controlled trial of folate treatment before conception to prevent recurrence of neural-tube defects

K. M. Laurence, DSC, FRCP(E), professor of paediatric research and clinical
  geneticist
Nansi James, MB, MRCP, fieldworker
Mary H. Miller, MB, DCH, fieldworker
*Department of Child Health, Welsh National School of Medicine, Cardiff*

G. B. Tennant, MSC, senior scientific officer
*Department of Haematology, Welsh National School of Medicine*

H. Campbell, FRCP, FRSS, professor
*Department of Medical Statistics, Welsh National School of Medicine*

## Abstract

A randomised controlled double-blind trial was undertaken in South Wales to prevent the recurrence of neural-tube defects in women who had had one child with a neural-tube defect. Sixty women were allocated before conception to take 4 mg of folic acid a day before and during early pregnancy and 44 complied with these instructions. Fifty-one women were allocated to placebo treatment. There were no recurrences among the compliant mothers but two among the non-compliers and four among the women in the placebo group. Thus there were no recurrences among those who received supplementation and six among those who did not; this difference is significant (p = 0.04).

It is concluded that folic acid supplementation might be a cheap, safe, and effective method of primary prevention of neural-tube defects but that this must be confirmed in a large, multicentre trial.

## Subjects and methods

Women resident in Glamorgan and Gwent who had had a pregnancy complicated by a fetal neural-tube defect (anencephaly, encephalocele, and spina bifida cystica)

Table 33.3 Outcome of pregnancy by treatment group

| Outcome of pregnancy | Folate groups | | Placebo group |
|---|---|---|---|
| | Compliers | Non-compliers | |
| Normal fetus | 44 | 14 | 47 |
| Fetus with neural-tube defect | 0 | 2 | 4 |
| All cases | 44 | 16 | 51 |

between 1954 and 1969 were traced. Those under 35 years of age at the time of study were visited in their homes by medically qualified fieldworkers.

During the home visit a questionnaire was completed giving details of the women's diet during the interpregnancy period and during her previous pregnancies. A simple diet sheet was used that provided a general pattern for meals and a check list showing the amount of food consumed during the average week and listing first-class proteins, dairy products, fresh vegetables and salads, cereals, and refined carbohydrates, paying special attention to those items rich in folic acid. Diets were judged as good, fair, or inadequate, those that were poor or fair but deranged by an excessive amount of fat and refined carbohydrates being judged as inadequate.[1] A sample of blood was taken from all women who were planning to have further children for estimation of serum and red-cell folic acid concentrations. Those willing to cooperate were asked to take twice a day a tablet containing either 2 mg of folic acid or placebo starting from the time contraceptive precautions were stopped. Women were allocated to receive treatment or placebo by random numbers and did not know the content of the tablets; we were also unaware of the treatment prescribed. Women were instructed to report to us within six weeks of a missed period and were revisited as soon as possible thereafter. Inquiries were made about the quality of the diet during the current pregnancy and about any anorexia or vomiting, drugs, or illness, and a further sample was taken for folate estimation and other investigations. The women were revisited at six months and again at the end of pregnancy, when details of the outcome of the pregnancy were available.

## Results

Altogether 905 women who had had a child with a neural-tube defect were seen by the fieldworkers, of whom 111 (12.3 per cent) agreed to take part in the prophylactic randomised controlled trial and achieved a subsequent pregnancy. Of these, 60 had been randomised to receive folate supplementation and 51 placebo.

Compliance in taking the folate tablets was monitored at the sixth to ninth week of estimated gestation; if the serum folate concentration at this stage was higher than 10 µg/l the woman's account of taking the tablets during the earlier part of the pregnancy could be accepted as valid. If the serum folate concentration was below 10 µg/l the woman was classified as a non-complier. None of the placebo group had a serum folate concentration above 12 µg/l. There were 16 non-compliers (27 per cent) among the 60 women allocated to receive folate treatment (Table 33.3). Compliance was not tested among the controls.

**Table 33.4** Numbers of women taking good, fair, or inadequate diets classified according to whether they received folate treatment and whether fetus was normal or had a neural-tube defect

| | Received folate | | Did not receive folate | | |
| | Normal | Neural-tube defect | Normal | Neural-tube defect | |
| Diet | Normal | defect | Normal | defect | All cases |
|---|---|---|---|---|---|
| Good | 17 | 0 | 26 | 0 | 43 |
| Fair | 17 | 0 | 24 | 0 | 41 |
| Inadequate | 10 | 0 | 11 | 6 | 27 |
| All cases | 44 | 0 | 61 | 6 | 111 |

**Table 33.5** Mean ±SD red-cell folate concentration (µg/l red blood cells) by treatment group and quality of diet

| | Folate groups | | Placebo group |
| Diet | Compliers | Non-compliers | |
|---|---|---|---|
| Good | 618 ± 60 (n = 17) | 277 ± 44 (n = 5) | 278 ± 25 (n = 21) |
| Fair | 847 ± 60 (n = 17) | 292 ± 23 (n = 6) | 298 ± 34 (n = 18) |
| Inadequate | 761 ± 85 (n = 10) | 193 ± 34 (n = 5) | 250 ± 26 (n = 12) |
| All cases | 738 ± 42 (n = 44) | 256 ± 22 (n = 16) | 278 ± 16 (n = 51) |

Six pregnancies resulted in a fetus with a neural-tube defect (Table 33.3): none in the compliers, two in the non-compliers, and four in the placebo group.

Table 33.4 shows the number of women taking a good, fair, or inadequate diet classified by outcome of pregnancy and whether they had received folate treatment. The proportion of women with inadequate diets was similar in the two treatment groups: 10 out of the 44 compliers and 17 out of the 67 non-compliers and women in the placebo group. All six of the recurrences of fetal neural-tube defects occurred in women taking an inadequate diet.

Table 33.5 shows the mean red-cell folate concentration in each treatment group by the adequacy of the diet. In each dietary group the compliers had a mean concentration at least twice that in the placebo group, and these differences were significantly different ($p < 0.001$).

## Discussion

None of the 44 women who received treatment had a recurrence, whereas there were six recurrences among 67 untreated cases. The probability of such a distribution, using Fisher's exact test with a single tail, was $p = 0.04$.

The specific effect of folate has to be separated from the non-specific effect of diet. There were no recurrences among the 84 women who received good or fair diets, but there were six recurrences among the 27 women receiving a poor diet (p < 0.0001, Fisher's exact test). As we have shown,[2] women who take poor diets are at an extremely high risk of a recurrence of fetal neural-tube defects. Within this high-risk group of women, however, there were no recurrences in the 10 who had taken folate supplementation but six recurrences in the 17 who had not taken supplementation (p = 0.04, Fisher's exact test). Thus although there may have been some bias owing to women who were receiving an inadequate diet also failing to comply, yet within this group receiving an inadequate diet the preventive effect could still be detected. We conclude that women receiving a poor diet who are at high risk of a recurrence of fetal neural-tube defects can reduce their risk either by improving their diet or by taking folate supplements.

The use of folate as an effective prophylactic regimen to prevent neural-tube defects in high-risk groups, communities with a high incidence of such defects, or even all women at risk of pregnancy should be further tested in a larger controlled trial conducted at several centres. Such a trial would be ethical as we found a probably biological beneficial effect, but the problem might be to consider an alternative regimen. A placebo could be justified by the argument that it is not normal practice to begin supplementation before conception is confirmed. As a result of the study by Smithells et al.[3] Pregnative Forte F without folate would seem to be a suitable alternative. With an expensive blunderbuss preparation of that type, which includes several agents in addition to folate, the specific beneficial agent and the hazards that might arise from the other constituents should be identified.

### References

1. Laurence, K. M., James, N., Miller, M. and Campbell, H. 'The increased risk of recurrence of neural tube defect to mothers on poor diets and the possible benefit of dietary counselling', Br. Med. J., 281, 1542–4 (1980).
2. Tennant, G. B. and Withey, J. L. 'An assessment of work simplified procedures for the microbiological array of serum vitamin B12 and serum folate', Medical Laboratory Technology, 29, 171–81 (1972).
3. Smithells, R. W., Sheppard, S., Schorah, C. J. et al. 'Possible prevention of neural tube defects by preconceptional vitamin supplementation', Lancet, i, 339–40 (1980).

The following (edited) letter appeared in the British Medical Journal on 30 May 1981.

## Trial of folate treatment to prevent recurrence of neural tube defects

Sir, We have been extremely interested to read the recent papers by Dr K. M. Laurence and others. We are puzzled by their use of the term 'double-blind' in their more recent paper, which can only have applied until six to nine weeks of gestation, when blood folate levels were estimated and 'non-compliers' were identified. The high rate of non-compliance must also have disappointed the authors. We entirely endorse their view that further studies are needed, directed towards the following ends:

1. To provide further confirmation that vitamin prophylaxis is effective.
2. To define further the role of folic acid and other vitamins.
3. To study carefully mothers who are enrolled for supplementation but who comply only in part.

There is considerable urgency. The medical correspondent of *The Times* has advocated (8 May) vitamin supplementation on the basis of our series and those of the Cardiff group. It can no longer be assumed that mothers not given vitamin supplements by research workers necessarily have none. There is also a danger of 'do-it-yourself' supplementation by mothers obtaining over-the-counter vitamin preparations, none of which contains folic acid.

R. W. Smithells, Sheila Sheppard, C. J. Schorah, N. C. Nevin, Mary J. Seller

---

The following (edited) article appeared in *The Guardian* on 10 December 1982.

## Specialists voice fear that some doctors and patients will boycott scheme to test vitamin theory

### Women to act as guinea-pigs in spina bifida trials, by Andrew Veitch

The controversial plan to find out whether vitamin supplements prevent mothers from having spina bifida babies is to go ahead, the Medical Research Council said yesterday. It involves denying the vitamins to hundreds of mothers known to be at risk.

Specialists said yesterday that it might be doomed from the start because not enough women or doctors would volunteer to take part.

The public controversy about the proposals – which reached a peak two weeks ago when the MRC secretary, Sir James Gowans, was accused of suppressing debate – and the mass of evidence of the merits of folic acid which had accumulated in the past two years, meant that few mothers would be prepared to volunteer for a trial in which they faced a one-in-two chance of not having folic acid and a one-in-four chance of receiving no vitamins at all.

Medical teams in Manchester, Leeds and Belfast have declined to take part in the trial. Teams in Liverpool and Chester are thought likely to follow suit. So the area with the highest incidence of spina bifida – the North-west – will not be represented.

Professor Norman Nevin, head of medical genetics at Queen's University Belfast, said that the MRC was not justified in giving some women a placebo. The trial was also condemned yesterday by the National Childbirth Trust. 'It is not ethical to withhold vitamins from some women', said the Trust's secretary, Ms. Hanna Corbishley.

---

The following (edited) article appeared in *The Guardian* on 13 December 1982.

## Wasted years, damaged lives

After two years of dithering the Medical Research Council has finally decided to go ahead with its plan to establish conclusively whether vitamin supplements prevent spina bifida in babies. In view of the large controversy these trials have generated, however, it is hard to see how they can now produce any evidence worth having. Medical teams in Manchester, Leeds and Belfast are refusing to take part, and it seems likely that Liverpool and Chester will follow suit. Moreover, it is hard to see how any woman would want to take part in these trials in the first place. Surely, any woman who has already had a spina bifida baby will reply that if there is even a slim chance that vitamins and folic acid will reduce the likelihood of another damaged child – and such supplements have no known toxic effects – then she would very much like to have them, please, and no, she wouldn't be prepared to run the slightest extra risk.

It is said that the Department of Health is reluctant to fund a national programme of vitamin and folic acid supplements until conclusive proof is provided. This means that, for the next five years, these supplements will not be available automatically to women at risk of producing a spina bifida baby – because of a trial whose conclusions are likely to be as dubious as its ethics.

The following (edited) letter appeared in *The Guardian* on 14 December 1982.

## Spina bifida: a new trial

Sir, I oppose the proposed trial both on ethical and practical grounds, and consider that it is unlikely to produce a more conclusive answer than is already available from the admittedly imperfect trials conducted by Professor Smithells and his colleagues.

Nevertheless, the results are so promising that to deprive women of a totally harmless vitamin cocktail seems unethical. I would find it difficult to persuade the mothers of any of my patients to have a placebo, when they could have something which is likely to be helpful.

It is true that we do not know which vitamins, or which combination of them, is likely to decrease the incidence of neural-tube defects, but I see no evidence that folic acid alone has shown itself to be of benefit. The data relating to this are based on very few pregnancies.

There is, however, an alternative and totally ethical way in which the question could be settled without difficulty. It is known that the incidence of neural-tube defects is 5 per cent after the birth of a baby with spina bifida or anencephaly. If, therefore, all women at risk are offered vitamin supplementation starting some three months before pregnancy is contemplated, within a very short time it will be apparent whether vitamin supplementation is helpful or not. It does not really matter which of the vitamins or their combination is helpful.

John Lorber
(Emeritus Professor of Paediatrics), Sheffield

The following abstract (i.e. summary) is taken from a detailed report of a major clinical trial, which was published in full in *The Lancet* in July 1991.

## Prevention of neural tube defects: results of the Medical Research Council vitamin study

MRC Vitamin Study Research Group

### Abstract

A randomised double-blind prevention trial with a factorial design was conducted at 33 centres in seven countries to determine whether supplementation with folic acid (one of the vitamins in the B group) or a mixture of seven other vitamins (A, D, $B_1$, $B_2$, $B_6$, C, and nicotinamide) around the time of conception can prevent neural tube defects (anencephaly, spina bifida, encephalocele). [In anencephaly, the brain does not develop. In spina bifida, the spinal cord is not fully enclosed in the bones of the spine. In encephalocele, the skull bones enclosing the brain do not join together properly.] A total of 1 817 women at high risk of having a pregnancy with a neural tube defect, because of a previous affected pregnancy, were allocated at random to one of four groups – namely, folic acid, other vitamins, both, or neither. 1 195 had a completed pregnancy in which the fetus or infant was known to have or not have a neural tube defect; 27 of these had a known neural tube defect, 6 in the folic acid groups and 21 in the two other groups, a 72 per cent protective effect (relative risk 0.28, 95 per cent confidence interval [CI] 0.12–0.71). The other vitamins showed no significant protective effect (relative risk 0.80, 95 per cent CI 0.32–1.72). There was no demonstrable harm from the folic acid supplementation, though the ability of the study to detect rare or slight adverse effects was limited. Folic acid supplementation starting before pregnancy can now be firmly recommended for all women who have had an affected pregnancy, and public health measures should be taken to ensure that the diet of all women who may bear children contains an adequate amount of folic acid.

The full article appeared in *The Lancet* on 20 July 1991, **338**, pages 131–7; it reports the work of a large number of investigators in several countries. The overall study co-ordinator, and the main author of the article is the epidemiologist Nicholas Wald, Professor of Environmental and Preventive Medicine at St Bartholomew's Hospital Medical College.

---

The following editorial appeared in *The Lancet* on 20 July 1991, and refers to the MRC Vitamin Study (1991), the abstract of which precedes this editorial.

### Folic acid and neural tube defects

Fifty years ago Gregg's classic observations linked congenital cataract to infection of the mother with rubella during pregnancy.[1] These findings were a huge advance in the difficult and unrewarding task of understanding and preventing birth defects. It could not be a more appropriate anniversary for the publication of the exciting paper in this issue [i.e. the paper whose abstract is reprinted above] which reports the prevention of neural tube defects by folate supplementation in a randomised clinical trial. The arguments over the role of micronutrients in this group of disorders have been to a very large extent resolved, at last.

A prevention trial of periconceptional supplementation with a vitamin and mineral preparation was planned in the 1970s by Smithells, but permission to carry it out was refused by an ethics committee who insisted that the design be altered to a study in which all women at increased risk of having an infant with a neural tube defect were offered the supplement.[2] In the interpretation of the modified study it was impossible to disentangle the apparent benefit of supplementation from possible differences in the risk of having a subsequent affected pregnancy between women who did take the supplement and those who did not.

The intervention of the ethics committee had other adverse effects. Given the findings in that study of a large difference in the recurrence rate of neural tube defects between the supplemented and unsupplemented groups the ethical difficulties of mounting a randomised trial became much greater. Yet the uncertainty about the efficacy of supplementation, and about which was the active component of the preparation, could not be resolved by repetition of the study with the same non-randomised design: the issue was not whether the results could be due to chance but whether they could be due to differences between the groups.

Those who argued for a trial pointed to other instances of apparent benefits in non-randomised studies that could not be detected when the same treatment was formally evaluated with random allocation: there are many examples in the perinatal domain.[3] Opponents believed that a randomised trial was redundant since the effect associated with taking supplements was so large that it was highly unlikely to be attributable to any known or unknown confounders. The arguments of those most closely involved and their comments on one another's views were made available at the time in a fascinating publication.[4] When the current trial was planned the debate became public and acrimonious. The trial was condemned by some as unethical: researchers with an interest in maternal and child health were asked to join the critics in trying to have the trial stopped.

Two factors seem to have been important in this reaction. One was the nature of the preventive agent: a multivitamin preparation was regarded as synonymous with good health. Even if it did not have the hoped for effect, it was perceived as being completely harmless. The term 'experimental drug' was not seen to apply here. Where an intervention is believed to be totally without risk, arguments about the need for certainty before it is widely prescribed are dismissed as academic. The second factor was the original ethics committee decision. If a randomised trial had been regarded as unethical even before the treatment had been tried how much more so was it afterwards? In the long term these factors probably slowed recruitment to such an extent that it took 8 years to accumulate enough participating women and enough pregnancies, despite the involvement of 33 centres. How many affected infants have been born during those years whose abnormalities would have been prevented if the trial had been completed sooner?

Several features of the current trial deserve special mention. The process for informing women about the trial, whereby they had time to consider whether they wished to take part, was careful and sensitive. The factorial design ensured that three-quarters of those taking part received folate or multivitamins or both. Assessments of compliance by counting the number of capsules at the regular prepregnancy and early pregnancy visits suggested that this particular intervention is highly acceptable to women at special risk of having a child with a neural tube defect; only 7 per cent of women stopped taking the capsules before they became pregnant and fewer than 1 per cent of the remaining women took less than half of their assigned capsules. Some commentators had predicted that participants would supplement themselves with folate or multivitamins in addition to the capsules given to them in the trial, but measurements of serum folic acid levels showed that this did not happen. The factorial design and the sequential analysis helped to limit the size of the trial, enabling the data monitoring committee to recommend that the trial be stopped after 1 195 pregnancies instead of the planned 2 000.

Supplementation with 4 mg a day of folic acid did not prevent all neural tube defects and the six unsuccessful cases were not accounted for by unusually low serum folic acid concentrations. This is a reminder of the possibility that the group of disorders may be heterogeneous in aetiology. The overall result was unequivocal. All analyses, whether based on the original allocation of the women (intention-to-treat), or restricted to women who were not already pregnant at the time of randomisation, or repeated after exclusion of women who stopped taking the capsules, showed the reduction in neural tube defects to be substantial with relative risks of the order of 0.28 to 0.17. Even the adjustments to the relative risk necessitated by the early stopping of the trial give a relative risk estimate of 0.33 – a two-thirds reduction – with a 95 per cent confidence interval of 0.06 to 0.80. The reduction was not as large as that found in the non-randomised studies.[5]

Thus the policy implications are clear. Women who have had an affected fetus should be offered folic acid supplements if they intend having another pregnancy and supplementation should begin before conception. Counselling services associated with prenatal diagnosis or the birth of infants with malformations will provide an appropriate place and setting for advice and prescription.

The unanswered questions will be less easy to resolve. Is 4 mg a day of folic acid the necessary dose or is the 0.36 mg a day contained in the original multivitamin preparation enough? How long before conception is supplementation needed? Perhaps the population-wide trial of primary prevention of neural tube defects currently under way in China can be modified to take up these two questions. Are there any risks in folic acid supplementation and if so are they the same at the two folic acid dosages? The present trial could not detect a harmful effect of the supplements but its capacity to do so was limited by the size of the groups. The collaborative birth defects monitoring programmes in Europe and worldwide may be able to devise a strategy for taking up the issue. Will the beneficial effect of folic acid be the same in populations with a much lower prevalence at birth of neural tube defects? It has been argued in the past that the determinants in such populations are likely to be different. Will the effect in women who are not at increased risk of having an affected child be the same as in the present trial? The authors argue that benefits can be expected but their magnitude cannot be predicted precisely. Compliance would probably be very different among women with no personal experience of the abnormality. Moreover, the practical difficulties of providing folic acid supplements to all women before pregnancy, and particularly to women before their first pregnancy, are formidable.

Can the requisite folic acid be eaten in food instead of given as a supplement? Green leafy vegetables are a good source, although the vitamin will dissolve in water with prolonged boiling; even then, raw green cabbage contains only 90 µg of total folic acid per 100 g. Can culturally appropriate dietary guidelines be prepared as a matter of urgency for all ethnic groups? Providing specific dietary advice about the prevention of malformations to women before pregnancy will be at least as challenging as providing supplementation.

The MRC Vitamin Study was built on almost 20 years of work on the possible role of folic acid and other micronutrients in human malformations[6] and on the increasing willingness of the perinatal community to collaborate in randomised trials to answer important questions of policy and clinical practice. It should lead to major benefits for infants, mothers, and the whole community.

## References

1. Gregg, N. M. 'Congenital cataract following German measles in the mother', *Trans. Ophthalmol. Soc. Aust.*, **3**, 35 (1941).
2. Smithells, R. W., Sheppard, S., Schorah, C. J., *et al.* 'Possible prevention of neural-tube defects by periconceptional vitamin supplementation', *Lancet*, **i**, 330–40 (1980).
3. Silverman, W. A., *Retrolental Fibroplasia: A Modern Parable*, Grune & Stratton, New York, p. 85 (1980).
4. Dobbing, J. (ed.) *Prevention of Spina Bifida and Other Neural Tube Defects*, Academic Press, London (1983).
5. Smithells, R. W., Seller, M. J., Harris, R., *et al.* 'Further experience of vitamin supplementation for prevention of neural tube defect recurrences', *Lancet*, **i**, 648–69 (1983).
6. Hibbard, E. D. and Smithells, R. W. 'Folic acid metabolism and human embryopathy', *Lancet*, **i**, 1254 (1965).

This editorial is reproduced in its entirety from *The Lancet*, 20 July 1991, **338** pages 153–4.

# 34
# Assessment of screening for cancer

## CARLO LA VECCHIA, FABIO LEVI, SILVIA FRANCESCHI AND PETER BOYLE

Screening has an important role in the control of cancer in developed countries. Estimates of the avoidable percentage of cancer deaths, for instance, indicate that a more rational use of screening for cancer of the cervix, uterus, and breast could lead to a 1 per cent reduction of all cancer deaths in the United States; this fraction is comparable to that achievable in principle, through a more rational use of available therapeutic advancements.[8] The speculative potential for reduction in mortality following screening by the year 2000 has been indicated as 60 per cent for cervical, 25 per cent for breast, 20 per cent for colorectal, and 5 per cent for oral and bladder cancers.[5] Any such estimate, however, is extremely imprecise and even more restricted and specific evaluation of any defined screening programme is hampered by several difficulties, among which the absence or paucity of randomized controlled studies is of particular relevance. Only the use of mammography for breast cancer screening has, in fact, been subjected to a number of randomized studies,[1,9,10] although the diffusion of the practice outside controlled interventions occurred before the publication of such studies. Thus, evaluation of mammographic screening for breast cancer was based at least in part on retrospective case control studies too.[2,7] The absence of controlled randomized studies does not *per se* invalidate qualitative as well as quantitative inferences in situations, such as cervical cancer, where the benefit from screening is substantial; but its absence is clearly of greater concern in relation to the issue of mass screening for other common neoplasms, such as the use of the haemoccult test to detect colorectal cancer, for which the benefit of various techniques is likely to be more limited.*

---

* 'Neoplasm' is a clinical term for a cancer (it means 'new growth'). The haemoccult test detects blood in faeces, a possible sign of cancer in the colon (large bowel) or rectum.

## Basic criteria for definition and evaluation of screening policies

The basic issue for the adoption of a screening programme is that diagnosis in the asymptomatic phase increases the duration and/or quality of life as compared with the best standards of clinical diagnosis. The likely benefit of a screening test must not only be clearly demonstrated but also set against its disadvantages. For instance, the improved prognosis of some cases of cancer detected by screening must be set against the longer morbidity for cases whose prognosis is unaltered; the less radical treatment to cure some early cases against the overtreatment of borderline, potentially nonevolving abnormalities; the reassurance for those with negative test results against the false reassurance for those with false negative results and the potential burden – in terms of budget, personnel, and other factors – on health services produced by false positive results.[4] In practical terms, it is essential to verify the existence of a certain number of prerequisites for a screening programme and to outline in advance the strategy for monitoring the effects.

### Screening prerequisites

It must be proven that the screening test is *effective* – that it reduces the incidence (whenever applicable) and certainly the mortality from the disease.

The effectiveness should be further evaluated in practical terms of applicability rather than simply on theoretical terms based on optimal conditions (*efficacy*). The assessment of effectiveness should be based on internationally accepted and consistent references, related to different studies and populations, or to consensus statements.

Furthermore, the cancer must be relevant from a public health viewpoint; the malignant condition should be common and the cause of substantial mortality and/or morbidity. Such evaluation can obviously lead to different conclusions across different countries and time periods. Some cancers (such as skin cancer, oesophageal cancer, and colon cancer) show order of magnitude variations in incidence in different areas of the world,[6] and thus represent very different public health priorities.

The target population of a screening programme must be well defined and selected in such a way that, given the likely sensitivity and specificity of the test, an acceptable predictive value will be achieved. Such a prerequisite has various implications, the first of which, more related to the biology of the cancer on screening, affects the selection of the truly high-risk population. Although for many malignant diseases, various characteristics and circumstances are known to enhance the risk of cancer significantly, generally the only ones suitable to be incorporated in differential screening recommendations are very simple variables such as sex and age and, subsequent to development of screening, a past history of screening itself. Features such as social class, occupational history, reproductive history, sexual habits, etc., although often epidemiologically relevant, do not generally allow a sufficiently simple definition of subgroups where the majority of cases actually occur. In addition, such characteristics depend heavily on individual self-perception and uselessly complicate the active call–recall system that is increasingly recognized as the crucial issue in the success of a screening programme. Furthermore, with certain obvious exceptions, the majority of cancers, in absolute terms, generally do not arise in high-risk groups as we currently understand cancer risk factors.

Because the purpose of this article is to show the extent to which screening programmes are complex activities, the issue of test validity will not be discussed in detail. It is, however, worth remembering that the sensitivity and the specificity of a test must be traded off against one another and that in many instances this trade-off should be resolved in favour of specificity because the monetary implications of anything but a very high specificity screening are generally unacceptable. In other words, the specificity of the test governs its predictive value because it operates on the vast majority of subjects, whereas the sensitivity operates on fewer, diseased people. In addition to being sensitive and specific, a suitable screening test should also be very reliable, that is, capable of giving the same result on repeat examinations of subjects, low in cost, convenient, painless, and safe.

A final prerequisite of a screening programme is a good agreement and availability on all the various steps subsequent to a test result: optimum frequency of recall plans for further evaluations following a positive test, classification and management of borderline and frankly malignant abnormalities, etc. Obviously, treatment protocols for screening detected cancers should be as conservative as possible.

Uncertainties about these areas will certainly be substantial, at least at the beginning of the screening programme. Making such uncertainties explicit and tackling them with appropriately designed investigations is an essential task of the screening programme.

### Criteria for the health service and society

The test must be *acceptable* to individuals and society. Further, it must be *affordable* in terms of costs, benefits, and allocation of resources for the health services and society as a whole. Apart, therefore, from general issues, the optimization of a screening programme depends heavily upon the characteristics of the area where it is carried out.

Whenever a screening procedure is recognized as effective, valid, and acceptable, it is important that the optimal criteria for its application in terms of costs and benefits are defined. The general issue is that all the target population should be screened at least once and thus that a specific effort is made to identify subjects who have never been screened. With this basic assumption in mind, a cost–benefit analysis within the broader framework of resource allocation should be taken into account before deciding on the optimal scheme of a screening policy.

An example of a cost–benefit analysis for screening for cervical cancer is given in Table 34.1.[3] Assuming that the theoretical optimal potential of cervical screening at yearly intervals for all Swiss women aged 35–64 is to avoid 150 deaths per year, there are only 4 additional deaths per year when a 3-year interval is chosen, but the number of tests (and, hence, the cost of the programme) is decreased by a factor of three. Obviously, the cost–benefit of screening in terms of allocation of available resources should be related to any specific population. For instance, the optimal scheme for a developed country may well be inapplicable to a developing one, where a longer interval may represent a more rational utilization of scanty available resources.[3]

## Methods for evaluating cancer screening

Some form of ongoing evaluation of established screening programmes is highly desirable to ensure that the programme is meeting its objectives and to assess the need for changes. Randomized controlled trials (RCTs) are, as in other medical fields, the

**Table 34.1** Application of estimated reduction in cumulative cervical cancer rates to Swiss mortality data, for women aged 35–64

| Interval between screenings | Reduction in cumulative rates % | Estimated reduction in total number of deaths per year | Number of tests |
|---|---|---|---|
| 1 | 93.5 | 150 | 30 |
| 2 | 92.5 | 148 | 15 |
| 3 | 90.8 | 146 | 10 |
| 5 | 83.6 | 134 | 6 |
| 10 | 64.1 | 103 | 3 |

Derived from the IARC Working Group Report.[3]

method of first choice, but other approaches can also be employed where practical or ethical constraints prevent a proper RCT from being carried out.[4]

*Non-randomized methods*

First, the yield of cancers from screening can be assessed. In itself, this tells nothing about the screening benefits but, assuming that the people screened have not previously been tested, gives an idea of the basic prevalence of cancer.

Subsequently, various comparisons of distribution of stages and survival rates of screening-detected versus non-screening-detected cancers can be made. Such comparisons, however, are affected by at least three different types of bias. 'Length-time bias' occurs because screening is likely to pick up a disproportionate number of slowly growing cancers with a good prognosis. 'Selection bias' depends upon the tendency of those who volunteer or accept invitations for screening to be younger and better educated. Such bias can be countered if the comparison is between the stage and survival distribution of all the cases of cancer occurring in a defined period in a group of people who have been offered screening, regardless of whether they accepted, and the corresponding distribution in a comparable group who have not been offered screening. 'Lead-time bias' applies to the comparison of survival rates and derives from the deliberate but unknown alteration of time from diagnosis to death obtained by advancing the date of diagnosis.

The foregoing is primarily clinical in its orientation. On a public health scale, the correlation of screening intensity with mortality or incidence rates has often been examined and has offered useful information if good routine health statistics are available, as in Nordic countries. In most countries, however, such an approach is hampered by inadequate knowledge of secular trends in the absence of interventions, interplay of possible confounding factors, and unsatisfactory recording of screening data, such as absence of reliable statistics based on people and not simply test-based data on screening.

Finally, when a screening test has already become widespread in a population, case control studies that contrast the histories of screening of people who have died of the illness at issue with those of a sample of controls drawn from the living population represent an interesting (and often the only practicable) alternative to RCTs.[4] Case control studies, at least if control of confounding is achieved, can provide results in a shorter time and with lower cost than can RCTs. Furthermore, they may yield information on the potential efficacy of a broad range of different screening frequencies and techniques, that is, all those actually experienced by the population, whereas in randomized trials, only one or a few screening schedules are usually tested.

*Randomized controlled trials (RCTs)*

In relation to screening, RCTs are more complex and costly than trials of therapy, involving follow-up of many thousands of healthy individuals for many years. Difficulties in the design, implementation, and analysis of such studies cannot be comprehensively listed here, but a few can be singled out as areas requiring emphasis:[4]

(a) the system for data management should be in place at the start, should be as simple as possible, and should be designed for long-term operation, with a gradual shift in task from screening to follow-up;

(b) the determination of sample size must account for compliance, contamination, and losses to follow-up;

(c) although the comparison of cause-specific death rates between the screening group and the control group is the primary aim of screening RCTs, the search for valid short-term outcomes must be also encouraged.

However lengthy and expensive they are, the potentials of screening RCTs to elucidate such aspects of the natural history of cancer as detectable preclinical phase, progression rates at various phases, etc., cannot be overemphasized.[4]

## Conclusions and prospects

In cancer screening, as in cancer treatment, it is unlikely that major technical breakthroughs will be available in the near future. In the past, new technology led to major advances in the screening for cervical cancer or in the treatment of leukemias or other lymphatic neoplasms, and demonstration of efficacy did not require controlled trials. Similar uncontrolled evaluation adopted for other neoplasms and measures, however, was not only unproductive, but caused substantial loss of time, information, and credibility.

The recognition of the limits of previous strategies should by itself lead to a less emotional, but more rational and carefully quantitative, approach to cancer screening that, in any case, is likely to remain a central (and increasingly important) instrument for controlling cancer in the near future. Substantial future progress depends on a number of factors, including possibly:

- increased ability of x-ray or other noninvasive procedures to detect smaller lesions and, wherever possible, reduction of the costs associated with such high-tech approaches as nuclear magnetic resonance [NMR];
- increased knowledge of the natural history of nonmalignant clinical conditions that may precede invasive disease;
- clearer identification of high-risk groups by use of biologic markers;
- development of more efficacious therapies for those neoplasms detected by screening, including a search for alternatives to severely mutilating treatment when early lesions are detected in a preclinical stage. In the last instance, if mammography were developed to detect very small, very early breast cancer, and if radical mastectomy

remained the only efficacious therapy, then this continued dependence on radical surgery would greatly hinder the uptake of the test among the general population.

Finally, in terms of assessing cancer screening, the ultimate evaluation of the costs and benefits of current and future strategies and programmes will increasingly rely on very large, carefully planned, controlled studies.

# References

1. Chu, K. C., Smart, C. and Tarone, R. E. (1988) 'Analysis of breast cancer mortality and stage distribution by age for the Health Insurance Plan Clinical Trial', *Journal of the National Cancer Institute*, 80, pp. 1125–32.
2. Collette, H. J. A., Day, N. E., Rombach, J. J. and de Waard, F. (1984) 'Evaluation of screening for breast cancer in a non-randomized study (the DOM project) by means of a case-control study', *The Lancet*, i, pp. 1224–6.
3. IARC Working Group on Evaluation of Cervical Cancer Screening Programmes (1986) 'Screening for squamous cervical cancer: Duration of low risk after negative results of cervical ontology and its implication for screening policies', *British Medical Journal*, 293, pp. 659–6.
4. Miller, A. B. (ed.) (1984) *Screening for Cancer*, UICC Technical Report, 78, UICC, Geneva.
5. Miller, A. B. (1986) 'Screening for cancer: Issues and future directions', *Journal of Chronic Disease*, 39, pp. 1067–77.
6. Muir, C., Waterhouse, J., Mack, T., *et al.* (eds) (1987) *Cancer incidence in five continents, volume 5*, IARC Scientific Publication 88, IARC, Lyon.
7. Palli, G., Rosselli Del Turco, M. *et al.* (1986) 'A case-control study of the efficacy of a non-randomized breast cancer screening program in Florence (Italy)', *International Journal of Cancer*, 38, pp. 501–4.
8. Peto, R. (1981) 'Why cancer? The causes of cancer in developed countries', *Times Health Supplement*, November 6.
9. Shapiro, S., Venet, W., Strax, P. *et al.* (1982) 'Ten-to-fourteen-years of screening on breast mortality', *Journal of the National Cancer Institute*, 69, pp. 349–55.
10. Tabar, L., Faberberg, G., Day, N. E. and Holmberg, L. (1987) 'What is the optimum interval between mammographic screening examinations? – An analysis based on the latest results of the Swedish two-country breast cancer screening trial', *British Journal of Cancer*, 55, pp. 547–51.

Carlo La Vecchia and Fabio Levi are at the Institut Universitaire de Médecine Sociale et Préventive and Istituto di Ricerche Farmacologiche 'Mario Negri'; Silvia Franceschi is at the Centro di Riferimento Oncologico, and Peter Boyle is at the International Agency for Research on Cancer. This article is an edited version of a longer text, which originally included details of the status of various screening tests in 1991. It was originally published in 1991 in the *International Journal of Technology Assessment in Health Care*, 7 (3), (1991) pp. 275–85.

# 35
# The global eradication of smallpox

## MARC A. STRASSBURG

On 8 May 1980, the 33rd World Health Authority Assembly declared the world free of smallpox. This followed approximately 2½ years after the last documented naturally occurring case of smallpox was diagnosed in a hospital worker in Merca, Somalia. A major breakthrough for the eventual control of this disease was the discovery of an effective vaccine by Edward Jenner in 1796. In 1966 the World Health Assembly voted a special budget to eliminate smallpox from the world. At that time, smallpox was endemic in more than 30 countries. Mass vaccination programs were successful in many Western countries; however, a different approach was taken in developing countries. This approach was known as surveillance and containment. Surveillance was aided by extensive house-to-house searches and rewards offered for persons reporting smallpox cases. Containment measures included ring vaccination and isolation of cases and contacts. Hospitals played a major role in transmission in a number of smallpox outbreaks. The World Health Organization (WHO) is currently supporting several control programs and has not singled out another disease for eradication. The lessons learned from the smallpox campaign can be readily applied to other public health programs.

The last documented case of naturally occurring smallpox in the world was diagnosed on 31 October 1977 in a 23-year-old male hospital cook living in Merca, Somalia. This was five days after rash had appeared and after exposure of friends, neighbors and other hospital staff members.[1]

To certify a country as smallpox-free, two years had to have elapsed without a case of smallpox being detected by an active and sensitive surveillance system. Almost two years to the day (26 October 1979) after this last case in Somalia, the (WHO) Global Commission for the Certification of Smallpox Eradication confirmed that smallpox also had been eradicated in Ethiopia, Somalia, and Kenya. Eradication efforts had been successful in this last endemic area, despite the ongoing war between Ethiopia and Somalia in the rugged and inaccessible Ogaden desert.

## History

The origin of smallpox probably predates written history. Epidemics of smallpox-like illnesses have been described in ancient Chinese and Sanskrit texts. Historical accounts beginning in the sixth century describe pandemics both in Europe and Asia. In the Americas, the disease was probably introduced during the 1500s by slave ships from Africa. Reported fatality rates for smallpox have varied between less than 1 per cent and 50 per cent. Differences in fatality rates were probably related to both the virulence of a particular strain (variola major and variola minor as well as intermediate strains have been described) and the nutritional status of the affected population.

Prior to the eighteenth century, few effective measures for the control of smallpox were known. Although quarantine proved useful for a number of diseases, the procedure had limited success in smallpox control, since the disease was communicable during the prodromal period before the onset of rash. Prior to Jenner's discovery of vaccination, a procedure known as variolation was used to confer immunity. Variolation was accomplished by obtaining material from the pustules of a smallpox patient and scratching the material onto the skin of a susceptible person. Many persons so variolated had symptoms of reduced severity, although they were capable of transmitting fully virulent cases of smallpox to others. Of special concern was that many of the variolated persons did not require bed rest, and thus they promoted a rapid spread of the disease. This practice, which originally had been described by the Chinese in 1000 BC, was still found in a number of countries in the twentieth century.[2]

## The vaccine

A major breakthrough in providing an effective measure for the control of smallpox occurred in 1796 when Edward Jenner[3] observed that persons who contracted cowpox, a relatively mild disease, developed immunity to smallpox. Jenner prepared a vaccine consisting of material from cowpox lesions. He fully understood the implication of the discovery of his new vaccine when he predicted that 'the annihilation of smallpox must be the final result of this practice.'

Despite the discovery of such an effective vaccine, it took nearly 200 years to bring about the eradication of smallpox. Several explanations for this delay may be offered. First, it was not until the 1950s that a heat-stable, freeze-dried vaccine was available. This important advance prolonged the viability of the vaccine in parts of the world where strict maintenance of the cold chain was difficult. Second, it was not until the 1960s that the bifurcated needle was developed. The bifurcated needle (used in the multiple-puncture vaccination technique) was easier to use, required less vaccine, and resulted in higher 'take' rates than other methods. Third, even with an improved vaccine and vaccination technique, not all countries were capable of carrying out a successful mass vaccination campaign. Although mass vaccination campaigns had been effective in eliminating smallpox in many Western countries, the limited resources and the organizational problems common to many health service systems in the developing world made complete vaccination coverage nearly impossible.

## The World Health Organization's program for eradication

In 1966 the World Health Assembly, which is the controlling body for WHO, voted a special budget ($2.5 million) to begin the global program aimed at eliminating smallpox from the world. Although it would seem that all involved in such a program would be highly motivated, many participants, both at national and local levels, were skeptical that smallpox or any other disease could be eradicated. One possible explanation for this lack of enthusiasm was that the WHO eradication program for another disease – malaria – was not succeeding.

In 1967, when the smallpox campaign began, more than 30 countries were considered endemic, with importations being reported in another 12 countries. At that time four major reservoirs existed: Brazil; Africa south of the Sahara; Asia, including Bangladesh, Nepal, India and Pakistan; and the Indonesian Archipelago. Although only 130,000 cases were reported in 1967, it was estimated that there were closer to 10 million cases.[2]

Of paramount importance to the success of the smallpox eradication program was administrative and logistical support. Under the able leadership of Donald A. Henderson of WHO, precise objectives and goals for each country were established. WHO trained both international and national epidemiologists and was responsible for securing additional supporting funds for the eradication program.

## New approach to eradication

A new strategy for smallpox eradication, one which did not rely on mass vaccination, was eventually adopted. This new strategy was called surveillance and containment and was developed by smallpox workers in West Africa. The development of this strategy was greatly influenced by a thorough knowledge of the following important elements in the natural history of smallpox.

1. The spread of smallpox was relatively slow, and a case usually infected only from two to five other persons.
2. Smallpox tended to cluster within villages or in a single area.
3. Man was the only reservoir of infection, and no carrier state was known.
4. Immunity was of long duration after either infection or vaccination.

Surveillance consisted of case-finding through systematic searches, improved reporting systems, and active source tracing. Many countries offered cash rewards to persons providing information leading to the discovery of a smallpox case. Containment efforts included isolation of patients and vaccination of all known or suspected contacts. The principal objective of this approach was to seal off outbreaks within specific geographical areas, thereby reducing transmission into unaffected areas. Although large-scale vaccination programs were still conducted, mass vaccination was no longer solely relied upon for control of the disease.

## The hospital's role in transmission

Important to the success of this new strategy was the development of effective isolation and quarantine measures. Historically, special huts, 'pest-houses', or isolation hospitals were principally used to remove affected persons from the community. It is probable that many of these early hospitals played major roles in smallpox transmission. This was well documented during the 1950s and 1960s when numerous hospitals were implicated as the principal source of spread in outbreaks. After analyzing 30 epidemics of smallpox in Western countries between 1946 and 1964, Thomas Mack of the Centers for Disease Control reported that, of 516 cases of smallpox, 280 had been hospital-acquired. The last major outbreak of smallpox in the United States, which occurred in January 1947, began after an immigrant with smallpox (from Mexico) was hospitalized at Willard Parker, the communicable diseases hospital in Manhattan. The first secondary cases included another patient and a hospital staff member. A total of 12 secondary cases resulted, and within 1 month over 6 million persons were vaccinated in New York City.[4] Common to many hospital-centered outbreaks was (1) misdiagnosis or late diagnosis of the smallpox case, (2) inadequate isolation of the patient, (3) spread among unvaccinated hospital staff, and (4) spread to the surrounding community.

In the Federal Republic of Germany (Meschede 1970 and in Monschau 1961) two unusual nosocomial smallpox outbreaks resulted from a hospitalized smallpox patient when transmission occurred without face-to-face contact. The study of these two hospital-centered outbreaks revealed that virus particles were disseminated by air over considerable distance within a facility. This unusual airborne transmission most likely occurred because (1) the source cases had extensive rash and cough; (2) the humidity in the hospitals was relatively low at the time; and (3) air currents were present that caused rapid spread of the virus.[5]

With the new emphasis on surveillance and containment, the necessity for effective isolation was even more critical to success. During 1975, I worked as a consultant in the Bangladesh Eradication Program in the crowded capital of Dacca City. At the Infectious Diseases Hospital there, it was necessary to post vaccinator guards around the clock to vaccinate routinely all persons going into the facility who did not have proof of a recent vaccination. In many countries the practice of hospitalizing smallpox patients was openly discouraged, and the patients remained at home accompanied by a vaccinator until the patient fully recovered.

Between 1967 and 1977 the eradication campaign moved steadily forward, with smallpox successively eliminated in Western and Central Africa, Brazil, Indonesia, Southern Africa, and finally in East Africa.

### Still cause for concern?

Although four years have passed without a reported case of naturally occurring smallpox, there are some who believe that smallpox may emerge from some hidden focus of infection, an unknown animal reservoir, or from some old smallpox crusts that are lying dormant somewhere in the world. This concern has been heightened by the recent discovery of a disease called monkeypox, which was first identified in a captive cynomolgus monkey in 1958 in Denmark. Monkeypox can be transmitted to man, although this is thought to be infrequent. Humans who have monkeypox present a picture clinically similar to humans with smallpox. Fifty cases have been reported for West and Central Africa between 1970 and 1980; however, in only five instances has secondary transmission possibly occurred. Both the low frequency of disease and the low transmission rate appear to indicate that monkeypox is not a public health problem of any significance. The source of human monkeypox is unknown but it is thought to be a zoonotic disease of rodents.

There may be some who believe that smallpox eradication will not be complete until those strains maintained in laboratory freezers are destroyed. Concern over the maintenance of such a virus was heightened by events in Birmingham, England. There, in August 1978, a photographer who worked above a laboratory housing the smallpox virus contracted the disease. Only one secondary case was reported – the photographer's mother.[6]

In 1976, 76 laboratories were known to stock smallpox virus; as of December 1981 there were four reporting that they still maintained the virus. Currently, one of the laboratories designated for WHO poxvirus research is the Centers for Disease Control, Atlanta.[7] Some scientists point to the present need to maintain the virus in the laboratory in order to help to investigate the ecology of monkeypox and other poxviruses,[8] and it is conceivable that some military personnel may want to keep this virus in their biological arsenals.

### What's next?

Now that smallpox appears conquered, many public health workers are looking for another candidate for eradication. Although not everyone agrees on a single definition of the word 'eradication', for smallpox it implied an absence of clinical cases of the disease on a continent, with little or zero likelihood of the disease reoccurring. In the selection of a new candidate for eradication, a number of factors need consideration: (1) the degree of understanding of the natural history of the disease; (2) types of appropriate control measures available; (3) mortality produced by the disease; (4) morbidity, including suffering and disability; (5) availability of adequate funding; (6) the cost–benefit of such an eradication effort; and (7) the probability of success within a given time period.

Many of these factors are interdependent. For example, malaria, which is considered by many as the leading cause of mortality in the world today, may require in excess of one billion dollars for the first years of an eradication program.[9] Similar expenses would accompany attempts to eradicate other diseases transmitted by arthropod vectors (e.g. yellow fever, trypanosomiasis, and onchocerciasis).

Zoonotic diseases are also difficult to eradicate because animal populations serve as principal reservoirs and are difficult to control. Possibly from the group of diseases that, like smallpox, is transmitted chiefly from person to person and for which man is either the principal or only reservoir of infection, a candidate can be found. From this group, measles clearly stands out as a potential candidate for eradication. Although the effect of measles on world mortality and morbidity may not be as great as was that of smallpox, the natural history of measles is well understood, there is a good vaccine (though not as heat-stable as the smallpox vaccine), and man is the only reservoir of infection. Thus measles would require a similar strategy and organization to carry out a successful eradication effort.

### References

1. Deria, A., Jezek, Z., Markvart, K., Carrasco, P. and Weisfeld, J. 'The world's last endemic case of smallpox: surveillance and containment measures', *Bull. WHO*, 58, 279–283 (1980).

2. WHO Expert Committee on Smallpox Eradication, World Health Organization Tech. Rep. Ser. No. 493 (1972).
3. Jenner, E. *An inquiry into the causes and effects of the variolae vaccine, a disease discovered in some of the western counties of England, particularly Gloucestershire, and known by the name of the cow pox*, Sampson Low, London (1798).
4. Weinstein, I. 'An outbreak of smallpox in New York City', *Am. J. Public Health*, **37**, 1376–1384 (1947).
5. Wehrle, P. F., Posch, J., Richter, K. H. and Henderson, D. A. 'An airborne outbreak of smallpox in a German hospital and its significance with respect to other recent outbreaks in Europe', *Bull. WHO*, **43**, 669–679 (1970).
6. Hawkes, N. 'Smallpox death in Britain challenges presumption of laboratory safety: peer review failed dismally', *Science*, **203**, 855–856 (1979).
7. 'Global eradication of smallpox', *WHO Weekly Epidemiol. Rec.*, **56**, 393–400 (1981).
8. Foege, W. H. 'Should the smallpox virus be allowed to survive?', *N. Engl. J. Med.*, **300**, 670–671 (1979).
9. Wood, C. (ed.) *Tropical Medicine: From romance to reality*, Academic Press, Inc., London, Chap. 5 (1978).

Marc A. Strassburg is an epidemiologist and, at the time that this article was written, he was head of program evaluation in the Department of Health Services, County of Los Angeles, California. The article is reprinted, with minor editing, from the *American Journal of Infection Control* (**19**, pp. 220–225, 1982), which is published by C. V. Mosby, St Louis, Missouri, USA.

# 36
# The epidemics of modern medicine

## IVAN ILLICH

During the past three generations the diseases afflicting Western societies have undergone dramatic changes. Polio, diphtheria, and tuberculosis are vanishing; one shot of an antibiotic often cures pneumonia or syphilis; and so many mass killers have come under control that two-thirds of all deaths are now associated with the diseases of old age. Those who die young are more often than not victims of accidents, violence, or suicide.

These changes in health status are generally equated with a decrease in suffering and attributed to more or to better medical care. Although almost everyone believes that at least one of his friends would not be alive and well except for the skill of a doctor, there is in fact no evidence of any direct relationship between this mutation of sickness and the so-called progress of medicine. The changes are dependent variables of political and technological transformations, which in turn are reflected in what doctors do and say; they are not significantly related to the activities that require the preparation, status, and costly equipment in which the health professions take pride. In addition, an expanding proportion of the *new* burden of disease of the last fifteen years is itself the result of medical intervention in favor of people who are or might become sick. It is doctor-made, or *iatrogenic*.

After a century of pursuit of medical utopia, and contrary to current conventional wisdom, medical services have not been important in producing the changes in life expectancy that have occurred. A vast amount of contemporary clinical care is incidental to the curing of disease, but the damage done by medicine to the health of individuals and populations is very significant. These facts are obvious, well documented, and well repressed.

### Doctors' effectiveness – an illusion

The study of the evolution of disease patterns provides evidence that during the last century doctors have affected epidemics no more profoundly than did priests during earlier times. Epidemics came and went, imprecated by both but touched by neither. They are not modified any more decisively by the rituals performed in medical clinics than by those customary at religious shrines. Discussion of the future of health care might usefully begin with the recognition of this fact.

In England, by the middle of the nineteenth century, infectious epidemics had been replaced by major malnutrition syndromes, such as rickets and pellagra. These in turn peaked and vanished, to be replaced by the diseases of early childhood and, some-what later, by an increase in duodenal ulcers in young men. When these declined, the modern epidemics took over: coronary heart disease, emphysema, bronchitis, obesity, hypertension, cancer (especially of the lungs), arthritis, diabetes, and so-called mental disorders. Despite intensive research, we have no complete explanation for the genesis of these changes. But two things are certain: the professional practice of physicians cannot be credited with the elimination of old forms of mortality or morbidity, nor should it be blamed for the increased expectancy of life spent in suffering from the new diseases. For more than a century, analysis of disease trends has shown that the environment is the primary determinant of the state of general health of any population: food, water, and air, in correlation with the level of sociopolitical equality and the cultural mechanisms that make it possible to keep the population stable.

Some modern techniques, often developed with the help of doctors, and optimally effective when they become part of the culture and environment or when they are applied independently of professional delivery, have also effected changes in general health, but to a lesser degree. Among these can be included contraception, smallpox vaccination of infants, and such nonmedical health measures as the treatment of water and sewage, the use of soap and scissors by midwives, and some antibacterial and insecticidal procedures. The importance of many of these practices was first recognized and stated by doctors – often courageous dissidents who suffered for their recommendations – but does not consign soap, pincers, vaccination needles, delousing preparations, or condoms to the category of 'medical equipment'. The most recent shifts in mortality from younger to older groups can be explained by the incorporation of these procedures and devices into the layman's culture.

In contrast to environmental improvements and modern nonprofessional health measures, the specifically medical treatment of people is never significantly related to a decline in the compound disease burden or to a rise in life expectancy. Neither the proportion of doctors in a population nor the clinical tools at their disposal nor the number of hospital beds is a causal factor in the striking changes in over-all patterns of disease. The new techniques for recognizing and treating such conditions as per-nicious anemia and hypertension, or for correcting congenital malformations by surgical intervention, redefine but do not reduce morbidity. The fact that the doctor popula-tion is higher where certain diseases have become rare has little to do with the doctors' ability to control or eliminate them. It simply means that doctors deploy themselves as they like, more so than other professionals, and that they tend to gather where the climate is healthy, where the water is clean, and where people are employed and can pay for their services.

## Useless medical treatment

Awe-inspiring medical technology has combined with egalitarian rhetoric to create the impression that contemporary medicine is highly effective. Undoubtedly, during the last generation, a limited number of specific procedures have become extremely useful. But where they are not monopolized by professionals as tools of their trade, those which are applicable to widespread diseases are usually very inexpensive and require a minimum of personal skills, materials and custodial services from hospitals. In contrast, most of today's skyrocketing medical expenditures are destined for the kind of diagnosis and treatment whose effectiveness at best is doubtful. To make this point I will distinguish between infectious and noninfectious diseases.

In the case of infectious diseases, chemotherapy has played a significant role in the control of pneumonia, gonorrhea, and syphilis. Death from pneumonia, once the 'old man's friend', declined yearly by 5 to 8 per cent after sulphonamides and antibiotics came on the market. Syphilis, yaws, and many cases of malaria and typhoid can be cured quickly and easily. The rising rate of venereal disease is due to new mores, not to ineffectual medicine. The reappearance of malaria is due to the development of pesticide-resistant mosquitoes and not to any lack of new antimalarial drugs. Immunization has almost wiped out paralytic poliomyelitis, a disease of developed countries, and vaccines have certainly contributed to the decline of whooping cough and measles, thus seeming to confirm the popular belief in 'medical progress'. But for most other infections, medicine can show no comparable results. Drug treatment has helped to reduce mortality from tuberculosis, tetanus, diphtheria, and scarlet fever, but in the total decline of mortality or morbidity from these diseases, chemotherapy played a minor and possibly insignificant role. Malaria, leishmaniasis, and sleeping sickness indeed receded for a time under the onslaught of chemical attack, but are now on the rise again.

The effectiveness of medical intervention in combatting noninfectious diseases is even more questionable. In some situations and for some conditions, effective progress has indeed been demonstrated: the partial prevention of caries through fluoridation of water is possible, though at a cost not fully understood. Replacement therapy lessens the direct impact of diabetes, though only in the short run. Through intravenous feeding, blood transfusions, and surgical techniques, more of those who get to the hospital survive trauma, but survival rates for the most common types of cancer – those which make up 90 per cent of the cases – have remained virtually unchanged over the last twenty-five years. Surgery and chemotherapy for rare congenital and rheumatic heart disease have increased the chances for an active life for some of those who suffer from degenerative conditions. The medical treatment of common cardiovascular disease and the intensive treatment of heart disease, however, are effective only when rather exceptional circumstances combine that are outside the physician's control. The drug treatment of high blood pressure is effective and warrants the risk of side-effects in the few in whom it is a malignant condition; it represents a considerable risk of serious harm, far outweighing any proven benefit, for the 10 or 20 million Americans on whom rash artery-plumbers are trying to foist it.

## Doctor-inflicted injuries

Unfortunately, futile but otherwise harmless medical care is the least important of the damages a proliferating medical enterprise inflicts on contemporary society. The pain, dysfunction, disability, and anguish resulting from technical medical intervention now rival the morbidity due to traffic and industrial accidents and even war-related activities, and make the impact of medicine one of the most rapidly spreading epidemics of our time. Among murderous institutional torts, only modern malnutrition injures more people than iatrogenic disease in its various manifestations. In the most narrow sense, iatrogenic disease includes only illnesses that would not have come about if sound and professionally recommended treatment had *not* been applied. Within this definition, a patient could sue his therapist if the latter, in the course of his management, failed to apply a recommended treatment that, in the physician's opinion, would have risked making him sick. In a more general and more widely accepted sense, clinical iatrogenic disease comprises all clinical conditions for which remedies, physicians, or hospitals are the pathogens, or 'sickening' agents. I will call this plethora of therapeutic side-effects *clinical iatrogenesis*. They are as old as medicine itself, and have always been a subject of medical studies.

Medicines have always been potentially poisonous, but their unwanted side-effects have increased with their power and widespread use. Every twenty-four to thirty-six hours, from 50 to 80 per cent of adults in the United States and the United Kingdom swallow a medically prescribed chemical. Some take the wrong drug; others get an old or a contaminated batch, and others a counterfeit; others take several drugs in dangerous combinations, and still others receive injections with improperly sterilized syringes. Some drugs are addictive, others mutilating, and others mutagenic, although perhaps only in combination with food coloring or insecticides. In some patients, antibiotics alter the normal bacterial flora and induce a superinfection, permitting more resistant organisms to proliferate and invade the host. Other drugs contribute to the breeding of drug-resistant strains of bacteria. Subtle kinds of poisoning thus have spread even faster than the bewildering variety and ubiquity of nostrums. Unnecessary surgery is a standard procedure. *Disabling nondiseases* result from the medical treatment of nonexistent diseases and are on the increase: the number of children disabled in Massachusetts through the treatment of cardiac nondisease exceeds the number of children under effective treatment for real cardiac disease.

Doctor-inflicted pain and infirmity have always been a part of medical practice. Professional callousness, negligence, and sheer incompetence are age-old forms of malpractice. The problem, however, is that most of the damage inflicted by the modern doctor occurs in the ordinary practice of well-trained men and women who have learned to bow to prevailing professional judgment and procedure, even though they know (or could and should know) what damage they do.

The United States Department of Health, Education and Welfare calculates that 7 per cent of all patients suffer compensable injuries while hospitalized, though few of them do anything about it. Moreover, the frequency of reported accidents in hospitals is higher than in all industries but mines and high-rise construction. Accidents are the major cause of death in American children. In proportion to the time spent there, these accidents seem to occur more often in hospitals than in any other kind of place. One in fifty children admitted to a hospital suffers an accident which requires specific treatment. University hospitals are relatively more pathogenic, or, in blunt language, more sickening. It has also been established that one out of every five patients admitted to a typical research hospital acquires an iatrogenic disease, sometimes trivial, usually requiring special treatment, and in one case in thirty leading to death. Half of these episodes result from complications of drug therapy; amazingly, one in ten comes from diagnostic procedures. Despite good intentions and claims to public service, a military officer with a similar record of performance would be relieved of his command, and a restaurant or amusement center would be closed by the police. No wonder that the health industry tries to shift the blame for the damage caused onto the victim, and that the dope-sheet of a multinational pharmaceutical concern tells its readers that 'iatrogenic disease is almost always of neurotic origin'.

## Defenseless patients

The undesirable side effects of approved, mistaken, callous, or contraindicated technical contacts with the medical system represent just the first level of pathogenic medicine. Such *clinical iatrogenesis* includes not only the damage that doctors inflict with the intent of curing or of exploiting the patient, but also those other torts that result from the doctor's attempt to protect himself against the possibility of a suit for malpractice. Such attempts to avoid litigation and persecution may now do more damage than any other iatrogenic stimulus.

On a second level, medical practice sponsors sickness by reinforcing a morbid society that encourages people to become consumers of curative, preventive, industrial, and environmental medicine. On the one hand defectives survive in increasing numbers and are fit only for life under institutional care, while on the other hand, medically certified symptoms exempt people from industrial work and thereby remove them from the scene of political struggle to reshape the society that has made them sick. Second-level iatrogenesis finds its expression in various symptoms of social overmedicalization that amount to what I shall call the expropriation of health. This second-level impact of medicine I designate as *social iatrogenesis*.

On the third level, the so-called health professions have an even deeper, culturally health-denying effect insofar as they destroy the potential of people to deal with their human weakness, vulnerability, and uniqueness in a personal and autonomous way. The patient in the grip of contemporary medicine is but one of mankind in the grip of its pernicious techniques. This *cultural iatrogenesis* is the ultimate backlash of hygienic progress and consists in the paralysis of healthy responses to suffering, impairment, and death. It occurs when people accept health management designed on the engineering model, when they conspire in an attempt to produce, as if it were a commodity, something called 'better health'. This inevitably results in the managed maintenance of life on high levels of sublethal illness. This ultimate evil of medical 'progress' must be clearly distinguished from both clinical and social iatrogenesis.

I hope to show that on each of its three levels iatrogenesis has become medically irreversible: a feature built right into the medical endeavour. The unwanted physiological social, and psychological by-products of diagnostic and therapeutic progress have become resistant to medical remedies. New devices, approaches, and organizational arrangements, which are conceived as remedies for clinical and social iatrogenesis, themselves tend to become pathogens contributing to the new epidemic. Technical and managerial measures taken on any level to avoid damaging the patient by his treatment tend to engender a self-reinforcing iatrogenic loop analogous to the escalating destruction generated by the polluting procedures used as antipollution devices.

I will designate this self-reinforcing loop of negative institutional feedback by its classical Greek equivalent and call it *medical nemesis*. The Greeks saw gods in the forces of nature. For them, nemesis represented divine vengeance visited upon mortals who infringe on those prerogatives the gods enviously guard for themselves. Nemesis was the inevitable punishment for attempts to be a hero rather than a human being. Like most abstract Greek nouns, Nemesis took the shape of a divinity. She represented nature's response to *hubris*: to the individual's presumption in seeking to acquire the attributes of a god. Our contemporary hygienic hubris has led to the new syndrome of medical nemesis.

By using the Greek term I want to emphasize that the corresponding phenomenon does not fit within the explanatory paradigm now offered by bureaucrats, therapists, and ideologues for the snowballing diseconomies and disutilities that, lacking all intuition, they have engineered and that they tend to call the 'counterintuitive behavior of large systems'. By invoking myths and ancestral gods I should make it clear that my framework for analysis of the current breakdown of medicine is foreign to the industrially determined logic and ethos. I believe that the *reversal of nemesis* can come only from within man and not from yet another managed (heteronomous) source dependent once again on presumptuous expertise and subsequent mystification.

Medical nemesis is resistant to medical remedies. It can be reversed only through a recovery of the will to self-care among the laity, and through the legal, political, and institutional recognition of the right to care, which imposes limits upon the professional monopoly of physicians. I do not suggest any specific forms of health care or sick-care, and I do not advocate any new medical philosophy any more than I recommend remedies for medical technique, doctrine, or organization. However, I do propose an alternative approach to the use of medical organization and technology together with the allied bureaucracies and illusions.

Ivan Illich is a theologian and philosopher who lives and works in Cuernavaca, Mexico. He is the author of several books including *Celebration of Awareness* (1969), *Deschooling Society* (1971), *Tools for Conviviality* (1973) and *Limits to Medicine* (1976). This article, which has been edited, originally appeared as the first chapter to the last mentioned book and was published by Marion Boyars, London. The extensive footnotes and references that accompanied the original version have been omitted here.

# 37

# The mode of state intervention in the health sector

## VICENTE NAVARRO

### Mechanisms of state intervention

Let us now analyze the specific mechanisms of state intervention in capitalist societies. And let us begin by somewhat arbitrarily dividing those interventions into primarily two levels: one of negative and the other of positive selection.

### A. Negative selection mechanisms

By negative selection, I mean that mode of intervention that systematically and continually excludes those strategies that conflict with the class nature of the capitalist society. This negative intervention takes place through (a) structural selective mechanisms, (b) ideological mechanisms, (c) decision-making mechanisms, and (d) repressive coercion mechanisms.

#### Structural selective mechanisms

These mechanisms refer to the exclusion of alternatives that threaten the capitalist system, an exclusion that is inherent in the nature of the capitalist state. In fact, the overall priority given to property and capital accumulation explains why, when health and property conflict, the latter usually takes priority over the former. For example, the appalling lack of adequate legislation protecting the worker in most capitalist societies (including social democratic Sweden) contrasts most dramatically with the large array of laws protecting private property and its owners.

This structural negative selective mechanism also appears in the implied assumption that all health programs and reforms have to take place within the set of class relations prevalent in capitalist societies. For example, in Britain, Bevan's Labour Party strategy of implementing the NHS (a victory for the British working class) assumed an unalterability of class relations in Britain. Indeed, the creation of the NHS was seen as taking place within the structure of capitalist Britain of 1948, respecting the class distribution of power both outside and within the health sector. Bevan relied very heavily on the consultants, who clearly were of upper class extraction and position, to break the general practitioner's resistance against the implementation of the NHS. As he proudly indicated, 'I bought them with gold.'[1] The strategy of using the nationalization of the health sector to break with the class structure outside and within the health sector, as Lenin did in the Soviet Union, was not even considered.[2]

Moreover, to reassure the medical profession in general and the consultants in particular, they were given dominant influence over the process of planning, regulation, and administration of the health sector.[3]

### Ideological mechanisms

These mechanisms insure the exclusion from the realm of debate of ideologies that conflict with the system. In other words, it is not only programs and policies, as indicated before, that are being automatically excluded, but, more importantly, conflicting ideologies as well. This is clearly shown in the lack of attention to and the lack of research in areas that conflict with the requirements and needs of the capitalist system. Reflecting the bourgeois bias of the medical research establishment for example, much priority is given to the assumedly individual causation of disease. One instance, among others, is that most research on heart disease – one of the main killers in society – has focused on diet, exercise, and genetic inheritance. On the study of these etiologies, millions of pounds, dollars, marks, and francs have been spent. However, in a fifteen-year study of aging, cited in a most interesting report prepared by a special task force to the Secretary of Health, Education, and Welfare in the US, it was found that the most important predictor of longevity was work satisfaction. Let me quote from that report:

> ... the strongest predictor of longevity was work satisfaction. The second best predictor was over-all 'happiness' ... Other factors are undoubtedly important – diet, exercise, medical care, and genetic inheritance. But research findings suggest that these factors may account for only about 25% of the risk factors in heart disease, the major cause of death. That is, if cholesterol, blood pressure, smoking, glucose level, serum uric acid, and so forth, were perfectly controlled, only about one-fourth of coronary heart disease could be controlled. Although research on this problem has not led to conclusive answers, it appears that work role, work conditions, and other social factors may contribute heavily to this 'unexplained' 75% of risk factors.[4]

But very few studies have investigated these socio-political factors. [...] In summary, the exclusion of ideologies which question or threaten the basic assumptions of the capitalist system is a most prevalent mechanism of state intervention, i.e. the exclusion as unthinkable of any alternatives to that system.

### Decision making mechanisms

The decision making processes are heavily weighted in favor of certain groups and classes, and thus against certain others. For example, the mechanisms of selection and appointment of members to health planning and administrative agencies in Britain and to the Health System Agencies in the US are conducive to the dominance over those bodies of individuals of the corporate and upper-middle classes, to the detriment of members of lower-middle and working classes.

*Repressive coercion mechanisms*
The final form of negative selection, repressive coercion mechanisms, takes place either through the use of direct force or, more importantly, by cutting (and thus nullifying) those programs that may conflict with sources of power within the state organism.

## B. Positive selection mechanisms

By positive selection, I mean the type of state intervention that generates, stimulates, and determines a positive response favorable to overall capital accumulation, as opposed to a negative selection which excludes anticapitalist possibilities. Offe distinguishes between two types of such intervention – allocative and productive.[5] In the former, the state regulates and coordinates the allocation of resources that have already been produced, while in the latter, the state becomes directly involved in the production of goods and services.

*Allocative intervention policies*
These policies are based on the authority of the state in influencing, guiding and even directing the main activities of society, including the most important one – capital accumulation. The policies are put into effect primarily (although not exclusively) through laws that make certain behavior mandatory and through regulations that make certain claims legal. In the health sector, examples of the former are laws requiring doctors to register contagious disease with the state health department and for employers to install protective devices to prevent industrial accidents, while an example of the latter is regulations determining that certain categories of people receive health insurance. Both laws and regulations are determined and dictated in the world of politics. As Offe indicates, in allocative functions 'policy and politics are not differentiated'. And, as such, those policies are determined by the different degrees of dominance of the branches of the state by pressure groups and factions primarily within the dominant class.

*Productive intervention policies*
As I have indicated, productive intervention policies are those whereby the state directly participates in the production of resources, e.g. medical education in most Western capitalist countries, production of drugs in nationalized drug industries, management of public hospitals, medical research, etc.
   Both allocative and productive policies have increased dramatically in all capitalist countries since World War II and, along with that increase, a shift has taken place from allocative to productive policies. An example of the latter is the production of medical knowledge, where there has been a shift in state intervention from an allocative function (e.g. subsidies, tax benefits) to actual production (e.g. nationalization of medical schools and research institutions). Similarly, there is a trend in the health sector to move from national insurance schemes (allocative) to national health services (productive). Britain in 1948, Quebec (Canada) in 1968, and Italy in the 1970s are each examples of that trend. In all capitalist countries, there has been an impressive growth of state intervention, primarily of the productive type of intervention, as measured by either public expenditures or public employment. Moreover, this growth has taken place mainly in the social (including health) services sector.

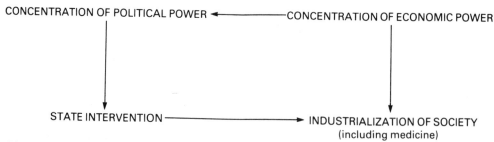

**Figure 37.1**   The dialectical relationship between concentration of economic power and industrialization of society (including medicine)

### The reasons for the growth of state intervention

The growth of the health sector in developed capitalist countries is due to the growth of social needs, which are determined by the process of capital accumulation and by the heightening of the level of class struggle. Let me expand on each.

*The growth of social needs as demanded by the process of capital accumulation*
A primary characteristic of that process of accumulation is, as indicated earlier, its concentration. Indeed, insurance, banking, manufacturing, and other sectors of economic life are in the hands of an increasingly small number of corporations that, for the most part, control the market in each sector. The consequences of that concentration are many but, among them, the most important is the type of technology and industrial development determined by and intended primarily to serve the needs of that concentration. And determined by that economic concentration and by that type of technological and industrial development are the following:

- *A division of labor, with a continuous demand for specialization* that fragments the process of production and ultimately the producer himself . . . In summary, and as expressed in Figure 37.1, increased economic concentration determines a growing concentration of political power and a greater need for state intervention to facilitate the type of industrialization demanded by that economic concentration – an industrialization that influences and determines the type of specialized medicine that is prevalent today.

  Let me clarify here that I believe the relationship among these categories to be dialectical, not linear, with a pattern of dominance that is expressed by the main direction of the arrow in Figure 37.1.
- *An invasion of all sectors of economic life by corporate capital.* Indeed, it is a tendency of the process of capital accumulation that the search for profits invades all sectors of economic life, including social services such as health, education, transportation, etc.
- *An invasion of the spheres of social life by corporate capital and its process of industrialization,* causing dislocation, diswelfare, and insecurity that state intervention, through social services (including medicine) is in turn supposed to mitigate. The most important example, of course, is the alienation that the industrialized process of production causes in the working population – an alienation that becomes reflected in psychosomatic conditions which medicine is supposed to care for and cure. Similarly, occupational diseases and environmental damage are, for the most part, also corporately caused, but, according to bourgeois ideology, individually cured through medical intervention.

- *An invasion of corporate capital into the spheres of private life*, with the commodification of all processes of interpersonal relationships, from sex to the pursuit of happiness. Indeed, according to corporate ideology, happiness depends on the amount and type of consumption, i.e. on what the citizen has, not on what he or she does.
- *An increased proletarianization of the population*, including the medical profession. As a result, the health professions have shifted from being independent entrepreneurs to becoming employees of private medical corporations (as in the US) or employees of the state (as in the majority of European capitalist countries). In both cases, that process of proletarianization is stimulated by the state, with the assistance of the corporate segments of the capitalist class.
- *An increased concentration of resources in urban areas*, and deployment of resources to those areas, required and needed for the realization of capital. This process of urbanization necessitates a growth in the allocative functions of the state (e.g. land use legislation and city planning) and of productive functions (e.g. roads and sanitation) so as to support, guide, and direct that process in a way that is responsive to the needs of capital accumulation. It is worth underlining in this context that the majority of infrastructural services are consumed by components of Capital and not by private households. For example, three-quarters of the US water supply is consumed by industry and agriculture (mainly corporate), while private households consume less than one-quarter. Water supply, however, is paid for largely from funds coming from the latter, not from the former.

Moreover, this process of economic concentration, and its concomitant industrialization determines a model of production and distribution in medicine that replicates the characteristics of the overall process of economic production and distribution, i.e. specialization, concentration, urbanization and a technical orientation of medicine. The nature of medicine, then, and its relation to the overall process of production determine in large degree its *characteristics*. And its position within that process of production explains its function, which is to take care of and solve the unsolvable – the diswelfare and dysfunctions created by that very process of production.

*The level of class struggle*
The tendencies explained in the previous section are the result of the growing needs of capital accumulation which take place within the context of a continuous conflict between Capital and Labor – a conflict primarily between the capitalist class and the working class. Indeed, the working class aims continuously at extracting significant concessions from the state, over and above what the state considers sufficient for the needs of capital accumulation defined in the previous section. For example, it is impossible to understand the creation of the NHS in Britain without taking into account the relationship of class forces in Britain and the wartime radicalization of the working class that had called into question 'the survival of capitalism'. As Forsyth has indicated:

> Rightly or wrongly the British Government at the outbreak of war could not be sure that large sections of the working class were entirely satisfied about the reasons for fighting the war . . . For the sake of public morale the Government tried to make it clear that after the war things were going to be very different from the heartbreak conditions of the 'thirties'.[6]

The much heralded consensus on the need for a national health service that existed among Labour and Conservative politicians was the result of the radicalization of the working class on the one hand, and the concern for the survival of capitalism by the capitalist class and the state on the other. Indeed, labor movements have historically viewed social services (including health) as part of the *social wage*, to be defended and increased in the same way that *money wages* are. In fact, Wilensky has shown how the size of social wages depends, in large degree, on the level of militancy of the labor movements.[7] Thus, contrary to popular belief, the size and nature of social benefits in terms of social services is higher in France and Italy than in Scandinavia or even in Britain. And I attribute this to the greater militancy of the unions in those countries and to the existence of mass Socialist and Communist parties (whose platforms are, at least in theory, anticapitalist) that force an increase of social wages upon the state. Another indicator is the percentage of GNP spent on social security which, in 1965, was 17.5 per cent in Italy, 18.3 per cent in France, but only 7.9 per cent in the US. The practical absence of a comprehensive coverage for social benefits in the US is also undoubtedly due to the lack of an organized left party.

In summary, then, the nature and growth of the state in contemporary capitalist societies can be attributed to the increased *social needs of capital* and *social demands of labor*. And in order to understand the nature of any state policy, including health policy, we have to place our analysis within those parameters. Having said that, let me clarify two points. First, there is no single-factor explanation of social policy. Rather, it is explained by the combination of factors already mentioned. And the nature and number of those combinations will depend on the *historical* origins of each factor, the *political* form determining the factor and its relation to others, and its *function* in that specific social formation. Second, there is no clear cut dichotomy between the social needs of capital and the social demands of labor. Any given policy can serve both. Indeed, social policies that serve the interests of the working class can be subsequently adapted to benefit the interests of the dominant class. As Miliband and others have shown so well, the 'bias of the system' has always insured that these policies can be deflected to suit the capitalist class. Indeed, history shows that concessions won by labor in the class struggle become, *in the absence of further struggle*, modified to serve the interests of the capitalist class.

In summary, I have aimed to show that if we are to understand the nature, composition, distribution and function of the medical care sector in Western developed capitalist societies, we must first understand the distribution of power in those societies and the nature, role, and instrumentality of the state. This understanding leads us to realize that (a) the assumedly transcended and diluted category of social class is a much needed category in understanding the distribution of power in our societies; and that (b) class struggle, far from being an outmoded concept of interest only to 'vulgar' Marxists, is most relevant indeed and as much needed today to understand the nature of our societies and of our health sectors as it was when Marx and Engels wrote that 'class struggle is the motor of history'.

Needless to say, this interpretation is a minority voice in our Western academic setting. It is in conflict with the prevalent explanations of the health sector, and this accounts for its exclusion from the realm of debate. Still, its veracity will be affirmed not by its 'popularity' in the corridors of power, which will be nil, but in its verification on the terrain of history. It is because of this that I dedicated this article to all those with whom I share a praxis aimed at building up a society of truly free and self-governing men and women – a society in which, as Marx indicated, the state (and I would add medicine) will be converted 'from an organ superimposed upon society into one completely subordinated to it'.[8]

## References

1. See Tudor Hart, J. 'Primary care in the industrial areas of Britain: evolution and current problems', *International Journal of Health Services*, 2(3), 349–365 (1972) and 'Bevan and the Doctors', *Lancet*, 2 (7839), 1196–1197 (1973).
2. For Lenin's strategy in health services, see 'Leninism and medicine'. In Navarro, V. *The Political Economy of Social Security and Medical Care in the USSR*.
3. For an excellent analysis of the professional dominance in the NHS, see Robson, J. 'The NHS company inc.? the social consequence of the professional dominance in the National Health Service', *International Journal of Health Services*, 3(3), 413–426 (1973). Also Draper, P. and Smart, T. 'Social science and health policy in the United Kingdom: some contributions of the social sciences to the bureaucratization of the National Health Service', *International Journal of Health Services*, 4(3), 453–470 (1974).
4. Special Task Force to the Secretary of Health, Education and Welfare, *Work in America*, M.I.T. Press, Cambridge, MA., pp. 77–79 (1973).
5. Offe, C. 'The theory of the capitalist state and the problem of policy formation'. In Lindberg, L. *et al.* (eds) *Stress and Contradiction in Modern Capitalism*, Lexington Books, London, p. 128 (1975).
6. Forsyth, G. *Doctors and State Medicine: A Study of the British Health Service*, Pitman and Sons, London, p. 16 (1973).
7. Wilensky, H. L. *The Welfare State and Equality*, University of California Press, Berkeley and Los Angeles (1975).
8. Marx, K. *Critique of the Gotha Program*, International Publishers, New York (1938).

Vicente Navarro is Professor of Health and Social Policy at The Johns Hopkins University, Baltimore, USA. This article is an edited extract from his book *Medicine Under Capitalism* which was published by Prodist, New York (1976).

# 38
# Priority setting in the NHS

## ALAN WILLIAMS

It is not only in Britain that health care systems are undergoing stringent scrutiny and radical reforms. All countries find themselves in the paradoxical situation that at a time when medical science and clinical practice both offer unrivalled opportunities to improve people's health, we seem to face ever more excruciating choices about what health care we can afford to provide, and what health care we have reluctantly to forego, at least for the time being. The reason for this dilemma is, of course, that the possibilities are expanding faster than the resources available to provide them.

Common sense tells us that if we cannot do everything we would like to do, we should concentrate our limited resources where they will do the most good. And in the NHS it is the Purchasing Authorities (mainly the District Health Authorities) that are charged with the task of deciding which of the many health care activities that providers (e.g. hospitals) *could* supply are actually worth buying, in order to make the health of the community they serve as good as it can be.

That has proved to be an extremely difficult task, and we need to explore *why* it is so difficult. Little problems like disagreement about objectives I will brush to one side! The unworthy suspicion that some people may not even be trying very hard to make the task of priority-setting easier I will likewise put on one side. I will even set aside the possibility that the whole idea of separating purchasers from providers was misguided in the first place. So what is left?

Well, what is left is the well-known fact that we currently know very little about the benefits (in health terms) of most NHS activities, and very little about their costs. The consequence is that we have only the vaguest idea what is good value for money and what is bad value for money. And since this is the crucial judgement that purchasing authorities have to make, this gap in our knowledge leaves a big black hole in the centre of their universe.

So let us take a big leap into the future and imagine that, for all NHS activities, we had information such as that set out in Figures 38.1–4. In each case there is measured along the horizontal axis a patient's life expectancy, and on the vertical axis

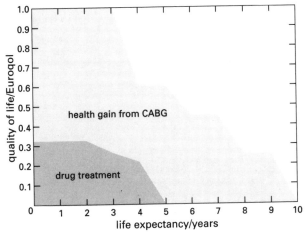

**Figure 38.1** Estimated quality and quantity of life with drug treatment or with *successful* bypass surgery for patients with severe angina (chest pain arising from obstruction of the coronary arteries, which supply oxygen and nutrients to the heart muscle). Coronary artery by-pass grafting (CABG) bypasses the obstruction with an artery grafted from elsewhere in the body; the procedure is fully discussed in another book in the *Health and Disease* series published by the Open University Press.[1]

an index of that patient's health-related quality-of-life. This index has as its anchor points 'being healthy' (valued at 1) and 'being dead' (valued at 0). (It is possible for states to be rated 'worse than being dead', and therefore to be assigned negative values, though no such states are included in the Figures.)

Figure 38.1 represents the situation of a patient with severe angina and left main artery disease (the most severe manifestation of coronary artery disease) facing a choice between continuing drug treatment or undergoing surgery (Coronary Artery Bypass Graft, or 'CABG'). The prospects with drugs are five years life expectancy, and steady deterioration of (already poor) quality of life. A successful CABG improves the patient's life expectancy to 10 years, and also beings about a dramatic improvement in the patient's quality of life, though this improvement tends to diminish again after a few years since the underlying condition continues to exact its toll. The health gain from a successful CABG is thus represented by the *lightly* shaded area in the diagram, and it will be seen that this is an amalgam of improved *length* of life and improved *quality* of life.

But things are not quite as simple as they seem. In the foregoing text I carefully specified that these gains were to be expected from a *successful* CABG. Not all surgery is successful (nor is all drug treatment, though I shall not pursue that point further here). CABG can be unsuccessful in two different ways. The least harmful way occurs when it simply fails to deliver the promised benefits, and the patient remains on the original prognosis (i.e. as if still on drugs), and this appears to be true of about 30 per cent of all cases undergoing surgery. Obviously nobody knows why this is so, or what it is associated with, otherwise such patients would not be offered surgery. But CABG can be unsuccessful in a much worse sense, namely that the operation may kill the patient, and this appears to be true of about 3 per cent of all cases. So a patient with this condition facing these choices could be seen as entering a lottery

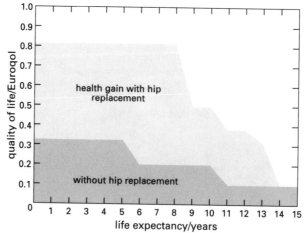

**Figure 38.2** Estimated quality and quantity of life for patients with or without total hip replacement surgery.

(and after all, we know that life generally is a lottery!) in which the patient opting for CABG has about a 67 per cent chance of winning a big prize (the *lightly* shaded area in Figure 38.1) by taking a 3 per cent chance of losing the *darkly* shaded area (the length and quality of life that would have been enjoyed if the drug regime had been chosen and the operation hadn't killed him). Needless to say most patients go for the surgery, with the encouragement of their doctors, because the balance is so advantageous for all but the extremely risk-averse.

I will deal more briefly with the other three figures, where similar considerations apply, though the probabilities are different (and they are also different for different types of patient even in the foregoing example). Figure 38.2 represents the case of total hip replacement, and the interesting feature of this diagram is that *all* the benefits are in the form of improvements in patients' quality of life. This treatment has no effect on life expectancy. Yet, as can be seen from the size of the *lightly* shaded area, the health gains from successful treatment are still very large, and may extend over many years.

Figure 38.3 deals with a very different situation, the surgical removal of subcutaneous lumps. These are mildly disfiguring and adversely affect people's quality-of-life to a very small extent, and they are not at all life-threatening. So here we have patients with quite good quality-of-life (especially compared with the two preceding cases) which can be made slightly better by successful simple surgery. Finally, Figure 38.4 deals with a rather less pleasant situation, where the patient has advanced lung cancer, has only two years life expectancy, with very poor quality-of-life. In this case successful surgery increases life expectancy by one year, but it takes its toll, by reducing the patient's immediate quality-of-life still more (since such patients are typically in poor shape). So the issue is whether the benefit of the increase in length of life is worth the sacrifice of immediate quality-of-life, taking into account also the attendant probabilities of a failed operation.

It will be noted that each of these cases illustrates a situation in which the precise nature of the health gains differs. But each is some amalgam of length of life and

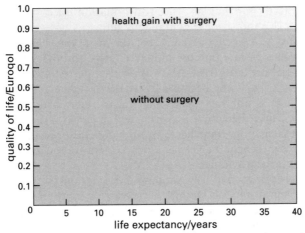

**Figure 38.3** Estimated quality and quantity of life for patients with or without surgical removal of subcutaneous lumps (just below the skin).

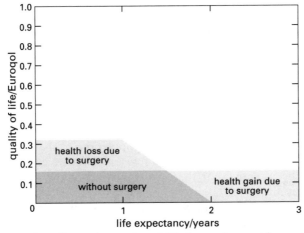

**Figure 38.4** Estimated quality and quantity of life for patients with or without surgical treatment of advanced lung cancer.

quality of life. It is therefore useful to have some overall measure of health benefit which embraces both of these elements. The '**Quality-adjusted life year**' (or **QALY**) is such a concept, the intuitive meaning of which is fairly simple to grasp, even though the actual measurements involved are quite tricky in practice. If by some treatment it were possible to give a patient an extra year of *healthy* life expectancy, that would be counted as 1 QALY (1 year at a quality-of-life rated at 1 on the index). But if, as is so often the case, the best we can do is offer people an extra year of *less healthy* life expectancy, then we would want to rate this health gain as less than 1 QALY, and assign it a lower value the worse it was. Equipped with this sort of measuring instrument, we could measure the area of the *lightly* shaded zones in Figures 38.1–4, since both are essentially based on 'quality' *times* 'duration' of life.

So far I have considered only the benefit side of the information-gathering task that health authorities face. But they also need information on costs, for it may be that although the surgical removal of subcutaneous lumps is not very beneficial in terms of the number of QALYs generated per person, it is very cheap to do, so it may nevertheless constitute good value for money relative to other procedures. CABG is much more beneficial (in terms of QALYs generated per person), but it is also much more expensive, so it will not necessarily be better value for money. Surgery for advanced lung cancer is not very beneficial, but is quite costly, so may well not be worth providing. Clearly the actual decisions will depend on the actual data, it is the general principle that is important here, and the general principle is that we need to know how much extra benefit we get per extra £ spent on each activity before we can judge which are worth providing.

But making decisions in this way requires information that we do not currently have, except in a few instances. Despite a century or more of clinical research conducted all over the world, we still know remarkably little about the effectiveness (let alone the cost-effectiveness) of most treatments upon the various kinds of patient getting them, cast in terms of the impact on a patient's life expectancy and quality of life. Moreover these gaps in our knowledge are not going to be filled in the foreseeable future from the results of properly conducted trials (though the more gaps that are so filled the better). So where is this information to come from?

Well, when in doubt about facts, a good strategy is to ask the experts. But who are they? I think we are going to have to assume that the medical practitioners are the experts, which is a very dangerous assumption for a variety of reasons, amongst which are that:

(i)   they differ from each other so dramatically in their policies and practices that they cannot all be right;

(ii)  their clinical experience differs greatly one from another, so their views are often based on rather peculiar subsets of the population;

(iii) unless they have had a strong research interest or native curiosity they will have had neither the incentive nor the opportunity to follow up their patients in a systematic way.

(iv)  for obvious reasons they tend to err on the side of optimism in assessing the success of what they are doing;

(v)   they are not impartial observers or reporters.

Despite all these important reservations I believe that we have no option in the short-run but to attempt to mine their clinical experience for whatever nuggets of information can be extracted from it, to enable us to proceed on a broad front with health outcome measurement.

My strategy would therefore be to take the 20 or 30 commonest things each clinician does, and ask each clinician to say what the typical state of the patient is (in terms of quality and expected length of life) before and after (and perhaps also during) treatment. If patients need to be divided into different categories for this purpose, well and good, and it would have to be accepted that it is the fairly short-term effects of treatment that need to be estimated to begin with. Estimates of longer-term effects would also be useful but would be more difficult to monitor. If necessary a range of different outcomes might be expected, since we know that people do not all respond to treatment in the same way (some are killed by treatments which do others a lot of good). The advantages of this strategy are that clinicians set their own norms (initially at any rate), and that it is rather difficult for them to admit that they have no idea what outcomes are in these terms, since they are advising patients to have these treatments, so must believe they have a beneficial effect on one or more of the health outcome parameters mentioned earlier. If they genuinely have no idea, then the initiative clearly shifts to managers, who must then make their own estimates from such data as they can lay their hands on.

But this descriptive profile needs to be converted into the single index of quality of life that I had on the vertical axis of Figures 38.1–4 so that different sorts of intervention can be compared. To do this we need ratings of each of these composite states indicating their goodness or badness relative to each other, and relative to being dead. One method of doing this is via the visual analogue scale in the form of a thermometer used by the Euroqol© group to get relative valuations from the general public. This thermometer is reproduced in Figure 38.5 at the centre of a sample page from the questionnaire. We have been conducting surveys for some years now on the citizens of Frome in Somerset seeking to elicit their ratings for various health states described in the Euroqol© manner. This descriptive system is reproduced in Table 38.1, together with an explanation of the five-digit codes that are used to make reference to each composite health state rather simpler.

**Table 38.1**   The Euroqol© Descriptive System (Version 12)

*Mobility*
1    no problems walking about
2    some problems in walking about
3    confined to bed

*Self-care*
1    no problems with self-care
2    some problems washing or dressing self
3    unable to wash or dress self

*Usual activities*
1    no problems with performing usual activities
     (e.g. work, study, housework, family or leisure activities)
2    some problems with performing usual activities
3    unable to perform usual activities

*Pain/discomfort*
1    no pain or discomfort
2    moderate pain or discomfort
3    extreme pain or discomfort

*Anxiety/depression*
1    not anxious or depressed
2    moderately anxious or depressed
3    extremely anxious or depressed

Note: For convenience each composite health state has a five digit code number relating to the relevant level of each dimension, with the dimensions always listed in the order given above. Thus 11232 means:
1   No problems walking about
1   No problems with self-care
2   Some problems with performing usual activities
3   Extreme pain or discomfort
2   Moderately anxious or depressed

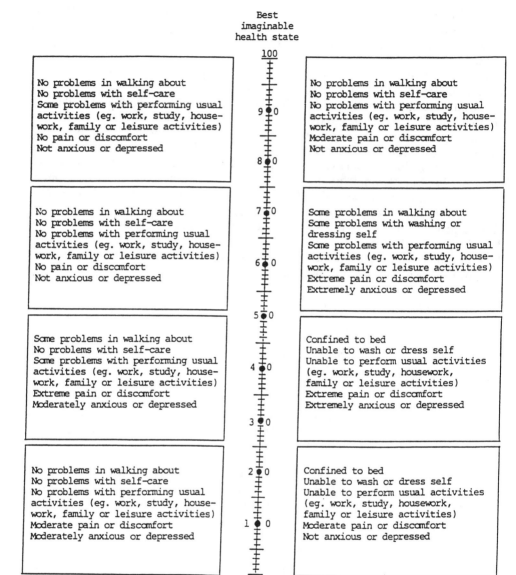

**Figure 38.5**   Scale developed for use with the Euroqol© Descriptive System (Table 38.1) to obtain quality of life measurements in surveys of the general public. Respondents are asked to draw one line from each of the eight boxes to intersect with the 'thermometer' at the point on the scale corresponding to their estimation of how high or low the state described in the box 'rates' in health terms. (You might like to do this yourself.)

**Table 38.2** A comparison of raw scores obtained in surveys using the Euroqol© analogue scale (Figure 38.5) and descriptive system (Table 38.1).

| Health state | Median score for health state | | | |
|---|---|---|---|---|
| | Frome (general population) | Sixth-formers | Health authority members | Belfast medical students |
| Own health | 85 | 80 | 93 | 90 |
| 11111a | 98 | 98 | 100 | 99 |
| 11111b | 97 | 98 | 98 | 98 |
| 11211 | 80 | 80 | 80 | 80 |
| 21111 | 80 | 70 | 62* | 69 |
| 11112 | 75 | 70 | 80 | 70 |
| 11121 | 75 | 70 | 74 | 70 |
| 12111 | 65 | 60 | 70 | 70 |
| 11122 | 60 | 50 | 45* | 55 |
| 21232 | 40 | 30 | 30 | 40 |
| 32211 | 40 | 32 | 40 | 30 |
| 22233 | 24 | 19 | 25 | 20 |
| 22323 | 20 | 20 | 20 | 20 |
| 33321 | 15 | 12 | 20 | 10 |
| Dead | 5 | 5 | 0 | 10 |
| Unconscious | 5 | 7 | 6 | 7 |
| 33333 | 2 | 1 | 5 | 2 |
| Number of respondents | 122 | 82 | 9 | 18 |

(Order of dimensions: mobility; self-care; usual activities; pain/discomfort; anxiety/depression)
* = Ratings which seem well out of line with those of the Frome respondents

The actual scores recorded on the questionnaire (the 'raw' scores) as derived from the Frome sample are set out in Table 38.2, together with those of three other groups: the members of a health authority in the south of England, some sixth-formers from different parts of England who were doing A level Economics, and some medical students in Northern Ireland. Despite some small differences here and there in the median scores, the overall impression is one of broad similarity of view between the three groups. But concentration on the medians obscures the variations that occur within each group, which are quite broad.

But the trouble with the 'raw' scores is that they are not on a scale in which 'healthy' equals 1 and 'dead' equals zero, so they have to be 'normalised' to bring this about. This requires people to value the state of being dead alongside other health states, which many people find difficult and some impossible. There is therefore some loss of respondents between Table 38.2 and Table 38.3, which shows these adjusted median scores. Again the similarities rather than the dissimilarities are the striking feature.

Having got this far we now have all the information needed to create diagrams such as Figures 38.1–4. It is admittedly crude and approximate, but when you are lost in a fog even a rough sketch map and a pocket compass constitute minor treasures. The great advantage of this way of thinking is that it provides a framework within which clinical data, managerial data, and financial data can all be brought together in a systematic way to bear on a problem that all three parties need to solve rather urgently; namely, how to establish priorities in health care in a rational, well informed

**Table 38.3**   A comparison of adjusted scores from Table 38.2 (on a scale from dead = 0, to healthy = 100)

| Health state | Median score for health state | | | |
|---|---|---|---|---|
| | Frome (general population) | Sixth-formers | Health authority members | Belfast medical students |
| 11111 | 100 | 100 | 100 | 100 |
| 11211 | 82 | 80 | 80 | 78 |
| 11112 | 79 | 68* | 70 | 72 |
| 11121 | 79 | 65* | 76 | 73 |
| 21111 | 69 | 68 | 61 | 68 |
| 12111 | 65 | 58 | 74 | 70 |
| 11122 | 59 | 47* | 50 | 51 |
| 32211 | 29 | 29 | 38 | 17* |
| 21232 | 26 | 21 | 28 | 23 |
| 22233 | 14 | 10 | 19 | 13 |
| 22323 | 10 | 10 | 15 | 6 |
| 33321 | 10 | 10 | 12 | 6 |
| 33333 | 0 | −5 | 11* | −6 |
| Unconscious | 0 | 0 | 4 | 0 |
| Dead | 0 | 0 | 0 | 0 |
| Number of respondents | 82 | 72 | 10 | 17 |

(Order of dimensions of health state: mobility; self-care; usual activities; pain/discomfort; anxiety/depression.)
* Ratings which seem somewhat out of line with those of the Frome respondents.

manner. The provision of such a framework for thought does not make the information gaps disappear, indeed it may make us aware of information gaps that we were not previously aware of, such as the need to get *valuations* of health gains as well as *descriptions* of them. But it shows us how best to use the information we do have, much of which lies untouched at present because it is not clear where it fits in to the overall picture, and it directs our attention to the key bits of information that we lack, so that our information-gathering activities can be directed in a more purposive way.

So I hope that those who are in a position to fill some of these gaps might feel motivated to try, in a small way, to do so, and to interest colleagues in contributing their mite to the enterprise, for this is too big and important a task to be left to the experts!

### Reference

1. Davey, B. and Popay, J. (eds) *Dilemmas in Health Care*, Open University Press, Buckingham, Chapter 9 (1993).

This article was adapted, by the author from a seminar presentation and appeared in the 'Reader Supplement for *Dilemmas in Health Care*', distributed to Open University students studying the course *Health and Disease* in 1993. It has not been previously published elsewhere. Alan Williams is Professor of Economics at the Centre for Health Economics, University of York.

# Part 5
## The social context of health care

### INTRODUCTION

Just as health is a contested concept (see the variety of conflicting perspectives in the articles chosen for Part 1 of this book), so health care means different things to different people in different places. The articles in Part 5 reflect some of this diversity, presenting both international comparisons and showing something of the variety of means by which health care is organized in the United Kingdom. A theme that runs through all of them is sensitivity to the social context in which health care is delivered. The organization of health care is not simply the straightforward application of scientific principles, but is influenced by history, social circumstances and cultural preferences.

In the United Kingdom and the USA, complex health care systems have evolved with time, and continue to change. Divergences have their roots in the social structure of the two countries in the last century, and even earlier, as the social historian Rosemary Stevens' article shows. 'The evolution of the health-care systems in the United States and the United Kingdom: similarities and differences', reveals that one distinguishing feature between the two systems lies in the degree to which medical practice is separated into specialties. In the United Kingdom there are numerous general practitioners (GPs), whose earnings derive from the State; they originated in the trade guilds of earlier centuries. The Royal Colleges of Physicians and of Surgeons catered largely for the upper levels of society, although they also practised in hospitals for the poor which were set up by charitable (often religious) organizations. By contrast, general practitioners had more humble beginnings in the traditional apothecary. The position of the general practitioner was secured when, in the early part of the twentieth century, the National Insurance Act provided for basic health care by GPs with referral to specialists – at least for men. However, in the USA at this time, the GP had all but disappeared. Medical practitioners in the USA had specialized early on (the system was based on competition), and this was associated with an emphasis on science as the basis for medical authority.

The limitations of the American health care system have been much publicized in recent years, emphasizing the lack of coverage for many people and spiralling costs. The health care reforms of the Clinton administration, planned to begin in 1995, are designed to address these problems. However, problems with the British system as it had developed since 1948 (the start of the National Health Service) were the subject of reforms initiated by Prime Minister Thatcher in 1989, and enacted in 1991. The cornerstone of the new policy was the introduction of an 'internal market' in health care to stiffen competition and improve efficiency, while (in theory) enhancing both the quality of care and the responsiveness of the health care system to consumers. 'Britain's health care experiment' is the subject of the second article in this part of the book, by the health policy specialists Patricia Day and Rudolf Klein, in which they describe the background to the reforms and assess their likely prospects of success. They point out that the administrative costs of the new arrangements are likely to be high, contrasting with the parsimony of what went before. However, they argue that one benefit of the market system is the incentive to scrutinize and make explicit the quality of care. In addition, they suggest that public discussion of what *cannot* be bought by purchasers (previously a matter hidden from view in the informal rationing practices of clinicians) is likely to place some pressure on central government to fund the service more generously. Overall levels of funding, they argue, may be more important than particular ways of organizing care in determining the success of the system. On the other hand, they point out that a central issue remains unresolved by the reforms – the reconciliation of a demand-led service fuelled by the requests of consumers, and a more centrally-planned service (which must inevitably mean disadvantageous treatment for some) with equity as a basic principle.

The consumer's view of the health care system is taken up by Fedelma Winkler, who worked for a number of years in Community Health Councils. Her article 'Transferring power in health care' contrasts the relative imbalance of power between users of the health service and providers of health care. She presents an impassioned argument for user 'empowerment', by encouragement of a system that monitors abuses of rights and responds to complaints, gives information about the quality of medical care to enable informed choices to be made, and fosters well-informed community representation. She is scathing about 'management-led' consumerism, with its manipulation of 'customer relations' to give the impression of democratic consultation. While her analysis is revealing, however, it does not address the point made by Day and Klein about the tension between equitable rationing and unbridled consumer choice.

David Werner then moves us to another continent, Latin America, but in 'The village health worker: lackey or liberator?' he maintains the focus on issues of power in health care. Werner is an American biologist and teacher who spent many years living and working in Mexico. His article suggests that health care workers should make a political alliance with the people they serve, to bring an end to the oppressive inequities that, amongst other things, lead to ill health. To this end, he argues for the more widespread use of village health care workers. He contrasts 'community supportive' with 'community oppressive' health care programmes: the former use people to control disease, while the latter use disease to control people. This theme is taken up, too, in an article by medical geographers Ramesh and Hyma, who describe 'Traditional Indian medicine in practice in an Indian metropolitan city'. They argue that traditional medical practitioners are closer to the Indian people's own conception of health than is Western medicine. However, the authors raise concerns about the continuation of traditional medicine, pointing to the submergence of this by a system modelled on Western medical practice.

Less passionate than the politicized accounts of Winkler or Werner, and firmly placed in the context of Western biomedicine, is the extract from 'A short cut to better services: day surgery in England and Wales', a report by the Audit Commission. Yet, when this is examined closely, it is revealed as also quite critical of some aspects of the health care system. Advocating the greater use of day surgery in the interests of cost savings and patient convenience, the report analyses obstacles to its wider use, identifying clinician's preferences for more traditional approaches as one obstacle amongst several. The report is aimed primarily at influencing hospital managers who have become increasingly responsible for setting the limits on, and influencing the nature of, the care provided by doctors and other health care workers under the reforms to the NHS described by Day and Klein. As in the relationship between consumers and providers, the relationship between managers and clinicians can be understood in terms of relative power to affect the delivery of health care. Thus even in this rational account, the social context in which health care is delivered is recognized as important.

# 39

# The evolution of the health-care systems in the United States and the United Kingdom: similarities and differences

## ROSEMARY STEVENS

I should like to present some ideas about the nature of the health-care systems of the two countries. For in the two systems there are some fundamental differences which long antedate the National Health Service in Britain or more recent Government initiatives here. Basic professional and social assumptions as they have evolved over the centuries, suggest that medical care itself means different things in different places. We are not always using common assumptions, rationalizations, or even definitions.

### Specialization: common developments

For 100 years we have been under the spell of a movement toward increased technical specialization in medicine. Now this movement is virtually completed. Specialized departments in hospitals sprang up on both sides of the Atlantic only in the 1870s and 1880s, marking organizational acceptance that specialization was here to stay. St Thomas's Hospital in London set up outpatient departments for ophthalmology in 1871, for otolaryngology in 1882, for dermatology in 1884.[1] Over here, the Massachusetts General Hospital was setting up its own departments of dermatology (1870), neurology (1872), laryngology (1872), ophthalmology (1873), and aural surgery (1886) during the same period.[2] While specialization was accepted reluctantly by leaders of the medical professions in both countries – the first neurologist appointed to the Massachusetts General Hospital was barely dignified by the title of 'electrician' – the movement toward specialization had become inevitable.

By the early 1900s it appeared in America that general practice was moribund, if not dead. While the role of the family doctor as adviser and counselor was idealized as the ultimate in the doctor–patient relationship after 1890, a certain aura of myth and nostalgia surrounded this idealization – as it has, indeed, to the present. The family physician, that 'chum of the old people, the intimate of confiding girlhood, the uncle and oracle of the kids',[3] had largely disappeared by 1915. Outpatient departments of city hospitals provided general services for the indigent masses. The American middle class was already going directly to specialists.

Even in England, where the general practitioner was more readily defined and firmly established, outpatient departments of general hospitals and the rise of special hospitals in the last quarter of the nineteenth century threatened the generalist's position. It has been estimated that, before the National Health Insurance Act of 1911, only 10 to 20 per cent of the British population had family practitioners.[4] Hospitals had become 'temples of research, and the avenues leading to additional medical knowledge'.[5]

By World War I the specialization movement was in full swing. New professions added vertical specialization to the horizontal specialization developing in medicine. Besides the great rise of the nursing profession, there were social workers, optometrists, X-ray technicians, laboratory workers, physical therapists, and (in the American Midwest) nurse-anesthetists. Medicine was no longer a single matter of a conference between two individuals: one patient and one practitioner.

Specialization demanded some response to the questionable relationship between the new specialists and general practitioners – if, indeed, the generalists were to survive. Generalist–specialist relations, transmitted later to questions of primary versus secondary (and tertiary) care, became one set of issues for discussion in the modern health-care system. A related set of issues concerned the emerging role of the hospital, that center of specialized knowledge and techniques. Was it to be the center of all medical care, the temple of service as well as scientific excellence? Such questions were engaging writers on both sides of the Atlantic well before World War I and became intense in the 1920s and 30s.

Other themes with which we still contend have been apparent over many decades. Problems of cost increases and cost containment in medical care have been discussed, particularly on this side of the Atlantic, for at least six decades. The distribution of medical services – questions of urban–rural distributions and the concentration of specialists in major cities – was already of concern in the 1920s. The medical profession, a rag-bag of individuals with varying training and from varying backgrounds on both sides of the Atlantic in the late nineteenth century, became homogenized, standardized, and middle class in the years between the two World Wars. As the status of the profession rose with its advancing techniques so, from World War I, did the social background of its students.

Yet, while some of the dilemmas of modern medicine are clear – the relationship between generalists and specialists, the role of the hospital, the nature of the 'physician', and the role of medical education – the specific responses to medical specialization in Britain and America have been, and may continue to be, quite different, because of the way each health system has developed.

## Professional distinction and social differences

Most of the basic characteristics of British and American medicine existed in embryonic form in the 1870s and were clearly evident by 1914. Differences existed in the relative development of professional patterns of medical practice in the two countries, in professional regulation and medical education, in general social attitudes toward the provision of medical care, and even in the behavior of patients.

A quite conservative student of the hospital scene, Henry Burdett,[6] noted with some criticism: 'Free relief has now become so general that the majority of the population in England consider it not only not a disgrace, but the most natural thing in the world, when they fall ill, to demand and receive free medical treatment without question or delay.'

In contrast, he commented, 'America, owing no doubt to the fact of its being a relatively new country, possessing few endowed charities, and an energetic population consisting largely of those who resort to it in the hope of earning an independence may be regarded as the home of the pay system.'

Most patients in American hospitals occupied pay beds or paying wards, in contrast to the largely charitable English hospital system. Moreover, patients were already characterized as being, in England, relatively passive recipients of medical care, while Americans were both more adventurous and more litigious.

Trying to explain the difference a generation earlier, a leading Californian physician had remarked: 'Patients in old countries are more timid: they are not anxious to be the subjects of experiments. In new countries, they bite at all new medicines.'[7]

But while this adventurousness might appeal to the desires of American physicians to show initiative, it resulted equally in 'serious annoyance' from malpractice claims. Modern Californians may be reassured to learn that malpractice claims similar to those of today were being made 100 years ago: 'A certain class of patients make it a business to extort money in this way, by the aid of a certain class of lawyers who go halves in the speculation'.[7]

There would inevitably have been differences in the type of medical organization developing for the small, densely populated, and relatively homogeneous population of Britain and the diverse population of America, scattered over a vast continent. But coupled with these topographical distinctions and with the more general distinctions between the rough and tumble of life in a rapidly growing country and one with centuries of social stability, there were already marked distinctions in patterns of professional organization in medicine.

Medicine in England grew from centralized professional guilds and from a professional system clearly stratified by social status. Before 1858, there were technically three recognized medical professions in England. The Royal College of Physicians, established in 1518, was the traditional domain of the educated elite. The Royal College of Surgeons, founded in 1800, represented the growing prestige of surgeons – well before the technological revolution in surgery made such a distinction functionally inevitable. Apothecaries formed a third strain. Systematic training of apothecaries for medical practice was achieved through an act of 1815, and the resulting apothecaries' license rapidly became the most popular way to become a licensed practitioner. In fact, the most common way of becoming licensed by the mid-nineteenth century was to become both an apothecary and a surgeon.[8]

The early existence of the guilds of physicians, surgeons, and apothecaries has left an enduring imprint on medical care in England. Physicians, as the elite of the medical profession, were a relatively small – if powerful – body, whose clientele during the nineteenth century was divided into two extraordinarily diverse groups. As private practitioners, members of the Royal College of Physicians catered largely to the upper segments of society, although they might function as general consultants to apothecaries when called upon to do so. Yet at the same time, because physicians had been instrumental in founding the great charitable hospitals of England in the eighteenth century, physicians were also the honorary medical staffs of the most prestigious hospitals – which, in turn, catered largely to the poverty-stricken.

Surgeon-apothecaries, on the other hand, found themselves a growing role during the nineteenth century as practitioners to the middle class in the expanding industrial cities. When the three branches of practice were combined into one medical register under the Medical Acts of 1858 and 1886, the earlier distinctions did not evaporate. There was now one medical profession, with a training supposedly designed for general practice, but distinctions remained at the graduate level. The elite of the profession (members of the Royal College of Physicians and fellows of the Royal College of Surgeons) continued to control major hospital positions. Indeed, the struggle for an honorary appointment could become the dominant motive of a doctor's career. In 1900, when American hospital building was in full swing and hospital appointments tended to be open to most recognized physicians, the British voluntary hospital was controlled by a small number of leading practitioners. Each was usually responsible for an identifiable group of beds in a particular ward and thus for the patients who occupied those beds. Surgeon-apothecaries, meanwhile, were general practitioners who worked almost entirely outside the voluntary hospital system.

National health insurance provided the final endorsement of this system in 1911 by creating a central role for the general practitioner. Members of the working population below a specified income level were now insured for the services of general practitioners, but not for hospital or specialist care.

General or family practice became, and has remained, central to the organization of the British system. It has been bolstered, it is true, by further government action: the National Health Service Act of 1946, which incorporated general practice as the basis of the health-care system, and changes in reimbursement following the profession's 'Doctor's Charter' of 1965, equalizing generalist and specialist incomes. But such actions would have been unthinkable had the earlier traditions not existed.

Modern medical care in Britain relies, in short, on the system of checks and balances which emerged from the prespecialization era. General practitioners control access to the health-care system; salaried hospital staff, the consultants (who are now, of course, all specialists), control access to hospital care. When each round of specialist treatment is completed, the patient returns to his family practitioner. The old social division between the branches of practice have been continued in the separate *functions* of primary and secondary care, and there continue to be far more general practitioners than specialists.

In the United States there were no guilds, no national focus for an elite such as London provided to British practitioners, and until the 1870s there were relatively few hospitals. American medicine was a profession without institutions. If the professional development of British medicine can be characterized as the history of guilds which eventually came together, establishing mutually acceptable positions, the development of American medicine for most of its history has been a search for *itself*, for identity and professional unity. Out of this movement was to come a medical profession committed to university-centered education and technological advancement, organizationally based on an array of specialists.

### Defining the practice of medicine

From time to time efforts were made to establish guilds on this side of the Atlantic. John Morgan was one of several Scottish-trained physicians returning to the Colonies who tried before Independence to establish the educated 'physician' as a separate rank of practitioner along British lines. But such efforts were doomed to failure in the competitive and social climate of the day. One continuing theme of American medicine was already evident. Even in the Revolutionary era there were relatively large *numbers* of doctors in America. Clearly medicine was felt to be a desirable occupation.

One estimate for New York in 1750 gives a ratio of one doctor to every 350 members of the population; in Williamsburg in 1730 there was one doctor to every 135 members of the population, relatively a far greater density of doctors than today.[9] It was just not practicable for the American doctor (unless he had considerable private income) to say he would do no surgery and dispense no drugs, but merely be an educated physician. Almost from the beginning, the American doctor has been an individual in a competitive market situation, dependent on his success – not on family connections or institutional affiliations (as is clearly the case of physicians in England), but on the exercise of his own initiative.

Even in the eighteenth century, any suggestion of a guild also suggested the imposition of a potentially dangerous monopoly. Social elitism in medical practice as in other fields has consistently been regarded as un-American. Early licensing laws were repealed in the 1830s and 1840s, leaving the field of medicine open to all comers. (Modern licensing laws date from the 1870s.) The rise of proprietary or profitmaking medical schools during the century added another component for untrammelled competition.

Instead of creating distinctions within the profession, medical societies arose in America to protect all 'regular' practitioners from the common threat of 'irregulars' or quacks.[10] The American College of Surgeons and the American College of Physicians, which followed in 1915, came much too late to direct basic patterns of the medical profession.

Probably the most important early impact of the College of Surgeons was its accreditation and upgrading of the standards of hospitals, which had sprung up like mushrooms from the 1880s in the American doctor's enthusiastic desire to do surgery. The British response to the technological possibilities or relatively 'safe' surgery in the post-asepsis, post-anesthetics era had been to exclude any remaining general practitioners from the staffs of hospitals, restricting operations to the small staff of consulting surgeons. But no such constraints existed in America, and there was a ready market for hospital construction in the expanding cities. Surgery, indeed, was so instantly popular that it was to become a lasting characteristic of American medicine: about a fourth of all American physicians have been surgeons in recent decades, a much larger proportion than in England. While England was consolidating the general practitioner, America was hailing the virtuosity of the surgeon and sometimes criticizing his excesses and deploring his greed.

But in all fields, compared with the individualism, exuberance, and ingenuity of

American medical practice at the beginning of this century, medicine in England seemed tame and settled. Abraham Flexner, reporting on England in 1912, found educational standards there low and medical education regarded among clinicians as merely a 'professional incident', with any interest in research mostly missing. The guild system was, he remarked, 'admirably calculated to protect honor and dignity, to conserve ceremony, and to transmit tradition'.[11]

While there were relatively large numbers of doctors in Britain in the first decade of the century, social and ethical structures in Britain precluded out-and-out competition. The British doctor, accustomed to working for the Poor Law and for public health authorities, might welcome National Health Insurance as a means of upgrading his financial status. In America, while there was also discussion of health insurance through the state, the mood was different. Fee-splitting was rife, there were kickbacks, usually from surgeons to referring practitioners. It was acknowledged that fees and services were related: the higher the fee, the better the care. The California state medical journal put forward as its primary objection to contract practice in 1913 *not* the argument that the rates paid were too low, but that patients for whom only 10 cents were paid would get only 10 cents' worth of treatment.[12] Cost and quality were inextricably combined, as indeed they have remained to this day.

Since there was no entrenched social structure for general practice, there was no ethical or other barrier against specialization or direct competition for patients by American physicians. There were both money and social advancement in specialism through private office practice – in contrast to the British system of social advancement through hospital positions. Virginia doctors, even in the 1870s, advertised in such areas as 'Speciality Surgery', 'Diseases of Females', 'Diseases of Urinary Organs', 'Diseases of the Ear and Eye'.[13] A formal social class system for medical education had failed in America; there was now an emergence of a self-proclaimed technological elite, competing directly with generalists for patients.

The standardization movement in American medical practice was well underway at the turn of the century. There was a gradual 'leveling up of the masses of the profession'.[14] The reorganization of the Harvard curriculum in 1870 had been followed by upgrading of standards in other schools, and the foundation of the Johns Hopkins school in 1893 provided a paradigm for the future development of scientific, laboratory-oriented medical schools based on universities.

The American Medical Association, unifying its scattered organization over the same period, rose on the banner of standardization. There was to be one American doctor, produced by medical schools of equivalent quality. While the profession in Britain was grappling with the problems of introducing general practitioner services under National Health Insurance in 1911, American medical education was set on the road to an increasingly scientific emphasis for medicine. The movement was rapid. By 1920, America had replaced Germany as the world leader of scientific medicine. Medical education was based on universities, with a strong research emphasis. It was not surprising that the graduates of these schools would turn increasingly to the specialities. Nor, indeed, was there any social structure such as National Health Insurance to encourage the continuation of general practice as a means of making a reasonable living; nor any ethical arrangement such as the referral system, which existed in England, to establish primary care as a central function of the emerging health system. In America generalists continued to compete with specialists, and one specialist with another.

## References

1. McInnes, E. M. *St Thomas's Hospital*, Allen and Unwin, London (1963).
2. Washburn, F. A. *The Massachusetts General Hospital: Its Development, 1900–1935*, Houghton Mifflin Co., Boston (1939).
3. Jacobi, A., quoted by Michael M. Davis 'Organization of medical service', *American Labor Legislation Review*, **6**, 16–20 (1916).
4. Titmuss, R. M. 'Trends of social policy'. In *Law and Opinion in England in the Twentieth Century*, Ginsberg, M. (ed.) Greenwood, London (1959).
5. Kershaw, R. *Special Hospitals: Their Origin, Development, and Relationship to Medical Education*, Pulman, London (1909).
6. Burdett, H. C. *Hospitals and Asylums of the World*, Vol. III, J. and A. Churchill, London (1893).
7. Gibbons, H. Annual Address to the California State Medical Society. *Transactions of the Medical Society of California*, privately printed (1872).
8. Newman, C. *The Evolution of Medical Education in the Nineteenth Century*, Oxford University Press, London (1957).
9. Shryock, R. H. *Medicine and Society in America 1660–1860*, New York University Press, New York (1962).
10. Kett, J. *The Formation of the American Medical Profession: The Role of Institutions 1760–1860*, Yale University Press, New Haven (1968).
11. Flexner, A. *Medical Education in Europe*, Carnegie Foundation, New York (1912).
12. *California State Journal of Medicine*, Editorial, **11**, 41 (1913).
13. Blanton, W. B. *Medicine in Virginia in the Nineteenth Century*, Garrett and Massie, Richmond (1933).
14. Mumford, J. G. *A Narrative of Medicine in America*, Lippincott, Philadelphia (1903).

Rosemary Stevens is in the Department of History and Sociology of Science, University of Pennsylvania, though at the time of writing the article she was at Tulane University in Louisiana. The article has been edited from a longer version that appeared in 1976 in *Priorities in the Use of Resources in Medicine*, Number 40 in the Fogarty International Center Proceedings, published by the US Department of Health, Education and Welfare.

# 40
# Britain's health care experiment

## PATRICIA DAY AND RUDOLF KLEIN

Britain's National Health Service (NHS) is at once the envy of the world and its butt. It is the envy of the world because it provides, with remarkable parsimony, a comprehensive service to the entire population. The service is tax-financed and free at the point of delivery, with remarkably low administrative costs. It is the butt of the world because the NHS provides care that, if usually high in quality, is delivered in an often dreary environment to patients trained to defer to the discipline of the queue and service routines. Since its creation in 1948, the British health system has always been undercapitalised and dominated by providers, who have defined the needs of patients rather than responding to the demands of consumers.

On 1 April 1991, the changes in Britain's NHS first announced by Prime Minister Margaret Thatcher's government at the beginning of 1989 came into full effect.[1] They represent an attempt to demonstrate that it is possible to combine the advantages of the National Health Service model (financial parsimony and social equity) and those of a market system (responsiveness to consumer demands): to show that the acknowledged weaknesses of the NHS – such as provider paternalism and waiting lists – are not necessarily inherent in its design.

### Pressure for change

Since its birth in 1948, the NHS has always been perceived as being under-funded, a perception encouraged by those working in it. All governments, Labour as well as Conservative, have sooner or later incurred the charge of starving the NHS of resources. In this respect, the 1980s were no different. What distinguished the decade was that the perception of an NHS tottering on the edge of collapse became so intense and pervasive that it pushed the government into its review of the NHS and the subsequent programme of reform. The political price of successful cost containment had become too high. This rising sense of crisis can perhaps best be explained by the interaction between three sets of facts. First, there were the actual budgetary constraints on the NHS. Second, public expectations were rising, in the shape of greater demands for health care responsive to individual wants rather than professionally defined needs. Lastly, the government's attempts to satisfy rising demands within constrained budgets led to greater pressure on NHS providers to increase productivity.

### Budgetary constraints

The 1980s were a decade of financial austerity for the NHS. Continuing a trend set by the previous Labour government in the late 1970s, following a series of economic crises, the Conservatives kept health care spending on a tight rein.

No one disputed that demands were on the increase. Britain's population, as is that of the United States, is ageing; technological innovation is extending the scope for medical intervention; and unexpected tragedies, such as acquired immunodeficiency syndrome (AIDS), create new calls for extra spending. The issue that emerged during the 1980s was whether such demands required an annual increment of 2 per cent in the budget of the NHS as previously assumed, or whether growth in services could be financed in other ways. The view taken by the Thatcher government was that service expansion could be financed by increasing the efficiency with which existing resources were used within the NHS. Throughout the 1980s the NHS did improve efficiency, productivity, and outputs. Lengths-of-stay were cut; costs per acute case fell. The number of patients treated in hospitals rose by more than 20 per cent over the decade, a far higher figure than would have been expected from either spending trends or demographic changes.

### Increased demand for care

The rise in the provision of services in the 1980s went hand in hand with a mounting perception of inadequacy. Waiting lists obstinately refused to decline despite a series of special government initiatives designed to reduce them. By the end of the decade, almost one million people were in the queue – mainly for elective surgery – instead of the usual 700 000 or so.

More convincing, if still ambiguous, evidence of frustrated demand is provided by the expansion of the private health care sector.[2] The number of people covered by private insurance rose from three and one-half million at the start of the decade to almost six million at the end – roughly 10 per cent of the total population. Overwhelmingly, if not exclusively, the private acute sector deals with quality-of-life procedures, such as arthroplasties or hernia repairs, while leaving the NHS to cope with life-threatening or chronic conditions. So, on the one hand, almost 20 per cent of the former procedures are carried out in the private sector. But, on the other hand, even the privately insured population use NHS facilities for over half of their hospital stays.

It is, in short, precisely what might be expected if one assumes that the NHS, given resource constraints, gives priority to life-threatening conditions over intervention designed to enhance the quality of life. In this respect, the 1980s conformed to the pattern set in the earlier decades of the NHS's existence. What appears to have changed is the attitude of a growing section of the population that is less tolerant of queuing.

### Pressure on providers

This transformation, while potentially threatening to the medical profession, was, in turn, accelerated by the attitude of the profession itself. The measures taken by the government in the 1980s to increase NHS productivity were increasingly persuading the medical profession to exploit public discontent. Following the 1983 Griffiths Report, the managerial structure of the NHS was greatly strengthened.[3] Central government set a series of productivity targets for health authorities. The balance between managerial and professional authority began to shift toward the former. As managerial pressure on the medical profession increased, so did the latter's discontent.

The medical profession reacted by questioning the budgetary constraints within which it had to work and denouncing the inadequacy of the NHS. Medical indignation was translated, in turn, into public dissatisfaction with the NHS. The culminating point came late in 1987, when the presidents of the Royal Colleges, representing the prestigious specialists, issued a public statement warning that the NHS was facing ruin. This statement, it is said, so infuriated Thatcher that she announced her review of the NHS to the surprise of even her own ministers and civil servants – a review that, against all precedent, excluded the medical profession. So began the process that was to end in the introduction of the programme of change.

## A new set of incentives

The dilemma in which Thatcher and her advisers found themselves when they started their review of the NHS had one obvious solution: to devise a new method for funding health care in Britain in line with its own ideological commitment to rolling back the frontiers of the state. Urged on by many of its own supporters, the Thatcher government investigated the possibility of moving toward an insurance-based system on the German or French models. But, predictably enough, it rejected this option (Klein, 1985).[4]

One option, clearly, was simply to soldier on: to continue with the policies designed to improve productivity by strengthening the management of the NHS. To a large extent, this was precisely what happened. But there was one crucial new element: the revolutionary notion (in the British context) of splitting responsibility for buying health care from that of actually providing services. Hitherto, these had been combined. District Health Authorities (DHAs) had been funded for running the services within their own boundaries. If those living in a district sought their health care in neighbouring health authorities or in prestigious London teaching hospitals, the resulting transfers of money did not reflect real costs. In short, the system of NHS finance did not provide any incentives to increase productivity, since greater activity simply added to costs without bringing in any corresponding revenue.

Since April 1991, the system is radically different. The roles of purchaser and provider are separated. DHAs will be funded according to the size and demographic composition of their populations, not according to the services for which they are responsible. Their function will be to buy the best services they can from a variety of providers. The key principle is that money follows patients. Patients can be treated in the district's own hospitals, in other NHS hospitals, in the private sector, or in NHS hospital trusts, a new category created by the 1989 review that allows hospitals to turn themselves, under certain conditions, into self-governing trusts.[5] This status gives hospitals considerable freedom to determine their own policies and salary scales, as well as to raise capital, provided they attract enough patients to generate sufficient income.

Although much of the rhetoric of *Working for Patients* was about making the NHS 'more responsive to the needs of the patient', the reality in the case of hospital services stopped well short of allowing consumer demand to drive the service.[1] Managers will continue to define the needs of patients, explicitly so in the case of the DHAs, which are charged with determining the needs of their populations when drawing up their purchasing plans. Managers also will have greater responsibilities (and powers) for calling the medical profession to account for their use of public resources. Medical audit is to become compulsory. Future consultant contracts will specify in far greater detail what is expected from the job holder. Distinction awards to consultants, which may double their salaries and greatly enhance their pension entitlements, will in the future no longer be based on clinical excellence alone. Managers will have a voice in making the awards, taking into account the contribution of candidates to the work of the NHS.

This challenge to the autonomy of the medical profession, as much as its manner of production, helps to explain the violent reaction to *Working for Patients*. Not only had the profession been excluded from Thatcher's review; the Prime Minister chose those she consulted precisely because they were not representative of the profession. But the results of the review appeared to present a direct threat to it. It was no wonder, then, that the medical profession fought the implementation of government's proposals, prophesying that they would create chaos and confusion.

### Reforming the primary health care system

Every member of the [UK] population is registered with a general practitioner (GP) and, on average, makes about four visits a year. The GP is the gatekeeper to the expensive hospital sector and the patient's agent in the choice of route into the complexities of specialist care. The Thatcher government's interest in reforming primary health care predates its programme of change in the hospital sector. A number of concerns drove the engine of change: primary health care spending is demand-driven and thus difficult to control; powerful voices were arguing for action to improve the quality of general practice; and there was a feeling that GPs should be made accountable for their use of public resources.

These concerns largely shaped the government's first set of proposals [in 1986], which were designed to provide incentives to improve quality and to introduce a tighter system of accountability, thereby giving a larger and more active role to managers.[6] The proposals also introduced a new policy theme, reflecting the Thatcher government's bias toward consumerism and the market principle. Although the system of remuneration introduced in 1948 maintained the principle of capitation payment first introduced in 1911, at the birth of National Health Insurance, this principle was subsequently eroded. By the mid-1980s, therefore, only 46 per cent of GP income was derived from capitation. The Thatcher government decided this trend should be reversed. With list sizes falling, the danger was no longer that GPs would accumulate excessive numbers of patients, but that they would be indifferent or unresponsive to consumer demands. Hence, they should derive a higher proportion of their income, say 60 per cent, from capitation fees to give them an incentive to compete for patients.

The profession viewed two new proposals for change that emerged from the review as particularly threatening. First, the review brought in the notion of 'indicative drug budgets' for individual GP practices, that is, a budget ceiling for prescribing costs. Second, the review introduced the idea of GP practice budgets: practices with more than 11 000 patients (subsequently reduced to 9 000) could opt for a budget, out of which they would buy a range of diagnostic and hospital services for their patients.

The new contract symbolised the changed status of GPs: accountable, at last, for what they did and with explicit obligations to carry out certain contractual tasks.[7] Under the previous contract, GPs had defined their own obligations.

## Implementation: the short term impact

### Hospital services

The timetable of change allowed little more than two years between the announcement of the programme of reforms and getting new machinery running. The notion of splitting the purchaser and provider roles not only meant developing a new grammar and language of management. It also meant creating a database capable of generating the information needed to operate the new system. Traditionally, the NHS has been information-poor, if awash with statistics. But if doctors were to be held more accountable, it was necessary to know more precisely what they did. If the money was to follow patients, it was essential to know how much they cost. Thus, a massive investment was needed to develop the NHS's primitive information system.

Change is being implemented incrementally; both purchasers and providers are exploring their new roles tentatively and interpreting them variously; there is, in effect, a series of experiments, reflecting local circumstances and understanding of what should be done. The point can best be illustrated by looking at how the principle of separating the roles of purchasers and providers is being interpreted in practice. This principle represents the key element in the new NHS. Moreover, it has also encouraged the myth that Britain has adopted the US model of competition in the health care market. In the outcome, there is not going to be much competition or much of a market. British purchasers (that is, the DHAs) are mostly going to stick to the hospitals in their own or neighbouring districts that have traditionally produced services for their populations. Most of the purchaser/provider service agreements are block contracts designed to ensure continuity in the provision of health care.[8]

If the move toward competition is going to be, at most, incremental and marginal, much the same is true of the transformation of NHS hospitals into self-governing trusts. Few proposals in the government's reform package have encountered more opposition. Self-governing status has frequently been denounced as privatisation by another name. The freedom of trusts to negotiate their own terms of service for their employees, instead of being bound by national agreements, has been seen as a threat by professional as well as trade union bodies. Right to the end, the process of setting up trusts was accompanied by demonstrations and opposition, often orchestrated by the Labour Party. Surprisingly, for those who thought that such trusts could turn out to be worker cooperatives dominated by consultants, the medical profession has been split. As often as not, consultants have voted against opting to set up trusts when managers have tried to set them up. There is therefore every opportunity for testing out the model before it becomes generalized.

Rather than a sudden plunge into a competitive health care system, the NHS's 'internal market' for hospital care will be a special kind of market, with managers trading with each other and with the consumer conspicuous by his or her absence. Thus it is not competition that is going to distinguish the new-style NHS. Rather, it is the move from the notion of trust to one of contract. The crux of the purchaser/provider relationship is precisely that, for the first time ever, the nature of the services to be provided in the NHS will have to be defined in the contracts or service agreements made. In the context of the NHS culture, this move from the implicit to the explicit, from trust to contract, is truly revolutionary and has perhaps the farthest-reaching long-term implications.

*General practitioners*
What goes for hospital providers also applies to general practitioners. The first impact of changes in the NHS may, paradoxically and perversely, blunt the incentives to compete and limit consumer choice. Most immediately, and perhaps most importantly, the change has been a financial bonanza for many (perhaps most) GPs who were already vaccinating, immunising, and screening most of their patients before the contract introduced bonus payments for meeting specific targets. Similarly, GPs who practice in inner cities – and thus qualify for the special 'deprivation payments' introduced by the new contract – get extra compensation for the difficulties involved in reaching these targets when dealing with a mobile population. Add to this the surge in spending on subsidies to GPs for employing practice staff, 70 per cent of whose salaries are met out of the public purse up to a limit of two per practitioner, and it is clear that they have emerged from their battle with the government a great deal richer if not happier.

There will also be some opportunities for entrepreneurial GPs to add to their incomes by engaging in fee-for-service activities made possible by the new contract, notably minor surgery and health-promotion clinics. Overall, however, it is clear that most GPs will have no pressing reason to engage in competition for patients. Similarly, it is likely that the most contentious component in the government's package – the introduction of budget holding[9] for GPs – will also dampen competition. Specifically, budget holding permits GPs to shop around, on behalf of their patients, for the kind of diagnostic and elective procedures that are the core of the waiting list issue. At the same time, it gives them an incentive to deal with patients' problems themselves, instead of passing them onto the hospital service. Budget-holding GPs thus will be forced to examine the financial implications of their clinical decisions. This caused the BMA, as well as the Labour Party, to pronounce anathema on the whole concept. The judgment of GPs, it was argued, would become corrupted. Instead of thinking only about the patient, they would be worrying about their bottom line. They would exclude expensive patients from their lists.

However, some 300 practices became budget holders in April 1991 – roughly 10 per cent of those eligible [i.e. with at least 9000 registered patients] – and this number is likely to double in April 1992.[10] In part, it reflects a realisation among GPs that budget holding gives them power. Instead of being dependent on the goodwill of hospital consultants, the situation may be reversed: consultants may actually come to see them as valuable customers and woo them accordingly.

## Future indefinite

What will Britain's health care system look like by the end of the 1990s? No confident answer can be given to that question, given that the NHS operates in a turbulent and uncertain economic and political environment. If Britain's economy prospers, so will the NHS budget. Conversely, if the economy remains sluggish, health care will continue to be on short commons. In this respect, the Conservative changes have done nothing to diminish the service's financial vulnerability to political decisions taken in the light of the government's overall policies of economic management.

Even if 1 April 1991 has not marked an immediate transformation of the NHS as experienced by its consumers, what will happen as the changes work their way through the system? Regarding costs, it is clear that spending on administration in the NHS – hitherto an extraordinarily parsimonious system – has risen and will continue to do so. Apart from the investment in information technology, probably justified in terms of improving services for patients, there will be the extra costs of billing under the contract system. More intangibly, the move toward demanding greater accountability from the medical profession could backfire if it leads to sullen resentment. Although the NHS may have relied excessively in the past on the relationship of trust between doctors and managers, this still remains one of its greatest assets. Much will therefore depend on whether ministers and managers succeed in their efforts to smooth down the ragged tempers of the medical profession.

The move toward explicit contracts is, nevertheless, responsible for some of the most immediate benefits that are emerging. It has forced into the open issues that have remained undiscussed for forty years. Thus, there has been an upsurge of interest in how to specify quality and how to ensure its delivery. Similarly, there has been a new-found zeal for devising standards for patient treatment. This, indeed, is a transformation, even if it will take some time before the effects trickle down to the patients. Again, the emphasis on prevention and health promotion in GP contracts marks a radical shift in public policy, although some of the enthusiasm for regular checkups and screening may be a touch promiscuous. It is not quite clear that it will have the hoped-for effect on health outcomes. In all of these (and other) respects, the NHS has become more self-critical and self-aware. Nothing will ever be quite the same, therefore, even if the programme of reform were put into reverse or on hold.

But there remains the question of whether the new-style NHS – whatever improvements it may bring – will actually meet the aspirations of its creators: whether, to return to the argument we began with, it will combine the advantages of the national health service model (financial parsimony and social equity) with those of a market system (responsiveness to consumer demands). Here the verdict must be an open one. For what is most significant about the new-style NHS – and the point most frequently neglected in discussions about it – is that it actually incorporates two different models. While the hospital model is management-and-provider-led, the primary health care model is much more consumer-led. Even if competition is going to be mainly conspicuous by its absence in both models – except at the margins – the nature of the markets will be very different. In the hospital model, purchasers are proxy consumers, while in the primary health care model, GPs are proxy consumers.

The two models are incompatible in at least one crucial respect. The responsibility of purchasing authorities is to determine the health care needs of their populations and to buy services accordingly. This is very much in the paternalistic tradition of the

NHS; equity has always been defined in terms of experts identifying needs and allocating resources accordingly. In this sense, the hospital model represents the apotheosis of the health expert. In practice, of course, things will be much less tidy; health authorities will also have to provide quick fixes in response to political or consumer pressures. But, quite clearly, the model is at odds with the demand-led, primary health care model. For if responsibility for buying services is to be diffused among GPs, not in accordance with some ideal population-based strategy but in response to the needs (and pressures) of patients as interpreted by individual practitioners, then population-based health care planning is in tatters. To the extent that the achievement of equity does indeed depend on sticking to a needs-based model, then clearly it cannot be combined with a market based on a plurality of buyers. Conversely, to the extent that responsiveness to consumer demands depends on a plurality of buyers, it cannot be combined with equity based on giving a purchasing power monopoly to expertise. So which model will win out?

Clearly, the big battalions are on the side of the monopoly-purchaser, hospital model. Hospital consultants have been remarkably slow to realise the way that general practitioner budgets could tilt the balance of power toward primary health care. But together with the equally threatened hospital managers, they form a potentially powerful coalition. They might therefore be expected to seek to abort the GP budget-holding experiment by a mixture of outright opposition and pre-emptive change, by demonstrating their willingness to adapt their practices to GP demands.

Another consideration is pulling in the opposite direction – one at the heart of the debate that prompted the Thatcher government's plunge into reform in the first place. This is the question of which model is most likely to ensure financial control. Here, on the face of it, the hospital model is a clear winner. Once a purchaser has decided what services to buy, within the constraints of the existing budget, expenditure is eminently controllable. In contrast, the primary health care model – as yet untested, in any case – diffuses spending decisions among GPs with no experience of budgetary control or tradition of public accountability. So, in terms of financial control, there would appear to be no contest.

However, the balance of argument changes when we turn to political considerations. Here the strength of the hospital model turns out to be its weakness, while the converse is true of the primary health care model. In the past, resource allocation decisions in the NHS have been largely implicit – part of the concordat between state and profession, which has left the individual doctor to ration at the point of delivery. The new system, however, forces purchasers to be more explicit about what services will be provided for their populations. The purchasing authorities will have to give visibility to decisions about what to buy and, more important, what not to buy. While the concentration of financial power and decision making reinforces control, it also increases the risk of political embarrassment. Without intending to do so, the government may have created a system that will add to the pressures for more public expenditure on the NHS. Conversely, while the primary health care model is weaker on financial control, it diffuses the decision-making process. It makes the consequences of resource constraints much less visible and, in this respect, would mark a return to the traditional British approach of making rationing largely invisible by leaving it to individual physicians and disguising it as clinical decisions.

So, in effect, two quite different futures for the NHS are on offer, apart from the possibility of muddling through with an unresolved conflict at the heart of health care policy. One would represent a reversion to tradition, modified at the edges; the other would mean a more radical break with the past. The present mix, however, is likely to prove unstable. The way in which future governments jump will depend on a variety of factors: the outcome of the present experiments, political ideology and expediency, economic prospects, and the attitude of the medical profession. Only one prediction seems reasonably safe: that Britain's health care system will continue to change before it reaches a stable state.

## References and notes

1. Secretary of State for Health, *Working for Patients*, Cmd 555, HMSO, London (1989).
2. Laing and Buisson, *Laing's Review of Private Health Care 1989/90*, Laing and Buisson Publications Ltd, London (1990).
3. Griffiths, Sir Roy, *NHS Management Inquiry*, DHSS, London (the 'Griffiths Report') (1983).
4. Klein, R. 'Why Britain's Conservatives Support a Socialist Health Care System', *Health Affairs* (**Spring**), 41–59 (1985).
5. In fact, trust status has been awarded to a wide range of health services beyond those provided by hospitals (e.g. community health trusts).
6. Secretary of State for Social Services, *Primary Health Care: An Agenda for Discussion*, Cmd 9771, HMSO, London (1986).
7. General Medical Services Committee, *NHS Regulations* (October), British Medical Association, London (1989).
8. NHS Management Executive, *Contracts for Health Services: Operating Contracts*, HMSO, London (1990).
9. Budget holding is more frequently referred to as 'GP fund-holding'.
10. Editors note: by 1994, the number of general practices responsible for their own budgets in England had risen to more than 1200; between them they provided primary health care for over 12 million people.

Rudolf Klein is Professor of Social Policy, and Patricia Day is a Reader in Social Policy at the University of Bath. This is an edited version of their original article which was published in the Autumn of 1991 in *Health Affairs* (**Fall**), 40–59, a leading American health services journal. We have altered some words to conform to English spelling.

# 41

# Transferring power in health care

## FEDELMA WINKLER

### Introduction

The stimulus for the discussion of consumerism, in the 1980s, came not from users themselves but from governments. For governments with an individualistic/market philosophy a policy that centres on individual choice is populist. Consumerism can be a useful vehicle for legitimating changes in work practices and for safely challenging the professional power structures. This may be in users' interests, but it can also be a mechanism to ration resources, by enhancing managerial control over the spending power of professionals.

Whatever the intention, this is undoubtably why customer relations are on the agenda of managers in Britain. It has shaped the response and language. It is also why managerial consumerism is viewed by users with a healthy dose of cynicism.

### The managerial response to consumer challenge

Managers discussing consumerism are therefore like landowners discussing land reform. It is their response to a real or perceived challenge to their power.

The response from health care providers in the past to real or perceived challenge to their power has been very different. It has been the response of any group whose power is threatened. These responses can be categorised as hostility, neutralisation, manipulation, making common cause.

#### Opposition

One of the few user groups which posed a threat to provider power was the women's health movement. The response to their challenge, and to the professionals who supported them, was one of outright hostility and opposition, irrespective of the health care system. Women involved in the pressure for change reported very similar responses to their challenges in whichever society they lived. This is not surprising given the similarities in professional socialisation across national boundaries. The responses took the form of vilification, attempts to discredit, marginalisation, and gradually cosmetic changes at the edges of issues. They got invitations to choose the curtains not the staff.

When the women's health movement did apparently succeed, it was in areas where they supported the dominant interests of professionals, for example the various screening campaigns, or when they set up independent services outside the mainstream systems.

### Neutralisation through diversionary activity

Inviting users to participate in planning is the most common response to users' requests for involvement. It seems less of a threat to managers than involving them in monitoring existing services. The invitation is made after long discussions about who is a user, and how representative any particular group is. Concern is frequently expressed about making the group too large so the numbers of user representatives has to be limited.

On committees users find themselves heavily outnumbered by professionals. The agenda is set by managers. Meetings are arranged to facilitate the paid employees. The user who wants to participate may have to take time off work or pay for child care. Unlike the professionals, they have no access to technical or peer support. Asked to comment on proposals, users' views are ignored unless they support dominant views. Users are expected to have one clear view, while professions may disagree amongst themselves. When users challenge the dominant interest, they are accused of unrepresentativeness.[1]

### Manipulation of users' views to managers' advantage

Management-led consumerism has been translated into customer relations. One of the instruments used is consumer satisfaction surveys. Their production has become a growth industry. They concentrate on the boxes in which treatments are packaged. Whether the questions are asked in Washington or London, the answers are very similar. Patients want a clean organised environment and palatable food, the hotel services that direct payment systems invest in.[2]

This activity has other functions than finding out what is already known. It enables the manager to demonstrate activity, to challenge professionals in the name of patient interests. It enables managers to join the doctors, nurses and trade unionists in claiming to represent patients' interests. If the manager does not like the results of a survey or finds it inconvenient, there are always easy ways of discrediting it – the methodology was flawed, the situation has changed.

Throughout the patient remains passive. The questionnaires are initiated by managers, questions are devised by managers and can be used by managers in battles with other interested parties.

### Sharing power

Some professionals and managers do seek the moral high ground as enshrined in The World Health Organisation's Alma Alta Declaration which proclaimed that

> The people have the right and duty to participate individually and collectively in the planning and implementation of their health care.[3]

So for these the search for ways involving users is an ongoing process and a struggle. Successful consumer initiatives need the support and commitment of professionals and managers. Professionals and managers often need considerable courage because siding with users can mean challenging other managers and professionals.

## Imperatives of consumerism

The principles which should form the cornerstone of consumerism are protection of the user and equality of access to services.

### Protection of users

The first step towards these principles must be to abandon the commercial analogies. Users of health care services are not like other buyers in the market place. Of course, we lack knowledge about the organisation, are ignorant about our own bodies, the status of carers, medical language, options for treatment. Most important, however, at the point of use we are often frightened or incapacitated. The fear and incapacitation may be short or long term. We have little option, but to trust the staff.

Patients' vulnerability must be recognised and protective mechanisms made central to the consumer's strategy.

### Equity of access

For many consumerism is synonymous with choice. Choice implies access. Social factors affect it. There is differential access between rural and urban populations, between differing income and age groups. The needs of acutely ill adults take priority over those with mental illness.

The ultimate test of any health care system is how accessible it is to its citizens and how equitable that access is. Measurement of access is a moral imperative for managers. The managerial imperatives on which to build consumerism are therefore:

- Abandon commercial analogies;
- Introduce measures to ensure equitable access;
- Make protection of users and promotion of human dignity key management goals.

All health care systems have the absence of these in common.

## Instruments for making consumerism real

### Rights

The aims of the organisation need to be clearly translated into statements of users rights.

Rights must be translated from the general principles to specific guarantees and shared with the users. In the most concerned institutions, users' rights are written into contract specification and can be as detailed as having facilities to shave daily, rights of access to telephones and uncensored mail. Contracts can also spell out the rights of patient advocates to visit and rights of patients' councils. I saw one contract which specified that not only must the facility be open to visits from relatives and advocates but the visits must be facilitated by the attitude of the staff. It is this attention to detail that guarantees patients' rights.

In the reorganisation of the National Health Service newly autonomous hospitals are trying to insert loyalty clauses in contracts to prevent staff raising issues that concern them publicly. The response from the Royal College of Nursing is to set up a whistle blower's hotline, a confidential telephone line for nurses to report their concerns.

Less than one quarter of the Health Authorities in Britain give guidelines to staff about how to raise issues of concern. Few actively encourage, let alone mandate staff, to report cases of suspected abuse.

The code of ethics for doctors in Britain even makes it a breach to 'disparage the professional skills, knowledge, qualifications or service of other doctors'. Managers do not even have a written code of ethics.

## Information

Information has a central role in informing people of their rights and protecting patients, in improving access to services and in redistributing power between providers and users.

Health care agencies are spending large sums of money on management information systems. In contrast, few resources are allocated to developing information packages for patients. Much of what is produced aims to market services or to gain compliance, not to empower users.[4]

Users lack knowledge about the availability of services, about clinical policies and above all about the quality of care and competencies of staff. Without this information, users cannot take responsibility for their own health decisions.

Institutions consider that they own the information. Sharing it means giving up a degree of power. Making information available, for example, on the success rates of particular procedures such as cardiovascular surgery would require not just the rates but supporting information on the criteria for the selection of patients. This requires an openness and a clarity of policy that is not currently characteristic of health care structures. It also requires a recognition that not all professionals have the same degree of competencies. Insiders use privileged information to select their therapist. Ways need to be found to systematise what is commonly called 'inside' information and share it with all users.

## Advocacy

The formulation of people's rights are important, but ensuring implementation is essential. Advocacy has a vital role to play in the implementation of rights and in making information available to users at point of impact.

Advocacy schemes were set up to empower users and to protect the weak. They were to do this through establishing and giving rights to users' representatives. In some countries, these schemes have been given legal backing, in others rights are locally negotiated. In all, the independence of the advocate from service deliverers is seen as crucial. Structurally, they must be located to aid identification with users. Access to information, to facilities, to users, and to the policy decision-making apparatus are crucial to their success.

The benefits of an advocacy scheme do not of course just go to users. They are a source of information for the manager, they are crucial to the development of bottom-up policy and they prevent or minimise patients' grievances.

*Redress systems*

A user-sensitive complaints and redress system is essential for any organisation which prides itself on the quality of its service. Complaints procedures are also an integral element of consumerism. The essential components of a good complaints procedure are accessibility, fairness, independence, power to rectify the problem and the right to trigger an independent review.

Most people feel inhibited to complain about personal service. The majority of dissatisfied people do not complain. A low complaints rate may not be the sign of a good service, but rather of an inaccessible or distrusted complaints procedure. I work for an agency that in five years had found the behaviour of only one family doctor unsatisfactory. This in no way reflected the quality of the service. Rather it reflected the interpretation by the organisation of what constituted a complaint. The interpretation was given to the organisation by professionals anxious to protect at all cost their own members. The complaints procedure was distrusted even by those working inside the organisation. A reformed procedure upheld complaints against three of the next five doctors it investigated. All of the complainants expressed surprise. They expected the doctors to be protected and had only pursued the complaints out of desperation.

Staff must have support and training in dealing with challenging comment not personal censure. An understanding of complainants' motivation could help make complaints less threatening. Staff's first response is often defensive with a tendency to blame the complainant. Yet altruism is frequently a factor in complaints. Complainants want to remedy a situation so that other people do not suffer. To gain access to information is another common reason. Compensation and desire for revenge can of course be the motivation but less frequently than staff think.

*Representation*

Representation is one aspect of consumerism that gives managers much angst. They enter into debates about who is the consumer, are they representative, how much information should they be given, can they be trusted to define their own needs?

Representation begins at the point of impact. Users should not have to stand alone right-less and unrepresented at the point of taking major decisions about their lives. Hence, the importance of information availability, advocacy and a culture of powersharing amongst deliverers of services.

These form the foundation for an informed representative movement. At the collective level more is required. Representation does not just happen. Resources have to be invested in providing support for representatives. Access to a panel of independent technical advisers needs to be established and facilities for training need to be available. Consumers must not go naked to the conference table.

The early 1970s saw the establishment of Community Health Councils, a national network of government funded agencies to represent users' interests in Britain. Their success has been mixed. They were handicapped by lack of information, technical advisers, resources and lack of accountability to their communities. They were a brave experiment and can teach us about representative or intermediary agencies.

Community Health Councils were most successful in areas of care easily understood by lay people. So their best work has been in representing the interests of people in long-stay hospitals. They were least successful in areas where clinical/technical expertise was at a premium. For this reason their contribution to the debate on rationing health services and defining needs has been largely confined to supporting medical and nursing demands for more resources. They also experienced most hostility when they became involved in clinical areas. Few managers or professionals welcomed their challenge, weak though it was, to their power.[5]

They were and are a vehicle for lay people concerned with health care issues to be involved with influencing, at however minimal a level, health care. They created a knowledgeable cadre of lay people prepared to challenge conventional power structures.

Representation must begin at point of use and be an integral part of the service. Managers must see that it is in their interests as well as in the interests of the users.

It means power holders sharing power with lay people, giving guarantees to deliver services according to the wishes of the community enabling them to participate in decisions about the allocation of resources and most importantly in monitoring services. It will be for each of us to find the path to popular democracy appropriate to our communities. Managers have yet to learn to value community involvement and to learn to use it for the benefit of the service and community.

Equally important, representation in health care should not be measured against some absolute 'Holy Grail' of representativeness. If so, it can only be found to be inadequate. Representation in health care will reflect the degree of involvement of citizens in all other areas of the democratic process. The inadequacy of the instruments should not be an excuse for not trying to seek ways of making it meaningful.

*Culture of the organisation*
The tendency of organisations to meet the needs of those who work within them, rather than the people they are supposed to serve is an international truism. Committed managers do not leave to chance the organisational responsibility for users' rights.

Ensuring that the organisation pulsates with commitment to its users and the community in which it is placed is the most important task of senior management. There is a lot of discussion about the need for a culture committed to users. There is little discussion about ways of involving users in creating this.

Doctors and nurses have convinced the public they have their individual patients' interests at heart. Managers have yet to convince their community that their first concern is the dignity and protection of patients' rights. Willingness to audit the openness of their institutions, to invest funds to aid the patient's voice would considerably increase credibility.

There are inspiring examples to be found where institutions have set about the process of turning themselves from provider-led to user-led services. The lessons are that it is a slow process, requiring total commitment from senior staff, a re-orientation of some staff and the liberation of others.

## Conclusions

The challenge from consumers themselves to managerial power has to date been relatively muted. There is a paucity of institutions, social and political, to represent users' interests. This is in contrast to the powerful establishments that represent the interests of professionals, managers and workers. The progress of consumerism through the 1970s, was described as crablike. It grew out of a philosophy that it was important to involve communities in decision making.

The 1980s was manager-led in response to political demands. It left us with, at its best, a customer relations definition of consumerism that relied on tokenism, or at its worst the market place philosophy of 'let the buyer beware'.

The 1990s will undoubtedly bring additional and different challenges – facilities owned and managed by the people who use them will be one such challenge. This in nascent form is already with us – users bidding for contracts to provide services for their members.

Managers in the future may well be judged by the degree to which they have involved users in decision making, and how accessible they have made information about decision making to the community and the users. Their performance may be measured on the degree to which they have taken users' views on board in policy making.

It would be a shame if this was seen as a threat and not an opportunity. Rights charters, information systems, advocacy schemes and accessible redress procedures are bits of the jigsaw to aid the empowerment of users. Managers now have the opportunity, the political backers and hence the power to put the jigsaw together and bind it with a culture committed to providing user-sensitive services.

That this involves transference of power needs to be recognised. Only when consumerist managers are the norm will we be able to speak of a partnership in care.

## References

1. Bold, M. 'Consultation forums with carers', pp. 29–40, in Winn L. (ed.) *Power to the People*, King's Fund, London (1990).
2. Winn, L. 'The arrival of consumerism', in Paine L. (ed.) *British Hospital Management*, Sterling Publications (1991).
3. World Health Organisation and United Nations Children's Fund, *Primary Health Care: International Conference on Primary Health Care*, Alma Alta, USSR (1978).
4. Winkler, F. 'Consumerism and information' in Winn, L. (ed.), *Power to the People*, King's Fund, London (1990).
5. Winkler, F. 'Can CHCs empower users?', *Radical Community Medicine*, Summer (1986).

This article was adapted by the author from a conference presentation and appeared in the 'Reader Supplement for *Dilemmas in Health Care*', distributed to Open University students studying the course *Health and Disease* in 1993. It has not been previously published elsewhere. Fedelma Winkler is the Director of Service Planning and Development at Barking and Havering Family Health Services Authority.

# 42
# The village health worker: lackey or liberator?

DAVID WERNER

Throughout Latin America, the programmed use of health auxiliaries has, in recent years, become an important part of the new international push of 'community oriented' health care. But in Latin America village health workers are far from new. Various religious groups and non-government agencies have been training *promotores de salud* or health promoters for decades. And to a large (but diminishing) extent, villagers still rely, as they always have, on their local *curanderos*, herb doctors, bone setters, traditional midwives and spiritual healers. More recently, the *médico practicante* or empirical doctor has assumed in the villages the same role of self-made practitioner and prescriber of drugs that the neighborhood pharmacist has assumed in larger towns and cities.

Until recently, however, the respective Health Departments of Latin America have either ignored or tried to stamp out this motley work force of non-professional healers. Yet the Health Departments have had trouble coming up with viable alternatives. Their Western-style, city-bred and city-trained MDs not only proved uneconomical in terms of cost effectiveness; they flatly refused to serve in the rural area. The first official attempt at a solution was, of course, to produce more doctors. In Mexico the National University began to recruit 5,000 new medical students per year (and still does so). The result was a surplus of poorly trained doctors who stayed in the cities.

The next attempt was through compulsory social service. Graduating medical students were required (unless they bought their way off) to spend a year in a rural health center before receiving their licenses. The young doctors were unprepared either by training or disposition to cope with the health needs in the rural area. With discouraging frequency they became resentful, irresponsible or blatantly corrupt. Next came the era of the mobile clinics. They, too, failed miserably. They created dependency and expectation without providing continuity of service. The net result was to undermine the people's capacity for self care. It was becoming increasingly clear that provision of health care in the rural area could never be accomplished by professionals alone. But the medical establishment was – and still is – reluctant to crack its legal monopoly.

At long last, and with considerable financial cajoling from foreign and international health and development agencies, the various health departments have begun to train and utilize auxiliaries. Today, in countries where they have been given half a chance, auxiliaries play an important role in the health care of rural and periurban communities. And if given a whole chance, their impact could be far greater. But, to a large extent, politics and the medical establishment still stand in the way.

## Rural health projects

My own experience in rural health care has mostly been in a remote mountainous sector of Western Mexico, where, for the past twelve years I have been involved in training local village health workers, and in helping foster a primary health care network, run by the villagers themselves. As the villagers have taken over full responsibility for the management and planning of their program, I have been phasing out my own participation to the point where I am now only an intermittent advisor. This has given me time to look more closely at what is happening in rural health care in other parts of Latin America.

Last year a group of my co-workers and I visited nearly forty rural health projects, both government and non-government, in nine Latin American countries (Mexico, Guatemala, Honduras, El Salvador, Nicaragua, Costa Rica, Venezuela, Colombia and Ecuador). Our objective has been to encourage a dialogue among the various groups, as well as to try to draw together many respective approaches, methods, insights and problems into a sort of field guide for health planners and educators, so we can all learn from each other's experience. We specifically chose to visit projects or programs which were making significant use of local, modestly trained health workers or which were reportedly trying to involve people more effectively in their own health care.

We were inspired by some of the things we saw, and profoundly disturbed by others. While in some of the projects we visited, people were in fact regarded as a resource to control disease, in others we had the sickening impression that disease was being used as a resource to control people. We began to look at different programs, and functions, in terms of where they lay along a continuum between two poles: community supportive and community oppressive.

## Community supportive programs or community oppressive programs?

*Community supportive programs*, or functions, are those which favorably influence the long-range welfare of the community, that help it stand on its own feet, that genuinely encourage responsibility, initiative, decision making and self-reliance at the community level, that build upon human dignity.

*Community oppressive programs*, or functions, are those which, while invariably giving lip service to the above aspects of community input, are fundamentally authoritarian, paternalistic or are structured and carried out in such a way that they effectively encourage greater dependency, servility and unquestioning acceptance of outside regulations and decisions; those which in the long run are crippling to the dynamics of the community.

It is disturbing to note that, with certain exceptions, the programs which we found

**Table 42.1** Primary health workers in Latin America

| Auxiliary nurses or health technicians | Health promoters or village health workers |
|---|---|
| At least primary education plus 1–2 years' training | Average of 3rd grade education plus 1–6 months' training |
| Usually from outside the community | Usually from the community and selected by it |
| Usually employed full time | Often a part time health worker supported in part by farm labor or with help from the community |
| Salary usually paid by the program (not by the community) | |
| | May be someone who has already been a traditional healer |

to be more community supportive were small non-government efforts, usually operating on a shoestring and with a more or less sub-rosa status. As for the large regional or national programs – for all their international funding, top-ranking foreign consultants and glossy bilingual brochures portraying community participation – we found that when it came down to the nitty-gritty of what was going on in the field, there was usually a minimum of effective community involvement and a maximum of dependency-creating handouts, paternalism and superimposed, initiative destroying norms.

## Primary health workers

In our visits to the many rural health programs in Latin America, we found that primary workers come in a confusing array of types and titles. Generally speaking, however, they fall into two groups (Table 42.1).

In addition to the health workers just described, many Latin American countries have programs to provide minimal training and supervision of traditional midwives. Unfortunately, Health Departments tend to refer to these programs as 'Control de Parteras Empíricas' ('Control of Empirical Midwives') – a terminology which too often reflects an attitude. Thus to Mosquito Control and Leprosy Control has been added Midwife Control. (Small wonder so many midwives are reticent to participate!) Once again, we found the most promising work with village midwives took place in small non-government programs. In one such program the midwives had formed their own club and organized trips to hospital maternity wards to increase their knowledge.

## Key questions

*What skills can the village health worker perform? How well does he perform them? What are the limiting factors that determine what he can do?* These were some of our key questions when we visited different rural health programs.

We found that the skills which village health workers actually performed varied enormously from program to program. In some, local health workers with minimal formal education were able to perform with remarkable competence a wide variety of skills embracing both curative and preventive medicine as well as agricultural extension, village cooperatives and other aspects of community education and mobilization. In other programs – often those sponsored by Health Departments – village workers were permitted to do discouragingly little. Safeguarding the medical profession's monopoly on curative medicine by using the standard argument that prevention is more important than cure (which it may be to us but clearly is not to a mother when her child is sick), instructors often taught these health workers fewer medical skills than many villagers had already mastered for themselves. This sometimes so reduced the people's respect for their health worker that he (or usually she) became less effective, even in preventive measures.

In the majority of cases, we found that external factors, far more than intrinsic factors, proved to be the determinants of what the primary health worker could do. We concluded that *the great variation in range and type of skills performed by village health workers in different programs has less to do with the personal potentials, local conditions or available funding than it has to do with the preconceived attitudes and biases of health program planners, consultants and instructors.* In spite of the often repeated eulogies about 'primary decision making by the communities themselves', seldom do the villagers have much, if any, say in what their health worker is taught and told to do.

## The political context

The limitations and potentials of the village health worker – what he is permitted to do and, conversely, what he could do if permitted – can best be understood if we look at his role in its social and political context. In Latin America, as in many other parts of the world, poor nutrition, poor hygiene, low literacy and high fertility help account for the high morbidity and mortality of the impoverished masses. But as we all know, the underlying cause – or more exactly, the primary disease – is inequity: inequity of wealth, of land, of educational opportunity, of political representation and of basic human rights. Such inequities undermine the capacity of the peasantry for self care. As a result, the political/economic powers-that-be assume an increasingly paternalistic stand, under which the rural poor become the politically voiceless recipients of both aid and exploitation. In spite of national, foreign and international gestures at aid and development, in Latin America the rich continue to grow richer and the poor poorer. As anyone who has broken bread with villagers or slum dwellers knows only too well: *health of the people is far more influenced by politics and power groups, by distribution of land and wealth, than it is by treatment or prevention of disease.*

Political factors unquestionably comprise one of the major obstacles to a community supportive program. This can be as true for village politics as for national politics. However, the politico-economic structure of the country must necessarily influence the extent to which its rural health program is community supportive or not.

Let us consider the implications in the training and function of a primary health worker. If the village health worker is taught a respectable range of skills, if he is encouraged to think, to take initiative and to keep learning on his own, if his judgement is respected, if his limits are determined by what he knows and can do, if his supervision is supportive and educational, chances are he will work with energy and dedication, will make a major contribution to his community and will win his people's confidence and love. His example will serve as a role model to his neighbors, that they too can learn new skills and assume new responsibilities, that self-improvement is possible. Thus the village health worker becomes an internal agent-of-change, not only for health care, but for the awakening of his people to their human potential ... and ultimately to their human rights.

However, in countries where social and land reforms are sorely needed, where oppression of the poor and gross disparity of wealth is taken for granted, and where the medical and political establishments jealously covet their power, it is possible that the health worker I have just described knows and does and thinks too much. Such men are dangerous! They are the germ of social change.

So we find, in certain programs, a different breed of village health worker is being molded ... one who is taught a pathetically limited range of skills, who is trained not to think, but to follow a list of very specific instructions or 'norms', who has a neat uniform, a handsome diploma and who works in a standardized cement block health post, whose supervision is restrictive and whose limitations are rigidly predefined. Such a health worker has a limited impact on the health and even less on the growth of the community. He – or more usually she – spends much of her time filling out forms.

In a conference I attended in Washington in 1980 on Appropriate Technology in Health in Developing Countries, it was suggested that *'Technology can only be considered appropriate if it helps lead to a change in the distribution of wealth and power.'* If our goal is truly to get at the root of human ills, must we not also recognize that, likewise, health projects and health workers are appropriate only if they help bring about a healthier distribution of wealth and power?

## Prevention

We say prevention is more important than cure. But how far are we willing to go? Consider diarrhea: each year millions of peasant children die of diarrhea. We tend to agree that most of these deaths could be prevented. Yet diarrhea remains the number one killer of infants in Latin America and much of the developing world. Does this mean our so-called 'preventive' measures are merely palliative? At what point in the chain of causes which makes death from diarrhea a global problem are we coming to grips with the real underlying cause? Do we do it ...

  ... by preventing some deaths through treatment of diarrhea?
  ... by trying to interrupt the infectious cycle through construction of latrines and
    water systems?
  ... by reducing high risk from diarrhea through better nutrition?
  ... or by curbing land tenure inequities through land reform?

Land reform comes closest to the real problem. But the peasantry is oppressed by far more inequities than those of land tenure. Both causing and perpetuating these crushing inequities looms the existing power structure: local, national, foreign and multinational. It includes political, commercial and religious power groups as well as the legal profession and the medical establishment. In short it includes ... ourselves. As the ultimate link in the causal chain which leads from the hungry child with diarrhea to the legalized inequities of those in power, we come face to face with the tragic flaw in our otherwise human nature, namely *greed*.

Where, then, should prevention begin? Beyond doubt, anything we can do to minimize the inequities perpetuated by the existing power structure will do far more to reduce high infant mortality than all our conventional preventive measures put together. We should, perhaps, carry on with our latrine-building rituals, nutrition centers and agricultural extension projects. But let's stop calling it prevention. We are still only treating symptoms. And unless we are very careful, we may even be making the underlying problem worse . . . through increasing dependency on outside aid, technology and control.

But this need not be the case. *If* the building of latrines brings people together and helps them look ahead, *if* a nutrition center is built and run by the community and fosters self-reliance, and *if* agricultural extension, rather than imposing outside technology encourages internal growth of the people toward more effective understanding and use of their land, their potentials and their rights . . . then, and only then, do latrines, nutrition centers and so-called extension work begin to deal with the real causes of preventable sickness and death.

### The village health worker

This is where the village health worker comes in. It doesn't matter much if he spends more time treating diarrhea than building latrines. Both are merely palliative in view of the larger problem. What matters is that he gets his people working together.

Yes, the most important role of the village health worker is preventive. But preventive in the fullest sense, in the sense that he helps put an end to oppressive inequities, in the sense that he helps his people, as individuals and as a community, liberate themselves not only from outside exploitation and oppression, but from their own short-sightedness, futility and greed.

The chief role of the village health worker, at his best, is that of liberator. This does not mean he is a revolutionary (although he may be pushed into that position). His interest is the welfare of his people. And, as Latin America's blood-streaked history bears witness, revolution without evolution too often means trading one oppressive power group for another. Clearly, any viable answer to the abuses of man by man can only come through evolution, in all of us, toward human relations which are no longer founded on short-sighted self-interest, but rather on tolerance, sharing and compassion.

I know it sounds like I am dreaming. But the exciting thing in Latin America is that there already exist a few programs that are actually working toward making these things happen – where health care for and by the people is important, but where the main role of the primary health worker is to assist in the humanization or, to use Paulo Freire's term, *conscientización* of his people.

### Misconceptions

I shall try to clear up some common misconceptions. Many persons still tend to think of the primary health worker as a temporary second-best substitute for the doctor

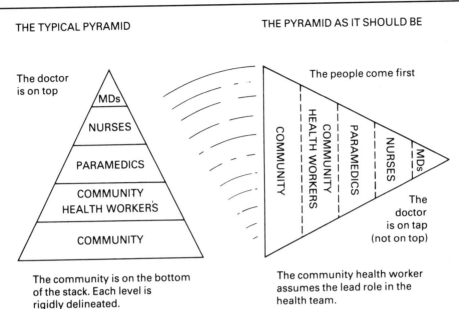

THE TYPICAL PYRAMID

The doctor is on top

The community is on the bottom of the stack. Each level is rigidly delineated.

THE PYRAMID AS IT SHOULD BE

The people come first

The doctor is on tap (not on top)

The community health worker assumes the lead role in the health team.

**Figure 42.1** Tipping the health manpower pyramid on its side.

... that, if it were financially feasible, the peasantry would be better off with more doctors and fewer primary health workers. I disagree. After twelve years working and learning from village health workers – and dealing with doctors – I have come to realize that the role of the village health workers is not only very distinct from that of the doctor, but, in terms of health and well-being of a given community, is far more important.

You may notice I have shied away from calling the primary health worker an 'auxiliary'. Rather I think of him as the primary member of the health team. Not only is he willing to work on the front line of health care, where the needs are greatest, but his job is more difficult than that of the average doctor. And his skills are more varied. Whereas the doctor can limit himself to diagnosis and treatment of individual 'cases', the health worker's concern is not only for individuals – as people – but with the whole community. He must not only answer to his people's needs but he must also help them look ahead, and work together to overcome oppression and to stop sickness before it starts. His responsibility is to share rather than hoard his knowledge, not only because informed self-care is more health conducing than ignorance and dependence, but because the principle of sharing is basic to the well-being of man.

Perhaps the most important difference between the village health worker and the doctor is that the health worker's background and training, as well as his membership in and selection by the community, help reinforce his will to serve rather than bleed his people. This is not to say that the village health worker cannot become money-hungry and corrupt. After all, he is as human as the rest of us. It is simply to say that for the village health worker the privilege to grow fat off the illness and misfortune of his fellow man has still not become socially acceptable.

The day must come when we look at the primary health worker as the key member of the health team, and at the doctor as the auxiliary. The doctor, as a specialist in advanced curative technology, would be on call as needed by the primary health worker for referrals and advice. He would attend those 2–3 per cent of illnesses which lie beyond the capacity of an informed people and their health worker, and he even might, under supportive supervision, help out in the training of the primary health worker in that narrow area of health care called 'Medicine'.

Health care will only become equitable when the skills pyramid has been tipped on its side, so that the primary health worker takes the lead, and so that the doctor is on *tap* and not on *top* (Figure 42.1).

David Werner is an American biologist and Director of the Hesperian Foundation in California, who has spent many years living and working in Mexico. This article previously appeared in *Health Auxiliaries and the Health Team*, edited by Muriel Skeet and Katherine Elliott and published by Croom Helm (1978).

# 43

# Traditional Indian medicine in practice in an Indian metropolitan city

## A. RAMESH AND B. HYMA

Practitioners of traditional medicine represent a vast human resource outside the official health services. This study restricted itself to examining the size, distribution and the current social, economic and political status and practice characteristics of traditional practitioners in the city of Madras, India. In India there are two parallel systems of medicine, the modern system commonly referred to as allopathy and homeopathy, and the Ayurvedic, Siddha and Unani system of medicine, commonly known as [the] indigenous system. Naturopathy and Yoga also attract followers for their therapeutic values. Of the three indigenous systems of medicine, Ayurveda is used all over the country.[1] Siddha is extensively used in the southern state of Tamil Nadu and in the neighboring states.[2] The Unani system is used predominantly in areas of Muslim culture.[3]

The Government is committed to promote and develop the indigenous system of medicine along with the modern medicine. The indigenous system of medicine is practiced by a large number of hereditary medical practitioners and by persons trained in teaching institutions run by the State Governments and other approved bodies. India now has a large number of qualified practitioners of integrated medicine and an estimated total of 7,000–8,000 professionally qualified practitioners of Ayurveda, Siddha, Unani and homoeopathy are entering the profession every year.

Carl E. Taylor has estimated that 'in India organized health services provide only 10 per cent of the medical care. Another 10 per cent is provided by qualified physicians in towns and cities. The balance is split between home medical care and indigenous practitioners.'

Madras is the fourth largest city in India with a population of nearly 3 million (1977 estimate), in which approximately 30 per cent live in 1,200 slums and squatter settlements where the basic needs of these people are not fully satisfied. Madras is also one of the major centers of modern medicine in India, with its established medical schools, numerous hospitals (both private and public), nursing homes, clinics, dispensaries and medical practitioners (general and specialists, etc.). It is also one of the centers of traditional medicine where numerous Ayurveda, Siddha, Unani and homoeopathy practitioners, clinical and pharmacological research centers and other clinics and dispensaries (both private and public) are found scattered at various parts of the city.

A heavy concentration (more than 50 per cent of the total IMPs [Indigenous Medical Practitioners]) has occurred in the old residential highly populated areas of the city followed by significant numbers clustered in the old commercial and manufacturing sectors in the northern parts of the city. In the newly developed residential neighbour-hoods their numbers are very low, below 0.1 per cent.

## An analysis of the questionnaire survey

[A sample of 95 IMPs (private and registered), were interviewed by a detailed questionnaire.]

### System of practice
Though there are three major types, Ayurveda, Siddha and Unani, still a number of practitioners practiced integrated medicine. The survey showed that 36.4 per cent of the IMPs belong to Siddha System, followed by Ayurveda (36.4 per cent), Unani (10.4 per cent) and Integrated (20 per cent) which clearly indicates the importance of Siddha and Ayurveda systems in meeting the basic health care needs.

### Practitioners' personal dimensions
The bulk of [practitioners] were male. Only a handful were females in all the three systems. These practiced mainly integrated medicine specializing in gynecology and obstetrics. Two-thirds of the practitioners interviewed were found in the age group between 40 and 60. The low figure in the age group between 20–40 clearly indicated that fewer practitioners have entered the profession in recent years in the city.

Though most of the IMPs belonged to the Hindu religious community, a small proportion were Muslims. Further, a fifth of the Muslims practiced Siddha and Ayurveda systems rather than Unani which is favoured by Muslim culture. About a third of the practitioners had college education. More than 50 per cent of the IMPs were born and brought up in Madras City itself, but of these the bulk practice Siddha medicine. About 16 per cent of the practitioners had a rural background and another 10 per cent came from outside the State of Tamil Nadu. Most of the practitioners who came from outside the state are engaged in Ayurvedic practice, indicating that a strong base for Ayurveda exists outside the State of Tamil Nadu.

Nearly half of the practitioners interviewed entered the profession because of its tradition within the family. A small proportion (15 per cent) of the practitioners indicated that some of their relatives also practiced Indian indigenous medicine.

### Practice
Most of the practitioners had not changed their location of practice since their reg-istration, indicating either the stability of their practice or lack of other alternatives! The location seems to be either older populated residential areas or economically viable areas. However, a quarter of the practitioners had their clinics in areas where they acquired them through hereditary practices. The high class and upper middle

class neighbourhoods did not seem to attract the IMPs. Further, the middle income group were concentrated mainly in the residential areas in the old congested parts of the city.

The general procedure (in contrast with modern medical practices) is to spend 10–20 minutes (25 per cent of the practitioners) or 20–40 minutes (35 per cent) per patient per day. In other words, this norm confirmed previous findings that 'the more traditional an indigenous medical practitioner was in his approach to diagnosis and treatment, the more likely he was to spend more than 10 minutes with a given patient.'

Most of the practitioners settled their fees with the patients at the time of each visit. A few of the patients received treatment on credit. The practitioners charge for their service on the ability of their clients to pay rather than conforming to fixed consultation fees.

*Diagnostic methods*
Few of the IMPs exhibited modern medical instruments such as stethoscopes, thermometers, blood pressure apparatus, syringes and needles. These were used mainly by those who practiced integrated medicine. These practitioners also occasionally sent their patients for laboratory tests for blood, stools, urine and X-rays. About 30 per cent said they performed minor surgery like stitching, incising or dressing wounds, etc. A quarter would not treat any cases relating to minor surgery.

Most of the IMPs use physical examination such as viewing the patient's body, touching and eliciting information by questioning. It appeared that nearly 50 per cent of the practitioners use pulse rates, 32 per cent diagnose by eye examination and 25 per cent by examination of hair and ears. However, pathological methods of diagnosis seem to still play a less important role in their method of practice.

*Prescription of medicine*
Less than 15 per cent of the practitioners said they prescribe Indian medicine as well as allopathy medicine. Nearly two-thirds of them said they prescribe only indigenous medicine. There were no responses from the rest. The prescription of medicine seems to be influenced to some extent by the hereditary formulae for preparing local herbs, powders, minerals, etc. and by local cultural knowledge and concepts related to the prevalent diseases in the area. Many methods and techniques employed are closely guarded secrets.

*Specialization*
There were some clear indications of the kinds of cases which the practitioners preferred to treat. Most of the practitioners were of the view that all types of diseases could be treated by indigenous medicine. In the most commonly treated diseases noted in our survey, ailments like coughs, diarrhoea, dysentery, fever, indigestion, etc. [were] given primary importance (by 80 per cent of the practitioners) followed by skin disorders (45 per cent of the IMPs treated these), ulcer (50 per cent), nervous disorders (42 per cent), rheumatism (24 per cent) and lung and bronchial ailments (24 per cent). About 5–6 per cent of the practitioners claimed that they can treat specific cases like anaemia, arthritis, colics, cellulitis, dermatitis, diabetes, jaundice, obesity, rheumatism, sexual disorders, menstrual disorders, mental diseases, children's diseases, infertility, impotence, etc.

There appears to be little formal specialization, in contrast with modern medicine. A handful of practitioners, however, claimed that they have developed special formulae in treating specific ailments like rheumatism, arthritis, children's diseases, skin diseases, etc. About 5 per cent claimed that they practiced witchcraft and black magic. However, there are no clear records of potent medicines and their effects on patients. No written records or files were maintained by the practitioners. Those few who did maintain some records were reluctant to produce them. So valuable information on types of diseases treated and the associated medicaments used is often lacking or unavailable to assess the efficacy of treatment.

## Discussion

The indigenous medical systems still remain a significant contributor to medical care of the people not only in rural areas but also in the cities. All three [systems] seem to provide fairly satisfactory solutions for common local ailments. However, observations indicate that in Madras city, Ayurvedic institutions and clinics in general continue to enjoy more public support than Siddha and Unani. The proportion of the total urban population receiving Ayurvedic care has steadily increased as evidenced by an increase in the sale of its popular products as well as expansion of some of its dispensaries.

Lack of standardized training and qualification of the practitioners is still evident, even though a large number are entering the profession every year. All grades and levels of training, with different knowledge, skills and sophistication of practice exist in the city. Most of the practitioners operate in isolation and their bargaining power is weak. This may be partly due to their inability or failure to form effective associations or societies or to belong to those few in existence so as to improve the quality of their services as well as to protect their interests.

Adoption of modern scientific and technical methods of practice is very incomplete. Techniques for preparation and preserving medical remedies are not standardized or inspected closely. Absence of toxicological and pharmacodynamic analysis is noted except for those conducted on a small scale in a handful of government and private research clinics and laboratories.

In the informal sector of the city, many of the IMPs seem much more secure and confident and continue to offer a useful public service in the city. Though not all IMPs may be suited for integration into modern health care organizations, certainly a sizeable number may be eligible for incorporation. Even where there is competition from modern practitioners in the same community, these IMPs are able to maintain stable practices and enjoy social prestige if not great economic prosperity. A number of favorable factors support them: they charge less for their services; they are located in centers where effective demand for their services still exists; they provide many dietary prescriptions which are expected by people of Indian culture when they are ill.

All indications are that indigenous medical systems will probably continue to provide services as long as the central and state governments continue to sponsor the indigenous systems officially. At present indigenous medical services freely cut across all socio-economic groups as well as rural and urban areas. However, they still continue to occupy an insignificant position under the programmes for health planning in the states. The possibility of bringing Indian medical practitioners into the national/

regional/local health care programmes needs to be continually evaluated especially in view of the shortages of trained health personnel to provide services for the development of rural as well as urban health care systems.

Strong governmental commitment, support and planning for this system are still lacking. State aid to institutions, dispensaries and private practitioners still remains a minor part of total health expenditures. The status of many of the private practitioners remains economically backward compared to allopathic doctors. Male domination to some extent may limit direct female access to health care in this system.

Given proper understanding, publicity and financial support, traditional systems of medicine can play a vital role in a country's health care delivery programmes. Understanding the complementarity of functions between the modern and the traditional medicine also awaits further exploration and research in the Indian urban setting.

This brings us to a final question as to whether one should advance the development of a dual health care system from which patients can select modern or traditional health services or an integrated system, where it is certain that traditional systems would occupy a subordinate role and lose their individual cultural heritage characteristics. This policy-implementation decision continues to pose a dilemma to many governments of developing nations.[4,5]

## Notes and references

1. Ayurveda is the traditional Hindu system of medicine based on Vedic scriptures; it utilizes herbs, minerals and diet restrictions in treatment of illnesses [and dates from] some time during the fifth century BC.
2. Siddha system of medicine in Tamil Nadu: this system is considered as an independent entity. Its antiquity is well recognized. The exact period of its origin is not known (some claim that it existed before [the] Vedic period). The therapeutics of Siddha medicine consist mainly of the use of metals and minerals, whereas in the earlier Ayurvedic texts there is no mention of metals. It has, however, many similarities with Ayurvedic medicine. It uses also products of vegetable and animal origins.
3. The Unani system, also known as the Greek/Arab system of medicine, brought into India by the Muslim conquerors, has also been in use for several hundred years. It uses herbs, minerals and metallic salts.
4. Birchman, W. 'Primary health care and traditional medicine – considering the background of changing health care concepts in Africa', Social Science and Medicine, 13B, 175 (1979).
5. Dunlop, D. W. 'Alternatives to "Modern" health delivery system in Africa: public policy issues of traditional health systems', Social Science and Medicine, 9, 581 (1975).

Professor A. Ramesh is Chairman of the Department of Geography in the University of Madras and B. Hyma is in the Department of Geography in the University of Waterloo, Canada. The article has been edited from a longer version that appeared in Social Science and Medicine, 15, 69–81, published by Pergamon Press, Oxford, UK (1981).

# 44

# A short cut to better services: day surgery in England and Wales

## THE AUDIT COMMISSION

### Introduction and background

Hospital patients may be classified into three main categories, in-patients, out-patients and day cases.

In-patients stay in hospital overnight. Out-patients come for minor procedures, investigations or consultations and leave as soon as they are over. Day cases do not stay in hospital overnight, but do need to stay for a short time after a procedure for recovery. Typically, day-case patients would stay in hospital for a morning or an afternoon. Exceptionally they might need to stay for the whole of the working day.

Day-case patients attend hospital at a pre-arranged time following an out-patient consultation, and know in advance what needs to be done. In contrast, 50 per cent of in-patients are emergency admissions. In England in 1985 (the latest year for which published data which specify operations are available) 794,000 operations and procedures were carried out as day cases. The 10 most frequent day-case procedures account for over 50 per cent of the total (Figure 44.1). Gastroscopy alone accounts for 15 per cent.

There are other procedures such as hernia repair, varicose vein surgery, cataract extraction and arthroscopy, which:

- are suitable for day surgery;
- are currently carried out extensively on in-patients;
- have long waiting lists.

This study is primarily concerned with the scope for more day surgery. There are also many medical procedures, such as some chemotherapy for cancer, for which a day-case setting is the most appropriate. In both cases substitution for in-patient care is likely to offer benefits to patients, such as shorter waiting times, and considerable potential for improved economy, efficiency and effectiveness.

Day surgery has been practised safely in this country for many years. Nicoll, a

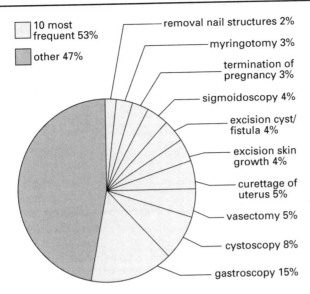

**Figure 44.1** The 10 most frequent day-case procedures accounted for over 50 per cent of day cases in England in 1985 (data from OPCS, 1985, *Hospital In-patient Enquiry*). [Myringotomy is an incision to drain fluid from the inner ear; three procedures use miniaturised viewing instruments ('scopes') to see inside different parts of the body – the rectum and large bowel (sigmoidoscopy), the bladder (cystoscopy), and the stomach (gastroscopy); curettage of the uterus is to remove excessive build-up of the lining of the womb; vasectomy creates a permanent obstruction of the tubes along which sperm travel from the testicles.]

surgeon in Glasgow, performed day surgery as early as 1906. But until the late 1960s, surgeons practising day surgery were lone pioneers. Interest in it from both managers and clinicians has increased considerably over recent years.[1]

Hospital expenditure on day cases, both medical and surgical, amounted to some £100 m in England and Wales in 1988–9. This is only 2 per cent of expenditure on in-patients and day cases combined, but it has almost doubled since 1978–9 (Figure 44.2), after adjusting for inflation (National Health Service (NHS) Pay and Price Index).

Three main factors have influenced the recent growth of day surgery:

(i) *Changes in clinical practice*: many clinicians are encouraging patients to become mobile again as soon as possible after an operation. This has contributed to a steady fall in the average length of stay of in-patients (Figure 44.3).

(ii) *Technological developments* are transforming the image of day surgery, as well as expanding its scope from minor routine procedures to relatively major operations. These include: faster acting, more precise anaesthetic drugs; better analgesics; lasers and fibre-optics, which have replaced major open surgery with less invasive procedures which can be done as a day case.

(iii) *Financial pressures*. In the UK financial pressure has been exerted mainly through reductions in in-patient beds.

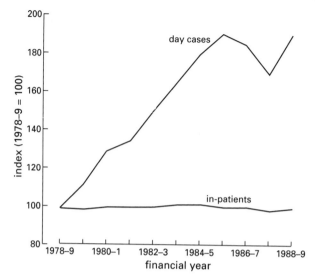

**Figure 44.2**   Change in estimated expenditure on acute in-patients and day cases (England – 1978–9 to 1988–9). Expenditure on day cases has nearly doubled over the past 11 years; that on in-patients has remained constant. Note: The sudden fall in 1987–8 is due to a change in the definition of day cases. 'Acute' is non-maternity, non-psychiatric patients. The figures are adjusted for NHS pay and price inflation.
*Source*: Department of Health

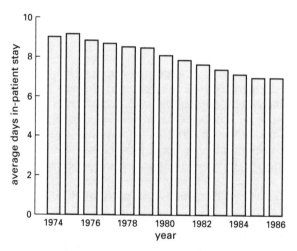

**Figure 44.3**   Average length of stay of in-patients in NHS hospitals: surgical specialities (England 1974–86). There has been a steady decline over many years.
*Source*: DHSS, NHS Hospital activity statistics, 1974–86.

The advantages of day surgery are:

(i) *It benefits patients.* This is because:
   (a) they are treated sooner than in-patients and suffer fewer last minute cancellations.
   (b) they spend less time away from home.
   (c) patient care is better. Specialised facilities offer the opportunity to provide a service which matches the needs of patients more closely.

(ii) *Costs are lower.* Two recent reviews[2,3] of academic studies of the average costs of day-case compared to in-patient treatment [largely in the 1970s] have shown that day-case treatment typically costs 40–50 per cent less, depending on the procedure being undertaken; 25–30 per cent may be a more realistic figure now. The majority of the differences in hospital costs reflect differences in the 'hotel' element (principally nursing and catering costs which account for about 40 per cent of a typical hospital budget), rather than the 'treatment' element.

There are some additional costs of day surgery outside the hospital which would not be incurred by in-patients. For example, those associated with community nursing services and additional visits by GPs. Few studies have looked at these in any detail. In none of the day-case units studied by the Audit Commission were there any routine arrangements for community support. As technology continues to increase the range of suitable surgical procedures, a greater need for community support may emerge.

Finally, there may be additional costs incurred by day-case patients and their families providing care at home. One study found that the households of day-case patients saved as much on hospital visiting and extra nightwear, as they spent on fuel, food, laundry and additional analgesics and dressings.[4] But there are other costs which are more difficult to quantify, for example, unpaid help at home provided by friends and relatives who may have to take time off work. There are also equally important unquantified benefits, not least a shorter waiting time for day-case compared to in-patient surgery.

In summary, the additional financial costs outside the hospital are small in relation to the likely differences in hospital costs. The additional non-financial costs which are largely incurred by patients and their families are more difficult to quantify, but are likely to be offset by the benefits they receive.

(iii) *Nurse recruitment and retention are easier.* The numbers entering the nursing profession have been falling steadily over recent years (Figure 44.4) due to a drop in the numbers of school leavers and changing preferences for other occupations. Day-case units provide more attractive working conditions than in-patient wards. They offer regular hours with no weekend work and a less stressful working environment. These conditions seem to be particularly attractive to mature trained nurses with families, an important source of staff which will need to be effectively tapped in the future.

## Problems in the development of day surgery

*Difficulties in assessing current performance, estimating the potential and monitoring change*
Day-case performance is difficult to assess because the available data often lack sufficient detail and are not consistent from one health authority to another. Without

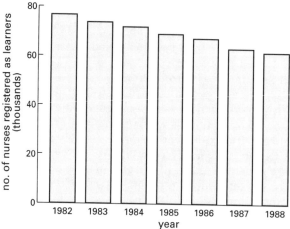

**Figure 44.4** Numbers of nurses registered as learners at 30 September each year (England 1982–8). There has been a steady decline in numbers entering the nursing profession over several years.
*Source*: Department of Health, 1989, *Health and Personal Social Services Statistics*

a clear assessment of the current position it is impossible to estimate the likely potential for expansion and to draw up firm plans for achieving it.

*Lack of specialist facilities*
Evidence collected by the Audit Commission's study team shows that most DHAs in England and Wales do at least have a dedicated day-case ward. About a third of these wards also have dedicated theatres. When these facilities are lacking, day cases, if treated at all, have to be treated on in-patient wards. This usually takes one of two forms:

(i) *Exclusive use of in-patient beds*. This offers none of the benefits to patients and nurses and is only likely to result in a minimal release of resources. It is no good replacing an in-patient stay with a day case and an empty bed overnight. No more patients will be treated and there will be no reduction in nursing costs.

(ii) *'Hot Bedding'*. In this case in-patients are asked to vacate their beds during the working day and wait in a lounge so that the beds can be used for day-case patients. This is unsatisfactory for two main reasons:
   (a) it offers a very poor quality of service to both in-patients and day-case patients;
   (b) it puts severe pressure on existing nurses, who are often expected to deal with more patients without additional nursing cover.

*Inappropriate and insufficient use of day-case units*
There are hundreds of different procedures carried out in a typical day-case unit. Some of them are entirely appropriate as day cases and would otherwise undoubtedly be in-patients. Others are relatively minor procedures, such as varicose vein injections, and in many hospitals are dealt with in a side room in the out-patient department. Between these extremes are procedures which have a varying need for full operating theatre facilities and post-operative nursing care, depending on such factors

as the severity and site of the pathology. For example, removal of a sebaceous cyst may be so minor a procedure that the patient can walk away immediately afterwards, or the cyst may be so positioned that it requires a general anaesthetic and prolonged surgery to remove it.

Inappropriate use of day-case units has two effects:

(i) Day-case performance statistics are artificially inflated compared to districts that carry out more of these procedures in out-patient settings.
(ii) Day-case unit capacity is taken up, rendering it unavailable for more appropriate cases.

### Poor management and organisation of day-case units

The low levels of utilisation (in some units) must in part be due to poor management and organisation of the units. The study team found examples of:

- lack of clear objectives and operational policies;
- inadequate managerial control with only superficial monitoring of activity;
- insufficient attention to the information needs of patients.

### Clinicians' preferences for more traditional approaches

The variation in day-case percentages between DHAs overlies a much greater variation between individual surgeons (Figure 44.5). The higher percentages for some procedures achieved by the 'pioneers' are swamped by their colleagues in the DHA aggregates. Evidence from interviews conducted by the Audit Commission study team indicates that the main disincentives for surgeons and anaesthetists to undertake day surgery include:

- more routine work considered by them to be of low status with no extra reward;
- a loss of their in-patient beds if resources are redeployed.

It is sometimes argued that surgeons are deterred from day surgery as it will, in the long run, reduce the number of patients seeking treatment privately. Nevertheless, many surgeons are keen to do more day surgery, as evidenced for example by a recent study which found that 55 per cent hold positive attitudes towards performing inguinal hernia repair as a day-case procedure, representing 5 times as many as currently 'often' operate in this way.[5]

The interviews carried out by the Audit Commission study team showed that of those surgeons and anaesthetists who do at least consider doing more day cases but choose against, the main reasons are:

(i) *Inadequate or poorly managed day-case facilities.*
(ii) *Fear that the outcome of the treatment will not be as good as that for in-patients.* The evidence from the available studies does not support this view.
(iii) *Lack of community support for patients.* Community support is not necessary for many of the procedures currently considered to be appropriate for day surgery.
(iv) *A belief that patients prefer to be treated as in-patients.* There is very little evidence on what patients think about day surgery. The few studies which exist are limited to patients' views about length of stay and are often based on small samples covering one hospital and one procedure.[3] The available evidence does not support the proposition that patients do not like day surgery. If anything, the

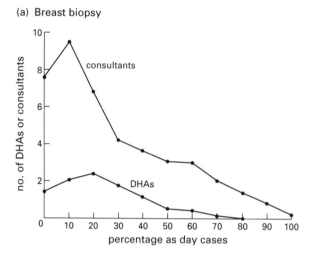

(a) Breast biopsy

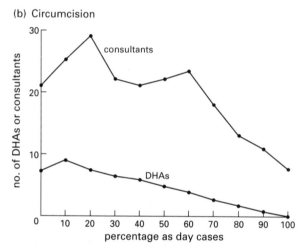

(b) Circumcision

**Figure 44.5** Variations in the percentage of operations carried out as day cases by DHAs and consultants. (a) Breast biopsy, (b) circumcision. The variation in day-case percentages between DHAs overlies a much greater variation between consultants. The higher percentages for some procedures achieved by the 'pioneers' are swamped by their colleagues in the DHA aggregates.
*Source*: Audit Commission analyses of data from 54 DHAs in England, 1988/9

tendency is in the other direction. But the evidence is poor and more work needs to be done.

(v) *The unsuitability of the patients they treat.* Clinicians often correctly point out that external factors can render patients unsuitable for day surgery. They may:
- be medically unfit (e.g. suffering from diabetes or being overweight);
- have no one to accompany them from the hospital or look after them at home;
- live in unsuitable accommodation (e.g. no telephone at home, too many steps to climb, inadequate heating);

- live too far from the hospital to travel home on the same day;
- have difficulty with transport arrangements.

These are all good reasons for not treating a patient as a day case, but they are only likely to apply to a minority of cases.

(vi) *Lack of proper training and experience in day surgery.* Good day surgery means using the most modern surgical and anaesthetic techniques. It also means that clinicians have to work to a strict timetable with little scope for the procedure to overrun its allotted time. Older surgeons and anaesthetists may not be familiar with some of the newer techniques.

*Managers' disincentives for change*
Managers face important disincentives for increasing the extent of day surgery. The main ones are:

- poor financial information which makes it very difficult to demonstrate that gains have been achieved;
- fear that moves towards more day surgery will inevitably lead to an increase in the number of cases treated, with little or no substitution of day cases for in-patients, and consequently increased difficulty keeping within a cash limit;
- worry that decisions on where surgery should take place are still viewed by many clinicians as entirely within their remit. Any attempt to 'meddle' in clinical matters will be met with resistance and is unlikely to achieve change.

These disincentives coupled with clinicians' preferences for the more traditional approaches have in the past developed into an impasse. Clinicians will not do more day-case work because the conditions are not right. Managers, on the other hand, are reluctant to encourage change because they believe their clinicians are basically against the idea and would not use any facilities they provide.

## Overcoming the barriers to change

Many of the barriers discussed [earlier] can be overcome. The Audit Commission has developed an approach to achieve this which it commends to managers and clinicians. The main elements of this approach, which will form the basis of local audits over the next year, involve:

- measuring performance, estimating the potential for more day surgery, developing plans and monitoring change;
- providing adequate facilities for day surgery;
- appropriate staffing of day-case units;
- efficient and effective use of day-case units;
- improving organisation and management of day-case units;
- changing clinicians' preferences;
- improving incentives for managers.

*Measuring performance, estimating the potential, developing plans and monitoring change*
Individual procedures should form the basis of performance comparisons at DHA and specialty level, but for operational planning and monitoring, it will be necessary to go to the level of individual consultants.

*Providing adequate facilities*
It is possible to carry out day surgery in various facilities. The two essential requisites are an operating theatre in which to perform the procedure and a ward for recovery. Dedicated wards are a minimum requirement for efficient and effective day surgery. Beyond this, having a theatre which is an integral part of the day-case unit results in:

- a better quality of service for patients (e.g. fewer last minute cancellations);
- lower running costs;
- higher capital and set-up costs.

*Efficient and effective use of day-case units*
Few units are utilising their capacity to the full and a number appear to be performing procedures which do not need the full facilities of a day-case unit.
    The Audit Commission recommends that:

(i) all cases should be treated in facilities with staffing levels sufficient for their needs, not in excess of them.
(ii) the capacity released as a result of the change, together with any existing unused capacity should be taken up with:
    (a) day cases currently being treated on in-patient wards;
    (b) new day cases identified as part of a planned overall increase in day surgery.

    Where the numbers of patients identified from these sources exceed the available capacity, additional capacity will be needed.

*Improving organisation and management*
There are three main aspects of good organisation and management:

- an operational policy;
- adequate managerial control;
- good management information.

*Operational policy.* Every day-case unit should have an operational policy setting out clear objectives, responsibilities and procedures for monitoring and reviewing each of its elements (Figure 44.6).

(i)   *Appropriate procedures.* A statement of which procedures are appropriate and inappropriate for the unit.
(ii)  *Booking of patients.* All patients should be given a firm appointment rather than be placed on a waiting list.
(iii) *Allocation of sessions/beds to consultants.* This is essential so that clinicians are clear how much day-case work they can do, and to ensure that capacity is fully used.
(iv)  *Admission procedures.* Admission of some patients can be staggered over the session to avoid unnecessarily long waits which often occur when all patients arrive at the same time.
(v)   *Discharge of patients.* Discharge should normally be carried out by nurses. This means that a major source of potential delay for patients – waiting for final approval for discharge from the surgeon or anaesthetist – is avoided. It does however mean that clinicians will need to delegate responsibility to nurses using written guidelines.

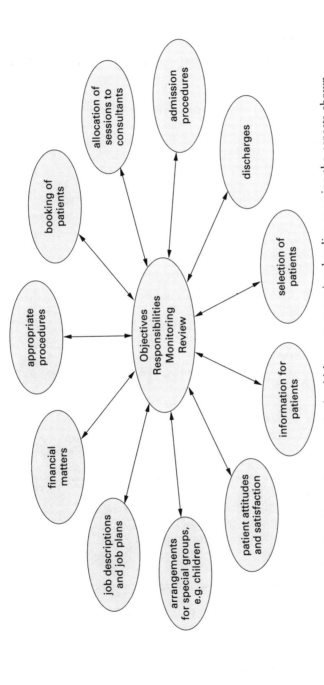

**Figure 44.6** Operational policy. Every day-case unit should have an operational policy covering the aspects shown.

(vi) *Selection of patients.* Patients need to be carefully screened for their suitability for day surgery at the time of their initial consultation. They should be screened for:
- medical fitness, including any necessary routine investigations;
- availability of someone to escort them to and from the day-case unit;
- provision of post-operative care at home;
- suitability of home circumstances (e.g. availability and accessibility of a telephone);
- distance they will need to travel after the procedure and having access to a suitable means of transport.

(vii) *Information for patients.* Patients need to have good written information about each stage of their treatment, backed up as much as possible orally.

(viii) *Patient attitudes and satisfaction.* Patients' perceptions need to be assessed and regularly monitored.

(ix) *Any special arrangements for particular groups of patients.* Children would certainly come into this category, and some mentally handicapped people might also be included.

*Management information.* The key to an effective operational policy and management control lies in good information. All day-case units should record:

- the length of time between the date a booking is made and the subsequent treatment or cancellation;
- the numbers of patients who do not attend for treatment;
- the numbers of patients who have to be admitted as in-patients at the end of each day, together with reasons;
- the extent of and reasons for post-operative emergency treatment and re-admission;
- patients' attitudes to and satisfaction with their treatment.

*Changing clinicians' preferences*
Adequate and well run day-case facilities are essential for good day surgery. Most of the fears held by clinicians will be overcome if:

(i)  the outcomes of treatments are regularly assessed as part of the medical audit procedures being set up in every hospital.

(ii) there are good patient-selection procedures. Problems such as patients being medically unfit, having no one to look after them at home, living in unsuitable accommodation or too far from the hospital, or a lack of adequate transport will be avoided. Their existence is insufficient justification for not doing day surgery at all.

(iii) patients' attitudes and satisfaction are regularly monitored.

Since the decision on appropriate mode of treatment is taken at the out-patient appointment, surgeons might be asked to indicate on a simple form why they are not opting for day-case, rather than in-patient treatment, for appropriate procedures. The reasons can then be recorded and discussed. But perhaps the chief effect would be that day surgery were considered as a possibility in every case. Surgeons may be more prepared to do this if they are given regular information on their own day-case activity in comparison with that of their colleagues. They might also be offered a direct incentive to treat more day cases if a proportion of the resources released by the substitution of day-case for in-patient treatment were retained for service enhancements.

*Improving incentives for managers*
Successful change depends on a good working relationship between managers and clinicians. It is important to ensure that:

• the views of both parties are clearly understood and taken into account.
• the objectives and the plans are mutually agreed.

Managers will have a greater incentive to develop day surgery if they can demonstrate benefits in the form of more patients treated or resources released for other purposes. The poor quality of financial information is a major problem.

Day surgery is often thought to be associated with an increase in surgery overall rather than with substitution for in-patients. Such an outcome is of course possible but the matter ought to be under the control of managers and clinicians. If in-patient beds are not closed when day surgery facilities become available, the tendency will be to treat more patients, which may of course be the intention. But if the aim is to substitute day-case patients for in-patients rather than expand, then clearly the in-patient beds should be closed.

## References

1. Bradshaw, E. G. and Davenport, H. T. *Day Care: Surgery, Anaesthesia and Management*, Edward Arnold, London (1989).
2. Royal College of Surgeons of England, Commission on the Provision of Surgical Services, *Guidelines for Day-Case Surgery*, July (1985).
3. Morgan, M. and Beech, R. 'Variations in lengths of stay and rates of day-case surgery: implications for the efficiency of surgical management', *Journal of Epidemiology and Community Health*, 44(2), 90–105 (1990).
4. Russell, I. T., Devlin, H. B., Fell, M., Glass, N. J. and Newell, D. J. 'Day-case surgery for hernias and haemorrhoids: A clinical, social and economic evaluation', *Lancet*, 16 April, 844–847 (1977).
5. Morgan, M., Reynolds, A., Swan, A. V., Beech, R. and Devlin, H. B. 'Day surgery for inguinal hernia repair: consultants' attitudes and clinical practices in four Regions', *paper submitted for publication*.

The Audit Commission was set up as an independent body in 1982 to promote the efficient use of resources allocated to the public services, while helping them to maintain effective standards. Its role was extended to the NHS in 1990, and the extract reproduced here is from its first report on the NHS, *A Short Cut to Better Services: Day Surgery in England and Wales*, HMSO, London (1990).

# Part 6
# Health work

The work of health care is conducted in a variety of locations and is done by a huge variety of people. These may include formally paid practitioners who have direct contact with their patients, ancillary staff who support formal health care workers but are at one remove from contact with patients, family members who care for sick people at home and, last but not least, sick people themselves, who may engage in a variety of self-care activities. This part of the book describes all these types of health care work; running through most of the articles is the theme of relative power – between workers and patients, and between different sectors of health worker.

Health work at home is described in an article by two health service researchers, Ann Bowling and Ann Cartwright, who describe the situation of people who are 'Caring for the spouse who died'. The practical problems of caring, social isolation and mental and physical effort in this very common form of health work are depicted. Although the vast majority of the people interviewed by Bowling and Cartwright wanted care to continue at home rather than in hospital, inevitably the burden was too great for some.

Hospital care for dying people is the subject of 'We didn't want him to die on his own', by David Field, who is a sociologist. He describes how nurses on one medical ward became emotionally close to their dying patients, providing care that broke down some of the impersonality which is often associated with hospital care. Field links nurses' capacity to do this with the existence of non-hierarchical relationships between health care staff, with doctors relinquishing power over the control of information. Freed to respond to patients' concerns about dying without worrying whether forbidden information is being disclosed, and supported by senior nursing staff, nurses provided care of such a quality that Field writes 'If I should die in hospital I hope it is on a similar ward.'

Thurstan Brewin, a cancer specialist, continues the theme of terminal illness, power and disclosure, arguing the case for a traditional, trusting and paternalistic relationship between doctors and terminally ill patients. In 'Truth, trust and paternalism',

Brewin argues that the doctor who tells everything to his or her dying patient, seeking authority from the patient to make decisions, discards half of the value of a consultation, which is for the patient to benefit from the doctor's experience and judgement.

In contrast, Ann Oakley, a feminist sociologist, shows how paternalism can easily become patronising and offensive in her critical account of the medical management of childbirth, 'Doctor knows best'. For her, the main effect of this has been to reinforce the oppression of women by a male-dominated medical profession. She argues that doctors often inflate their expertise, questioning the reliability of women's own accounts of their pregnancies. More than a decade later it is, perhaps, encouraging to see the House of Commons Health Committee in the 'Second Report on Maternity Services', supporting Oakley's critique of medical dominance in this area of health work, and making practical suggestions to redress the balance. Significantly, this involves adjusting the balance of power between midwives and doctors, a suggestion that parallels Field's account of terminal care, where he argued that nurses left to make decisions themselves provided more responsive care. In the extract included in this book, the House of Commons Health Committee, like Oakley, argues against treating pregnancy as an illness, against paternalism and for patient choice, in favour of midwives taking greater powers to assist women in childbirth.

Within the medical profession there is a formal hierarchy of grades; there is also a less formal hierarchy of medical specialisms, with casualty work once being considered a fairly unpopular area (although this may now be changing). The sociologist Roger Jeffery's classic article 'Normal rubbish: deviant patients in casualty', describes the work of three casualty departments, showing how medical staff differentiate between 'good patients' and 'rubbish' as they get through the work. Jeffery's account links with Goffman's account of mental illness in Part 2, where he distinguishes between sufferers from physical illness – who have an easier time in defining themselves as sick – and people with mental illness, where blame for the condition and doubts about malingering concern the health workers who treat them.

Perhaps lowest in the hierarchy of hospital work are ancillary staff, whose position is reflected in poorer rates of pay and a low degree of autonomy. Elizabeth Paterson, a sociologist, provides an account of 'Food-work: maids in a hospital kitchen', which reflects the struggle by such workers to maintain self-esteem and control over their working conditions by carving out areas where discretion is exercised. Paterson shows how such discretion is, paradoxically, centred on distinguishing between clients of varying social prestige. Medical staff and private patients are given the newer, shiny containers; ordinary patients get 'any bashed object.' In the hospital kitchen, lettuce is bad, macaroni cheese is good, and this has nothing to do with their taste, everything to do with the work context in which these objects are processed. Most of the articles in this part of the book show how hierarchy and value are implied by categorizing people and the work they do; Paterson's article shows how this can also be extended to food items.

# 45
# Caring for the spouse who died

## ANN BOWLING AND ANN CARTWRIGHT

This article is based on a study of experiences and attitudes of over 360 elderly widowed men and women, their general practitioners and their relatives, friends and neighbours.

### The last illness

Widowhood is occasionally a sudden event with no prior warning, but more usually, especially among older people, it is the climax of a period during which life has revolved around caring for a sick spouse. It is the final stage of the role of wife or husband. Indeed, for women, eventual widowhood can realistically be regarded as a normal part of the process of ageing.

Two-fifths of the widowed said the death was expected as far as they were concerned. An illustration of such a death is:

> He was treated for two years with gastro-enteritis and pains in his back. He had primary cancer in his stomach and spleen – he had them removed but it had gone too far. The doctors gave him two months but I kept him alive by nursing him for eighteen months, and they sent me no nursing help at all.

Coping with illness over a long period may make the surviving spouse tired and, if they do not get adequate support, resentful. But it can give them an opportunity to prepare for the changes ahead. One widower commented that he had few problems now as he had had time to prepare himself for the death and adjust to new roles:

> No problems really. If she'd gone suddenly it would have been much more of a blow.

Expected deaths were more common if the cause was cancer, 56 per cent; for bronchitis, or other respiratory diseases, 53 per cent; whereas it was 34 per cent for deaths from other causes. And, as might be predicted, the death was more often expected if the person had been ill for a long time. Roughly a third were ill for less than a year, a third for between one and five years, and a third for longer.

It was not only the length but also the nature of the illness which contributed to the distress of both the person who died and the surviving spouse. A symptom which gave rise to much concern and anguish for their relatives was confusion. Just under a third, 30 per cent, of the deceased were said by the widowed to have been mentally confused before they died. Almost two-thirds, 63 per cent of the widowed whose spouses were mentally confused found this 'very distressing', and 12 per cent found it 'fairly distressing'.

> He used to have brain storms, at least that's what I'd call them because he tried to strangle me a couple of times and he said he was going to poison me.

> He used to lose his way home, and one day he moved all the dandelions from the side alley and planted them in the front garden. He didn't know. I had bad nerves and I used to lean on him, but when he became so ill I had to be the one to do everything.

Two-fifths of the widowed said the deceased had other symptoms or problems which they themselves had found distressing. These included pain, depression, sleeplessness, incontinence, inability to move, vomiting, loss of appetite, difficulty breathing or talking, and difficulty eating or feeding.

> He couldn't hold his knife to eat. Things kept shooting off his plate. Vomiting all the time. He was all dirty and my daughters used to clean him up, all sick and blood.

So widowhood for most, three-quarters, was preceded for a period of six months or more when their spouse was ill, and this was often accompanied by distressing symptoms. What help did they get during that time?

Just over half, 53 per cent, of the deaths in our sample took place in hospital. In addition, 44 per cent of those dying at home were admitted to hospital at some time during the last year of their lives. Just over two-fifths, 42 per cent, had ten or more consultations with a general practitioner in the year before they died, and almost three out of ten, 29 per cent, had ten or more home visits.

Nearly half of all those who died had needed help while at home with dressing or undressing and a similar proportion with bathing, while two-fifths had needed some help at night. A relatively high proportion of those dying from cancer, 80 per cent, and those whose deaths were ascribed to pneumonia or influenza, 79 per cent, had needed some sort of help while at home. And Table 45.1 also shows the heavy demands of those who had been confused.

In over a third of instances where any help was given, 38 per cent, the widowed person had done everything, and in a further third, 39 per cent, they had helped mainly. For 17 per cent the care was equally shared between the widowed and others, and for 6 per cent the care was given mainly or entirely by people other than the widowed. There was no difference between the widows and the widowers who said this care had fallen mainly or on them. Apart from the spouse the main person who gave help when it was needed was a relative, 31 per cent, a professional person, 25 per cent, and a friend or neighbour, 6 per cent. A fifth of the widowed felt that their

**Table 45.1** Care at home by whether or not the person had been mentally confused at all before death

| | Mentally confused before death | | All deaths % |
|---|---|---|---|
| | Yes % | No % | |
| *Type of care given:* | | | |
| Dressing and undressing | 65 | 38 | 46 |
| Getting in or out of bath | 64 | 39 | 47 |
| Washing or shaving | 53 | 35 | 41 |
| Being lifted | 65 | 34 | 43 |
| Getting to lavatory | 60 | 32 | 41 |
| Help or care at night | 61 | 33 | 42 |
| Other care of this sort | 28 | 15 | 19 |
| None | 18 | 42 | 35 |
| *Number of deaths (= 100%)* | 106 | 252 | 359 |

spouse or they themselves could have done with more help; help with lifting being the most frequent need, by one in eight.

The burden on those widowed who had cared mainly or entirely for their spouses often seemed considerable:

> He had a stroke three years ago. It left him paralysed and he never spoke afterwards. He was like a baby. I managed to look after him all the time. He was able to use the one leg if I helped him to . . . I would get him out into the sun sometimes. It was a struggle but I did it. In fact I dropped him several times when I had to lift him, he was ten stone!

## Attitudes to care

The widowed were asked what they felt about the care and treatment their spouse had from their general practitioner before their death and then to sum up whether this care was 'very good', 'fairly good', or 'not very good'. We have already noted that 8 per cent had no contact with a general practitioner in the year before their death. For the others, in two-thirds the care was felt to be 'very good', a quarter of the widowed described it as 'fairly good', and a tenth as 'not very good'.

We asked the widowed whose spouses died at home whether they would rather the person had been in hospital or whether they were glad he or she had died at home. The majority, 91 per cent, said they were glad their spouse had been at home when he or she died:

> I'm glad he was in his own home and I was there.

Among the five who said outright that it would have been better if the person had been in hospital were two who were somewhat critical of their general practitioners.

> They didn't bother with him. I don't suppose they could do much for him. They were very nice, but they're busy aren't they? I didn't dare send for him. He came

once and said 'There's nothing I can do for him'. We couldn't lift him. He was a dead weight – even the nurse said it was too much. It used to be terrible. She said he ought to be in hospital in a special bed. He had terrible back sores. They did their best to get him into hospital.

## Restrictions on the surviving spouse

Some of the widowed had been under a great deal of strain in caring for their ill spouse. The following examples are of widows who cared for their husbands entirely on their own. They both said the could have done with help:

He wasn't able to get into a bath. I used to have to wash him all down. He couldn't even stand in the shower for that length of time. I had to lift him up the bed. He used to pull the door and hang onto the door-handle and I'd help him up.

I was exhausted when he passed away after looking after him. The nurse promised to bring me a stool so I could put it on the bath. She kept promising but they never came. They sent a night commode but that was only suitable for a lady. My husband was fifteen stone, he couldn't sit on it.

Also, many of those who said no help, or no more help, was needed with caring for their husband or wife went on to say that this was because they would not have accepted help from anyone other than the widow or widower.

He didn't want to be exposed to the nurses, he was a modest sort of man.

He didn't want anyone else to do things for him – it's private and personal. I used to rush my shopping so I could get back to him. I had not had a full night's sleep for eighteen months.

Similarly, one of the familiars commented that the deceased had preferred his spouse to help with nursing care as he found personal help from others embarrassing:

He would get embarrassed, with me being his daughter, and wouldn't let me help except at the very end. The night he died he let me clean him. He said 'Fancy you having to do this'. Ten minutes later it was the end.

Even when professional nursing care was given the widowed sometimes commented that it was inadequate because it was hurried or infrequent. In one case the nurse came just fortnightly to bath the deceased, and in another the nurses visited but asked relatives to help as they had such little time:

We had a very hard time. My daughter and I had to help him with everything at the end – eating and everything. My daughter helped so much with him – she washed him, cleaned him. The nurses came every day but they were often in a rush so they often used to ask my daughter to take over.

We asked the widowed if they had given up or done less of anything during the time of the deceased's illness. Thirty-six per cent had not, more, 53 per cent, had given up something, and 11 per cent had done less of something. The activities they cut down on were: visiting friends or relatives for 45 per cent of all the widowed;

going out to other social activities, 46 per cent; going on holiday, 41 per cent; entertaining people at home, 31 per cent; going to work, 12 per cent. Restrictions on other activities were mentioned by 10 per cent. Many of those who said their activities were not, or only a little, restricted, said this was because they had no outside activities to be disrupted. For example:

Social wise we never went out anyway, so that didn't matter.

The strain imposed by caring for the dying spouse was greater when the surviving husband or wife was not robust. The proportion who said their activities had been severely restricted increased from 21 per cent of those who rated their own health as excellent or good, to 31 per cent of those who rated it as fair, and 44 per cent of those who regarded it as poor. It was not that those in poor health were more likely to have given up visiting relatives or friends, or entertaining people at home, but that they apparently became too exhausted to do even ordinary activities. One widow said:

I was an ill person over eighty with a heart complaint and yet they sent a dying man home to me with no help at all. I had a bed downstairs for him but he was always messing it. He had no control over his legs. When he fell I had a twelve stone man to lift – and I've got a heart condition! I was so tired my ankles were enormous at night. I had to sleep in the chair in the end as I was too tired to go up and down stairs.

Restrictions on the activities of the spouse were rather greater for cancer deaths than for others. Thirty-six per cent of the widowed whose spouse had died of cancer said their activities had been severely restricted compared with 23 per cent of other deaths. At the same time the longer the illness the more likely it was to restrict the spouse's activities; 53 per cent of those whose spouse was ill for less than six months had been restricted in some way, compared with 65 per cent when the illness lasted between six months and two years, and 76 per cent for longer illnesses.

The more restricted their lives had been the more likely the widowed were to wish something could have been done differently. The proportion wishing this rose from 18 per cent of those who were not restricted to 33 per cent of the severely restricted.

I couldn't go far. I couldn't go anywhere – just down the road, shopping. I couldn't leave him for any length of time. It made me confused and ill at times – looking after him for so long. For the past few months I had to carry him to the bathroom.

I didn't go out – it caused my blood pressure. I used to like a drink at the pub but I couldn't leave her, or ask anyone to stop in whilst I went for a drink. You can't do that can you?

In addition to restrictions on physical activities, the widowed often mentioned the mental strain they suffered in the period before the death:

It was nerve-racking – living with the knowledge that he could die any day. When he was choking I was on my own and there was no-one to help me – I never saw a nurse. I had to be awake at night because of the choking. I wasn't given any advice as to what to do for him. [Died from cancer of the stomach.]

In some of these cases an element of relief at the death was expressed. One woman who died of multiple sclerosis was described as mentally confused and depressed. She had been ill for twenty years and her husband had retired early to look after her:

Friends and relatives would come in and see her sitting there in her chair, all clean and cheerful, she always had a smile for them, they didn't realize what I had to do to keep her like that. I think the doctor and the nurse realized that I was on the edge of a breakdown myself. She kept calling at night, I never got no sleep.

The widowed often seemed to accept the burden of caring that had been placed on them as their duty. Two widows said:

It was like living in a vacuum really, it was all unreal, but I would not have had it any other way.

When you marry someone it is for life so it was my place to look after him.

The feeling that they themselves, not only professionals, had done all they could, and that their husband or wife had been well looked after, may help reduce feelings of guilt after the death. As one widow said:

The only thing that goes through my mind is 'Did I do everything to help, did I do enough?' It keeps going through my mind.

Almost a quarter of the widowed, 24 per cent, said their spouse's ill-health had affected them financially. This proportion was higher for widows, 28 per cent, than widowers, 18 per cent. Although no differences were found with place of death or length of illness, deaths from cancer and bronchitis had more effects on finances than other deaths, 32 per cent in comparison with 21 per cent. It was pointed out earlier that cancer deaths also imposed the most restriction on the spouse's activities.

Those classified as working class were more likely to say they had been affected financially, 26 per cent, than those classified as middle class, 15 per cent. Forty-three per cent of those who said they were affected financially received no financial help. Altogether, 23 per cent received supplementary benefit before the death and 9 per cent received a disability pension, 9 per cent an attendance allowance, and 10 per cent received help from a relative or other sources. One widow whose husband was chronically ill with bronchitis for twelve years and whom she nursed intensively for about six months was discouraged from claiming the attendance allowance by her general practitioner. She said the doctor told her:

It wasn't worth it, he wouldn't be here long enough.

As 26 per cent had said their activities were severely restricted and 19 per cent said they were fairly restricted because of the deceased's illness, probably more than the 9 per cent receiving an attendance allowance were eligible for it. Those who were affected financially mentioned the cost of extra food, clothes, and heating as being the main problems:

I had to keep getting him trousers, the others were falling off him. I had to get baby foods, Complan, and the nurse told me to get Ovaltine. The gas bill was high, we had to burn that night and day, same as the lights.

It is clear that the care of dying people at home often imposes severe physical, financial, and psychological strains on their relatives. Wives and husbands generally take on this task willingly but often they do it unaided when appropriate help and support could mitigate the physical hardship, the social isolation, and the mental distress.

The authors of this article are both medical sociologists. Ann Bowling was formerly a Research Officer and Ann Cartwright was, until her retirement, Director at the Institute for Social Studies in Medical Care in London. This is an edited extract from a chapter in their book *Life After A Death: A Study of Elderly Widowed*, published by Tavistock (1982). Ann Bowling is currently a Reader in Health Services Research, at St Bartholomew's Hospital Medical College, London.

# 46

# 'We didn't want him to die on his own' – nurses' accounts of nursing dying patients

DAVID FIELD

Over half of all deaths in the United Kingdom occur in National Health Service hospitals (Wilkes, 1980), a situation which has prevailed for over two decades. Cartwright *et al.* (1973) writing with reference to 1969 estimated that nearly a third of all hospital beds were occupied by patients who were dying, or who would die within the year. While for dying patients and their relatives their experience is unique and problematic, for hospital staff care of the dying is part of their work. As such it is shaped in various ways by the organizational demands and routines of hospital life. The two groups of hospital staff most directly concerned with such work are doctors and nurses, with the everyday care and close contact with the dying falling to the latter. In this paper I look at nurses' accounts of their experiences of nursing dying patients and their attitudes towards nursing the dying. I suggest ways in which the organization of their work influences such experiences and attitudes.

The study was based on interviews with all of the nursing staff working on day shifts in a 28-bed general medical ward at a general hospital in the Midlands. Nurses received practical and psychological support from other team members when they experienced difficulty in their work, and also received such help from other members of the ward staff. The ward as a whole was run along team lines, with authority delegated widely among the trained nursing staff. For example, charge nurse duty rotated among all qualified staff rather than being based simply on seniority. A policy of 'open disclosure' existed on the ward which meant that nurses could inform patients about their diagnosis and prognosis – including that of terminality – without first having to seek permission to do so from the consultants. The nursing staff were encouraged by the Nursing Officer and Ward Sister to follow the open disclosure policy, and were helped by them in implementing this policy.

Informal audio-taped interviews were conducted by the author with each nurse in the vacant night sisters' office. Interviews lasted from 15 to 50 minutes, were transcribed by the author, typed up, and a copy of the transcript sent to the nurse after all interviews had been completed. The ward sister, seven qualified nurses, nine nurses in training and two nursing auxiliaries were interviewed. All but two of the nurses were female, and their experience ranged from trainees on their first ward placement to one nurse with 20 years experience of nursing. Most of the nurses (14) were between the ages of 20 and 25 years old.

## Awareness contexts

A central concern of the study was to examine nurses' views of various awareness contexts (Glaser & Strauss, 1965). At one extreme is the situation of 'open awareness' where all parties, including the patient, know that the patient is dying and know that such knowledge is shared. At the other extreme is the situation of 'closed awareness' where the doctors know that the patient is dying but the patient does not. Other staff and relatives may also be aware of the impending death. Between these extremes are the self-explanatory 'suspicion' and 'mutual pretence' situations. The majority of nurses who expressed a preference chose 'open awareness';

> ER: . . . it's far easier to cope with a patient that's dying and knows they're dying (unprompted).
> For the nurses in training such a view was largely anticipatory, although two of them had experienced 'suspicion awareness' and found this difficult to cope with. They were tentative in their choice, and even for trained staff the preference for 'openness' was not unproblematic, as this experienced staff nurse indicates:
> DF: So you have no difficulty talking to them?
> RL: Oh no. Sometimes I find it difficult if they don't know they're dying, and the relatives have expressed a wish that they're not to be told and the doctors haven't told them yet. You know, . . . the time when they first get to know, I find that a bit difficult still. It's alright when they know. It's alright if they don't know. It's the in between bit when they're getting to know and they're asking some difficult questions.

As this shows, *getting* to the situation of open awareness may be hard – especially for the unqualified nurse. It was in this phase of their relationship with the dying patient that the qualified staff saw their ward sister as playing an important role as the 'broker' who negotiated the transition to open awareness when they could not do so. (Both the sister and the nursing officer told me that they saw this as an important part of their work.) Despite the difficulties of achieving open awareness all of the qualified nurses indicated that they had developed strategies for 'telling' patients the truth about their terminality.

> EW: If the patient asks you outright if they're dying and you know then I think a student nurse or a pupil nurse might sort of hedge 'Of course you're not going to. Ask the doctor'. They may sort of hedge. But, it depends . . . sister does allow us to use our own judgement, but just the same you've got to be very careful what you say.
> DF: Can you think of anyone you've actually told?

*EW:* I've never actually said to someone 'Yes, you are dying'.

*DF:* But there are ways of saying you're dying.

*EW:* I remember a lady saying 'Well I'm not going to get better am I?, and then I said 'Well no, I don't think so. But nobody knows for sure' . . . 'If it's left to us, if it's left to our care you will go home'.

*DF:* So, you always try to be positive?

*EW:* Yes. You try to be positive as well because nobody can say 'yes, you are doing to die'.

(EW returns to this issue without prompting at the end of the interview): I try not to lie or pretend to them. Try not to disguise. I try not to kid them along. I try not to say 'Oh no you're not going to die', try not to do that. That's wrong. They still need the same sort of – they still need nursing. It's just your approach to them. I think you should be as honest as you can. If you can't then I think you should get somebody else to talk to them who can be.

As these extracts show, important elements of the strategies developed were the need to be positive, and a stress on being honest with the dying patient.

### Emotional involvement

Given the strong preference expressed by these nurses for 'open awareness' it is perhaps not surprising that nearly all of them (16) said that they were or had been emotionally involved with dying patients, often to the extent of crying and grieving at their deaths. All of the qualified staff and five of the trainees felt that such involvement was inevitable and unavoidable. For the qualified nurses such involvement was not seen as particularly problematic, and five felt it was positively beneficial and rewarding for them. Unqualified staff were not as positive with five expressing problems. A student nurse gave a very full account of her experience of nursing an 80-year old terminally ill woman with whom she had become very emotionally involved. The woman had died two weeks before the interview and the student had shared the death with the woman's husband. Both of them had cried after the death.

*SH:* Well I shouldn't really have done that. I shouldn't have got involved so much probably, but it's hard to draw the line. And – particularly with somebody like her. She was so kind to everybody. And I thought 'well, this isn't a very good example for the younger nurses walking out crying with the husband' but I thought 'well they obviously know it's an upsetting thing even though they weren't involved'. And they said afterwards they were glad they weren't involved at all because it would have made them cry. But I wasn't the only one in tears so I didn't feel so bad. It wasn't as if it was just me who was involved with her.

*DF:* Do you feel it is bad to cry when a patient's died?

*SH:* Not really. Not if the relative's there and – he said then 'She wasn't just another lady was she?' 'No', I said. 'None of them are. Everybody's an individual here'.

Another indicator of the high level of emotional involvement which these nurses seemed to have with their dying patients was the continued contact which some of them maintained with the relatives of patients who had died and with terminally ill patients who had been discharged. The most dramatic example of such behaviour was provided by the sister. She told DF that she kept in contact with many relatives even though she didn't always want to:

> Sr: ... because they are a terrific drain. And very often ... you want to forget about work and it's forced upon you. I always have this terrible feeling that they expect so much of nurses, that you are representing every nurse. So to be unkind or to be curt, or not to have time would, well have a devastating effect on them. They feel they could be next. And so you're obligated to give them every consideration, and yet I don't always want to ... and I think that possibly the only common denominator with all these people is that they want to talk about their deceased. I have known them, probably in quite an intimate way. You can't nurse a dying patient without – well you *can*, but obviously it isn't desirable to keep them at a distance – and so you *do* get to know them very well. And this is what they're really after. They want to talk about the person, not the death ... I can never bring myself to cut them off, and they may not be able to do this with anyone else.

One nurse said that she got pleasure from nursing the dying:

> DF: You said you got pleasure from nursing the dying patient.
> EW: Well, well perhaps that's the wrong thing – *satisfaction*. I don't mean pleasure: satisfaction. You can *see* results from nursing a patient that's a long term patient or dying. You can see what you're doing for them. ...
>     You can make time to sit and talk with them. And obviously if they're dying the physical condition is going to deteriorate so you've got to be that extra bit careful keeping them clean and comfortable, bathing and things like that. And to me that's nursing.

As this extract shows, nursing the dying may be satisfying for the nurse because it allows them to fully implement their ideal of nursing care.

## Discussion

What emerges very clearly is a consistent set of predispositions to act in particular ways. Namely; to become emotionally involved with the patients they are nursing (and their relatives), especially if they are long-term patients; to disclose rather than to withhold information about dying when this is sought by the patient; to be honest in their dealings with patients (and relatives); to accept individual responsibility for patients while working as part of a team; to help and support each other. In short a predisposition to provide 'total nursing care' for the 'whole person'. I suggest that these predispositions *are* likely to be acted upon in the ward which was the focus of this study for a number of reasons.

General medical wards differ from other wards in a number of ways with respect to patient flow and rhythms of work, and with respect to the characteristics of their patients. They are generally geared towards less intensive therapeutic intervention than acute surgical wards or coronary care units; their patient turnover is on average lower with a concomitant longer term stay; and their patients are older. Patients are typically mature adults rather than children or teenagers. Further, deaths are usually predictable to nursing staff and relatively infrequent when compared to some other settings. Most patients recover or are discharged in an improved condition. Thus, nurses may have more extended contact with patients and so have a greater chance to get to know them, and are dealing with deaths which are less problematic and less frequent than those found in other settings. During the second week of my study period the mean age of the 33 patients who spent time in the ward was 57, ranging from 15 to 96 years in age, and a standard deviation of 23. There were 63 deaths on the ward during 1982.

Despite the high level of bed occupancy, the rhythm of work on the ward appeared to be generally relaxed. During the 'slack times' (when most of my visits occurred) nurses could typically be found chatting to patients. The democratic and 'permissive' leadership style of the sister was very evident, and the attitude that nursing work meant *doing* something *to* patients (Clarke, 1978) was noticeably absent. Trainees were fully involved with patient care, and were not relegated to performing only routine tasks. As I remarked earlier, the ward very clearly worked as a cohesive team involving all of the nursing staff. The sister's role appeared to be in large part devoted to supporting the rest of her team, facilitating their interpersonal relationships with patients (and trying to develop their skills) where necessary, and mediating between nurses and patients and the medical staff. Her leadership style and strongly expressed attitudes were central to the ethos of patient care enacted on the ward.

### Doctor–nurse relationships

A crucial structural characteristic of ward organization is the nature of doctor–nurse relationships. In a previously studied acute surgical ward (Knight & Field, 1981) these were very formal and hierarchical, with consultants and other surgical staff talking only to the sister or charge nurse. This hierarchy was mirrored by a similar formal ranking of the nursing staff. Nurses on this ward were forbidden to disclose their prognosis to dying patients. On the present ward, relationships were much less formal, with nurses allowed a good deal of autonomy. Cases were discussed between medical and nursing staff, and nurses reported that a good relationship existed between them.

> DF: Do you have reasonably good relations with the doctors on this ward?
> ER: Most of the time, yes. It's very friendly, all of the doctors and nurses are on first name terms. If you ask them 'Will you do me a favour? Mr so-and-so wants a chat' – he hasn't asked for the doctor, just got you in a bit of a predicament – and they go off. They are quite good.

With respect to care of the dying, medical staff had less active involvement and might withdraw almost entirely once the transition from 'therapeutic cure' to 'relief care' (Saunders 1978) had been decided upon. Medical staff were willing to accede to nurses' views about the desirability of 'disclosure'. For example, a case was recounted where medical staff felt that a patient should not be informed that she was terminally ill whereas the nursing staff felt that she should be. It was agreed that the Sister would tell the patient who, when told, thanked the Sister and made arrangements to ensure that a planned holiday occurred whilst she was well enough to go.

The predisposition to care is, one suspects, an important characteristic of entrants to the health care professions. Studies of medical students suggests that it may quite quickly become transformed as they lose their 'idealism' (Becker & Geer, 1958), develop 'detached concern' (Fox, 1957), and in many other ways change their earlier commitment to caring for 'whole people'. A similar process may also affect nurses (Clarke, 1978, Melia, 1972). Such change is not inevitable, but induced during the course of nurse training and early ward experiences as a qualified nurse. The predisposition to care for the 'whole person' and the derivation of satisfaction and reward from such caring nursing can flow from the type of arrangement identified above. This is to the mutual benefit of nurse and patient, and can pertain, it seems, even in such an apparently negative situation as nursing the dying.

## Coda

RE: We had a patient who was here over a year – and we were all very close to 'C'. I saw him from when he came in, to getting really better, then going down again. It was awful because there was nothing I could do; I just had to sit and hold his hand. At that time we were all taking it in turns to sit with him as long as we could 'cos we just didn't want him to die on his own. Nobody wanted just to go in and find him dead. Which I think goes for most patients that you know are on their last legs. You *don't* want to leave them on their own. . . . I remember very clearly a patient on geriatrics. I had nursed him on nights, and I went back on to days – he was a double-sided CVA. He was very incoherent. By some miracle could just whisper words. And at night he couldn't sleep because he was so uncomfortable so I used to spend a lot of my nights sitting and talking to him and holding his hand. When I went back on to days I went behind the curtains – and he was really on his last legs. So I just sat with him and held his hand. And I remember the staff nurse coming in and asking me if I had nothing better to do. So I said 'No. Not at this moment, no.' So she said 'would you mind going and finding something to do?' I remember it so clearly. I really hated her, because this man was dying. I'd been with him all this time, and why should he die alone? All she was content with was giving him BPO's and he still had an enema the day he did die. Well he died that afternoon. I felt awful – this poor little man – and just as I went behind the curtains he just said – he grabbed hold of my arms (he got very little movement in that hand), and he just put his hand on mine and whispered 'I love you'. And then he died in the afternoon. I thought 'well it's all worthwhile' because at least he realized that somebody cared.

## Acknowledgments

A number of people have commented on various versions of this paper and it is impossible to say who has contributed what to the final product. I thank them all. I also thank the nursing officer of the medical unit, the ward sister, and especially the nursing staff on the ward for their courtesy, friendliness, and frankness. If I should die in hospital I hope it is on a similar ward.

## References

Becker, H. S. and Geer, B. S. 'The fate of idealism in medical school', *American Sociological Review*, **23**, 50–56 (1958).

Cartwright, A., Hockey, L. and Anderson, J. C. *Life Before Death*, Routledge and Kegan Paul, London (1973).

Clarke, M. 'Getting through the work'. In *Readings in the Sociology of Nursing* (eds Dingwall, R. and McIntosh, J.) Chapter 5, Churchill Livingstone, Edinburgh (1978).

Fox, R. C. 'Training for detached concern'. In *The Student Physician: Introductory Studies in The Sociology of Medical Education* (eds Merton, R. K., Reader, G. G. and Kendall, P. L.) Harvard University Press, Cambridge, Mass. (1957).

Glaser, B. G. and Strauss, A. L. *Awareness of Dying*, Aldine, Chicago (1965).

Knight, M. and Field, D. 'A silent conspiracy: coping with dying cancer patients on an acute surgical ward', *Journal of Advanced Nursing*, **6**, 221–229 (1981).

Melia, K. M. '"Tell it as it is" – qualitative methodology and nursing research: understanding the student nurse's world', *Journal of Advanced Nursing*, **7**, 327–335 (1982).

Saunders, C. (ed.) *The Management of Terminal Disease*, Ch. 1, Edward Arnold, London (1978).

Wilkes, E. *Terminal Care: Report of a Working Group Standing Medical Advisory Committee*, SMAC, London (1980).

David Field is a medical sociologist and at the time of writing this article he was a lecturer in the Department of Sociology, University of Leicester. He is currently Professor of Sociology at the University of Ulster. This article is an edited version of the original, which appeared in the *Journal of Advanced Nursing*, **9**, 59–70 (1984).

# 47
# Truth, trust and paternalism

## THURSTAN B. BREWIN

Let's be a little more honest about the importance of 'being honest'. We need to strike a balance between 'informed consent' and 'paternalism'. The idea of the first as a great good and the second as a great evil is today in danger of being carried to absurd lengths. Yet few doctors dare say so (at any rate in public) for fear of being called paternalistic, old fashioned, arrogant – or worse.

Communication is of crucial importance in medicine. Partly to inform, explain, and advise. And partly – especially when a patient is frightened, ill, weak, or otherwise vulnerable – to raise morale, give confidence, encourage, and protect. Whether or not we call this 'paternalism', the fact is that to try and abolish it would be a sure way to add greatly to the sum total of human suffering.

Unfortunately, as so often in life, one aim may conflict with the other. To compromise makes us feel uncomfortable. We would prefer to be guided by some noble moral principle. But such principles – pure and inspiring though they seem at first sight – are liable to give contradictory advice. Sanctity of life is a precious concept, but most people feel that it has to be restrained at times, if it is not to cause excessive suffering or distress. The rights of the individual may have to be curtailed in the interests of the community. Similarly, though we all prize truthfulness, there are times when the thought of 'telling someone the truth' – or a particular part of it – may seem so cruel and pointless that most of us (whether doctors or not) will decide against it.

It is easy to denigrate compromise of this kind. But sometimes the only alternative is to embrace one noble principle and murder another. Which seems even worse. So we compromise; but, we hope, in a civilised and humane manner.

Two new books provide good examples of the tendency to stress the first aim of communication at the expense of the second. One, written jointly by a journalist and a doctor,[1] covers all kinds of ethical dilemma (abortion, embryo research, confidentiality, resource allocation, and so on) and is recommended for the fair and thorough way it deals with most of them. However, when it comes to 'informed consent' both this book and the other (written by a journalist on her own[2]) give views which, I would guess, will be judged by future generations to be lacking in balance. The advantages of trying to explain risks and options to all patients are well set out, but the serious limitations and disadvantages are too often played down or ignored.

Here are two uncompromising extracts from the first book:[1]

> Consent is meaningless unless it is informed. And it is not possible for the patient to be informed unless he has been told the whole truth about himself. (p. 144)

> The patient's most important safeguard is for the doctor to tell the truth – not simply never to lie, but not to withhold information . . . for without information there can be no consent to treatment. (p. 173)

This sort of thing sounds fine until we come down to earth and think it through, in terms of practical everyday life. Is consent really to be judged 'meaningless unless it is informed?' What about trust? If I seek the help of an accountant, builder, lawyer, or cobbler, my consent to what he does with my money, my house, my reputation, or my shoes is likely to be based on a blend of information and trust. Of course, I may want to discuss certain options and risks. But the more trust the less need for me to ask a lot of searching questions. Thus saving both his time and mine.

As soon as the expert that I consult sees what the problem is, may I not just trust him to do his best and get on with it? Does he have to keep explaining to every client or customer why he prefers his own particular way of doing things? Or how he has been lately trying out new methods? Or how somebody in a similar situation once finished up worse off instead of better off? And if he 'deliberately conceals' such things (partly because if he tried to explain everything to everybody he could never get on with his work) is he being unethical? Is his failure to tell the whole truth to be judged morally equivalent to telling a lie?

What happens when the element of fear is injected into a non-medical situation? Most people facing death or danger during a hijack, the failure of an aircraft, or some other disaster will feel safer if there is some leadership. A good leader behaves in a very similar way to a good doctor in a medical crisis.[3] Much will depend on his personality, but he must not be too optimistic, nor too pessimistic. He must be blunt enough to get everyone's confidence, but he will often keep to himself certain grim possibilities and certain areas of doubt or confusion. Nearly everyone will see this as part of his job and will not think any less of him for it. Nobody calls him a paternalist just because he uses his discretion. Words of encouragement that cut no ice with people who are not unduly frightened may greatly help those who are. If he does a good job he can improve morale immeasurably. Above all, he does not just blindly dish out 'complete honesty' and tell everybody everything that they 'have a right to know'. It is not that easy. Nor will he – if he has a grain of sense – ask each person to choose if they want to know the full facts or not. What are they supposed to say? And what will be the subsequent state of mind of someone who replies that he prefers not to know? Will he not just feel a coward and worry about what others have been told?

Moreover, trust is a marvellous time saver. Whether we are speaking of medical or non-medical problems, discussions of risks and options may, of course, have a high priority. On the other hand, it does not make sense to allow lengthy low-priority explanations to encroach too far into available time, leading to less work done and fewer people helped. How strange that this obvious and important point regarding priorities is so seldom mentioned by those who urge patients and others not to take so much on trust. They seem to imagine that vast chunks of time can be plucked out of thin air without any damage to general standards of care and efficiency.

Trust also means less risk of those misconceptions that experience teaches us can arise so easily when detailed information is given. Phillips and Dawson, the authors of the first book I am quoting, believe that 'to argue that detail equals confusion is an example of the worst kind of paternalism'. But any doctor who asks a patient or relative at the end of a lengthy interview (or even a brief one) 'what will you say if someone asks you what I have told you?', soon discovers how common are immediate misconceptions – quite apart from how much is remembered later. Evidence confirms it.[4] And this is hardly surprising. Picture a doctor in his own home discussing complicated matters with his plumber. How will he get on if he tries to repeat it all to a friend a week later? And supposing experience has taught the plumber that, although some doctors understand what he is talking about, others don't – and suppose that the plumber (especially when he is busy) says to the customer 'you will just have to trust me to do the best job I can'. Is that arrogant paternalism?

True, there are patients getting too much paternalism and not enough explanation. But when it is the other way round it is much less likely to be reported. No patient is going to complain that he was told too much. Nor that when he was frightened nobody held his hand.

Fortunately for general standards of medical care, a fair amount of trust and a limited amount of information about risks and options still suits many patients very well (including many doctors when they are ill) – at least in the United Kingdom. Others (again including many doctors, who vary just as much as anyone else) prefer a lot of information and are greatly reassured by it. Knowledge can improve morale. So can trust. Sometimes it is right to discuss painful choices with the patient, even though they will distress him. Sometimes it seems better not to. As in ordinary life, only a very insensitive person believes that what is best for one patient is necessarily best for another. Moreover, the very same person may need much more protection (paternalism if you like) at one stage of his illness than at another.[3]

Such a regard for individual variations seems to worry some anti-paternalists almost more than consistent paternalism. All patients should be treated alike, they seem to say. Not to do so is arrogant.

Also very common is a remarkable ambivalence towards this question of whether or not the doctor should use his discretion. Here are some examples from the second book (Faulder[2]). On the one hand we are told that 'The medical consensus . . . is that remote risks do not need to be revealed . . . the patient will be told only what the doctors think it is fit for her to know . . . this outrageous paternalism has been endorsed in case after case in the English courts'. And that, 'Either a moral right [the right to informed consent] exists or it does not. If it does, then it is universal and no-one has the right to deny it to anyone'. Also that, 'Informed consent . . . is neither a concession nor a courtesy to be granted by well disposed doctors as and when they see fit, but an inalienable human right . . .'. Yet on other pages we read that 'A doctor has to tread very carefully. Some information he must volunteer, but if he sees that the patient is shutting herself off from hearing too much, although agreeing to his proposals for treatment, then he is justified in presuming that she is giving her consent . . . this kind of signalling from the patient is usually expressed tacitly'. And elsewhere that 'It is equally a denial of autonomy to force unwanted information on those who have clearly indicated, not necessarily verbally' (my emphasis) 'that they do not want it'. We also read that, 'Doctors argue with some truth that it is all very well for the strong and healthy to cry shame, but paternalism is still what the vast majority of their patients thrust upon them'. And that 'It is far too easy for the outsider to condemn doctors for not telling the truth'.

Phillips and Dawson[1] would presumably disagree with this last comment. 'We feel', they say, 'that the importance of telling the truth cannot be over-estimated.' But, like many other fine principles, we all know in our heart of hearts that this is not so. It can be overestimated. Easily. 'Truth', in fact, can sometimes create havoc. One distinguished American journalist learnt this during his own illness and was not afraid to say so afterwards. 'Most doctors', he said, 'are panic producers without realising it ... they under-estimate the extent to which their truths become death sentences.'[5]

Many friends and relatives curse the clumsy insensitivity of doctors who needlessly tell patients grim or frightening facts about proposed treatment. 'That stupid doctor', they say, 'why did he have to tell my mother – frightened enough already – about something terrible, if it is very unlikely that it will ever happen?'

Of course, it is another story when those with the benefit of hindsight express indignation that the unfortunate victim of some remote risk was never warned about it. It would be interesting to know how consistent such critics are. When they visit friends or elderly relatives in hospital do they treat them all alike? Do they consistently discourage trust and urge them all to question staff closely in order to make sure that they are fully aware of all remote risks?

We may perhaps speak of 'anti-paternalists' as either extreme or moderate. The moderate group often imagine that they are in conflict with traditional medicine. Their criticism serves a useful purpose, but what they are really doing is little more than tilting at windmills. They ignore the fact that all good medical teachers have always spoken out against arrogance, insensitivity, discourtesy, or failure to take a proper interest in a patient's real problems and lifestyle – which is apparently what they mean by paternalism. What they should really be accusing us of is failing to live up to our ideals.

The extreme anti-paternalist, on the other hand, hates trust. Probably in his private life he is secretly very pleased when somebody trusts him. But he doesn't like to see other people being trusted. It worries him. He is even not too happy about people being given advice. He would prefer them just to be given facts and then to make up their own minds. This is in order to preserve their 'autonomy'. He forgets that if any of us in any situation (medical or non-medical) takes advantage only of an expert's skill and knowledge – not his experience and judgment – we are throwing away half the value of the consultation.

What we need is better communication; more explanation for those who need it, less for those who don't; and greater empathy and understanding of the patient's real needs, fears, and aspirations. What we don't need is unhelpful rhetoric; a wholesale attack on trust; excessive emphasis on 'fully informed consent' and 'autonomy'; and a serious distortion of priorities with a consequent fall in standards of care.

For two reasons there has to be compromise. Firstly, because noble principles often give contradictory advice. Every patient has a right to full information. He also has a right to be treated with compassion, common sense, and respect for his dignity – a respect that is not usually enhanced by asking him, 'Do you want us to be frank about all the risks or not?' Secondly, because we are all the prisoners of time, the more time we spend trying to explain things, the less there is for other aspects of patient care.

Who should make the compromise? Presumably it should be those members of society who have most experience of all the subtle and paradoxical ways in which human beings may react to illness and to fear; and who have had the greatest opportunity of learning, from first hand experience, when to speak out and when to keep silent. In other words, doctors and nurses, rather than philosophers or experts in ethics.

Provided, of course, that we are at least as concerned for the welfare of patients as are the rest of society. Which is not for us to judge. But even Bernard Shaw, in the famous preface to *The Doctor's Dilemma*, observed that 'doctors, if no better than other men, are certainly no worse'.

## References

1. Phillips, M. and Dawson J. 'Doctors dilemmas: medical ethics and contemporary science', 230, Harvester Press (1985).
2. Faulder, C. 'Whose body is it? The troubling issue of informed consent', *Lancet*, ii, 75, Virago Press (1985).
3. Brewin, T. B. 'The cancer patient: communication and morale', *British Medical Journal*, ii, 1623–7 (1977).
4. Joyce, C. R. B., Caple, G., Mason, M., Reynolds, E. and Matthews, J. A. 'Quantitative study of doctor-patient communications', *Quarterly Journal of Medicine*, 38, 183–94 (1969).
5. Cushner, T. 'A conversation with Norman Cousins', *Lancet*, ii, 527–8, Virago Press (1980).

This article first appeared, in the form reproduced here, in the 31 August 1985 issue of *The Lancet*, pages 490–492. Until his retirement, Thurstan B. Brewin was a consultant oncologist (cancer specialist) in practice in Scotland, who has published a number of articles in the medical press on communicating 'bad news' to cancer patients.

# 48
# Doctor knows best

## ANN OAKLEY

> You decide when to see your doctor and let him confirm the fact of your preg-
> nancy. From then onwards you are going to have to answer a lot of questions
> and be the subject of a lot of examinations. Never worry about any of these.
> They are necessary, they are in the interests of your baby and yourself, and none
> of them will ever hurt you.[1]

These admonitions, from a British Medical Association publication on pregnancy, are
intended to console. Their tone is patronizing and their message clear: doctors know
more about having babies than women do. (An alternative, and less charitable, construction would be that women are fundamentally stupid and doctors are inherently
more intelligent.)

Obstetrics, like midwifery, in its original meaning describes a female province. The
management of reproduction has been, throughout most of history and in most
cultures, a female concern; what is characteristic about childbirth in the industrial
world is, conversely, its control by men. The conversion of female-controlled community management to male-controlled medical management alone would suggest that
the propagation of particular paradigms of women as maternity cases has been central to the whole development of medically dominated maternity care. The ideological
element, as would be expected, is not part of the agenda in conventional medical
histories chronicling the rise of male obstetrics – for example H. R. Spencer's *The
History of British Midwifery from 1650 to 1800.*[2] Spencer terminates his discussion
in a tone characteristic of the genus when he says:

> In conclusion it may be said that during the hundred and fifty years since Harvey
> published his 'De Generatione Animalium', a great advance had been made in the
> science and art of midwifery. This was due chiefly to the introduction of male
> practitioners, many of whom were men of learning and devoted to anatomy, the
> groundwork of obstetrics.

The achievements of male obstetrics over those of female midwifery are rarely argued empirically, but always *a priori*, from the double premise of male and medical superiority. More recent investigations of this argument are now revealing a different picture, in which the introduction of men into the business of reproductive management brought special dangers to mothers and babies. The easier transmission of puerperal fever in male-run lying-in hospitals is one example; the generally careless and ignorant use of technology another.[3,4] In Britain in the eighteenth and early nineteenth centuries many of the male midwives' innovations were often fatal for both mother and child. The forceps, in particular, which are frequently claimed to be the chief advantage of male medicine, were not used in more than a minority of cases attended by male midwives, and had little effect on infant mortality, except perhaps to raise it further.[4] In the 1920s in America, where female midwifery was to be most completely phased out, doctors had to contend with the fact that midwifery was obviously associated with less mortality and morbidity than the interventionist character of the new obstetrical approach.[5]

Improvements in knowledge and technique do not in retrospect justify male participation in midwifery during the eighteenth and nineteenth centuries, and if they did so at the time it was the ideological power of the claim to greater expertise that had this effect. The success of the claim seems to have had a great deal to do with the propagation of certain notions of womanhood. The nineteenth century was a crucial period both for the evolution of modern woman's position and for the consolidation of the male obstetrical takeover. Medical writing about women's diseases and reproductive capacity during this period was characterized by a curiously strong 'emotionally charged conviction' in relation to women's character.[6] Women were also seen as the 'carriers' of contagion, an intrinsic threat to the health of society. Class intersects with sexism here, for it was working-class women who were seen as 'sickening' in this sense.[7]

'It is almost a pity that a woman has a womb', exclaimed an American professor of gynaecology in the 1860s.[6] This statement neatly summarizes the low regard in which the medical profession held its female patients; through its ideological construction of the uterus as the controlling organ of womanhood, it effectively demoted reproduction as woman's unique achievement to the status of a pitiable handicap. Such a construction presented women essentially as reproductive machines, subject to a direct biological input. It enabled physicians to assert a role in the mechanical management of female disorder, thus justifying the particular techniques of drastic gynaecological surgery and obstetrical intervention, and therefore establishing the 'need' for a male medical ascendancy over the whole domain of reproductive care.

All sorts of claims were made about the womb, and its associates, the ovaries, as the site and cause of female inferiority, from physiological pathology to mental disorder, from personality characteristics to occupational qualification (or, rather, disqualification). It was not simply the process of reproduction that was perceived as disabling, but the possession of the apparatus, which evidenced its presence in a monthly flow of reminders about the incapacity of women to be anything other than slaves to their biology.[5]

Doctors contended that a woman's reproductive organs explained her femininity in a double-bind sense: women were ill because they were women, but also if they tried to avoid being women by choosing to follow masculine occupations. Medicine thus outlined the contours of woman's place – in nature, not culture, safely outside the limits of masculine society.

How and why male medicine came to assume control over the care of women in childbirth in Britain and America over the last hundred years is, of course, a complex question. But its general location is within this framework of medical concerns about the essential character of women. There are important parallels between medical and social ideologies of womanhood, yet medicine plays a particular role as social ideology. The reason for this is that the theoretical foundations of patriarchy lie in the manipulation of women's biology to constitute their social inferiority. Medicine, as the definer of biology, holds the key to its 'scientific' interpretation, and thus its cultural consequences. The power of medical ideology stems from the incorporation of social assumptions into the very language of physiological theories. The sent and received message hence has a holistic appearance.[8] To deduce the ideological component is a difficult exercise.

Ehrenreich and English[9] demonstrate how the exclusion of women from obstetrics followed a long process of staged decline in the female community health care function. They argue that male medical hostility to women is based on a fear of female procreative power – hence the corroding impact of male obstetrics on female midwifery, whether to its virtual extermination, as in North America, or to its definition as a secondary status health profession, as in Britain. Barker-Benfield's thesis is that the assault on midwives, the rise of eugenic interest in women as breeders, and the coterminous development of destructive gynaecological surgery, can only be understood as aspects of 'a persistent, defensive attempt to control and shape women's procreative power'. Among the many pungent anecdotes included in Barker-Benfield's book is his account of how J. Marion Sims 'discovered' the speculum. Sims said 'Introducing the bent handle of a spoon into a woman's vagina I saw everything as no man had ever seen before . . . I felt like an explorer . . . who first views a new and important territory.' And a contemporary commentator caught up the colonial metaphor: 'Sims' speculum has been to diseases of the womb . . . what the compass is to the mariner'. Sims saw himself as a Columbus; his New World, and that of his male gynaecological successors, was the vagina.

The tools used by traditional female midwives lack documentation, but it seems likely that they also used an instrument such as the bent handle of a spoon to examine the vagina and cervix. But the routinization of the speculum-assisted vaginal examination by doctors facilitated an opposition between male medical knowledge of women's bodies and women's own knowledge. Throughout obstetricians' long fight to establish themselves as experts, in possession of *all* the resources necessary to the care and control of women in childbirth, this clash has remained the most vulnerable link in the chain of medical command.

The conflict between reproducer as expert and doctor as expert may have five outcomes: the reproducer may accept the doctor's definition of the situation; the doctor may accept the reproducer's; the reproducer may challenge the doctor's view; the doctor may challenge the reproducer's; or the conflict between them may be manifested in a certain pattern of communication between doctor and patient that indicates the presence of unresolved questions to do with what has been termed 'intrauterine neocolonialism'.[10] In a large series of doctor–patient encounters observed for the Transition to Motherhood study, this latter outcome was much more common than direct confrontation. The woman's status as an expert may be accorded joking recognition:

*Doctor*: First baby?
*Patient*: Second.
*Doctor*: [laughing]: So you're an expert?

Or:

*Doctor*: You're looking rather serious.
*Patient*: Well, I am rather worried about it all. It feels like a small baby – I feel
   much smaller with this one than I did with my first, and she weighed under
   six pounds. Ultrasound last week said the baby was very small, as well.
*Doctor*: Weighed it, did they?
*Second Doctor* [entering cubicle]: They go round the flower shows and weigh
   cakes, you know.
*First Doctor*: Yes, it's a piece of cake, really.

But frequently, patients concur in the doctor's presentation of himself (most obstetricians are male) as the possessor of privileged information:

*Male Doctor*: Will you keep a note in your diary of when you first feel the baby
   move?
*Patient*: Do you know – well, of course you would know – what it feels like?
*Doctor*: It feels like wind pains – something moving in your tummy.

At the same time, a common feature of communication between doctor and patient
is a discrepancy between their labelling of significant symptoms. The medical dilemma
is that of discerning the 'presenting' symptoms of clinically significant disorders; the
patient's concern is with the normalization of her subjective experience of discomfort.
Of 677 statements made by patients, 12 per cent concerned symptoms of pain or
discomfort, which were medically treated either by being ignored, or with a non-
serious response, or through a brief and selective account of relevant physiological/
anatomical data.

*Doctor*: Feeling well?
*Patient*: Yes, but very tired – I can't sleep at all at night.
*Doctor*: Why is that?
*Patient*: Well, I'm very uncomfortable – I turn from one side to the other, and
   the baby keeps kicking. I get cramp on one side, high up in my leg. If I sleep
   on my back I choke myself, so I'm tossing and turning about all night long,
   which isn't very good.
*Doctor*: We need to put you in a hammock, don't we? [Reads case notes] Tell
   me, the urine specimen which you brought in today – when did you do it?

*Patient*: I've got a pain in my shoulder.
*Doctor*: Well, that's your shopping bag hand, isn't it?

*Patient*: I get pains in my groin, down here, why is that?
*Doctor*: Well, it's some time since your last pregnancy, and also your centre of
   gravity is changing.
*Patient*: I see.
*Doctor*: That's okay. [Pats on back]

Such abbreviated 'commonsense' explanations are one mode in which doctors talk to patients. The contrasting mode is to 'technicalize' – to use technical language as a means of keeping the patient in her place. In maternity consultations this interactive pattern particularly characterizes those encounters in which a patient contends equality with the doctor:

> *Doctor*: I think what we have to do is assess you – see how near you are to having it. [Does internal examination] Right – you'll go like a bomb, and I've given you a good stirring up. So what I think you should do, is I think you should come in.
> *Patient*: Is it possible to wait another week, and see what happens?
> *Doctor*: You've been reading the *Sunday Times*.
> *Patient*: No, I haven't. I'm married to a doctor.
> *Doctor*: Well, you've ripened up since last week and I've given the membranes a good sweep over.
> *Patient*: What does that mean?
> *Doctor*: I've swept them – not with a brush, with my finger. [Writes in notes 'give date for induction']
> *Patient*: I'd still rather wait a bit.
> *Doctor*: Well, we know the baby's mature now, and there's no sense in waiting. The perinatal morbidity and mortality increase rapidly after forty-two weeks. They didn't say that in the *Sunday Times*, did they?

A second classic area of dispute between reproducers and doctors is the dating of pregnancy. Six per cent of the questions asked and 5 per cent of statements made by mothers in the antenatal clinic concerned dates, mothers usually trying to negotiate the 'correct' date of expected delivery with the doctor, who did not see this as a subject for negotiation – as a legitimate area of maternal expertise. The underlying imputation is one of feminine unreliability.

> *Doctor*: Are you absolutely sure of your dates?
> *Patient*: Yes, and I can even tell you the date of conception.
> [Doctor laughs]
> *Patient*: No, I'm serious. This is an artificial insemination baby.

> *Doctor*: How many weeks are you now?
> *Patient*: Twenty-six-and-a-half.
> *Doctor* [looking at notes]: Twenty weeks now.
> *Patient*: No, twenty-six-and-a-half.
> *Doctor*: You can't be.
> *Patient*: Yes I am, look at the ultrasound report.
> *Doctor*: When was it done?
> *Patient*: Today.
> *Doctor*: It was done today?
> *Patient*: Yes.
> *Doctor* [reads report]: Oh yes, twenty-six-and-a-half weeks, that's right.
> [Patient smiles triumphantly at researcher]

Perhaps it is significant that increasingly the routine use of serial ultrasound cephalometry is providing an alternative medical technique for the assessment of gestation length. A medical rationale for the inflation of medical over maternal expertise is thus provided. Unbridled medical enthusiasm for new techniques is a general feature of modern medicine and it may be not so much that obstetrics is a special case but that medical attitudes see female reproductive patienthood as a particularly passive and appropriate site for their introduction.

# References

1. 'You and your baby, Part 1: From pregnancy to birth', *Family Doctor Publications*, BMA, p. 8 (1977).
2. Spencer, H. R. *The History of British Midwifery from 1650 to 1800*, John Bale, Sons and Danielsson Ltd., London (1927).
3. Oakley, A. 'Wise woman and medicine man: changes in the management of childbirth'. In Mitchell, J. and Oakley, A. (eds) *The Rights and Wrongs of Women*, Penguin, Harmondsworth (1976).
4. Versluyen, M. 'Men–midwives, professionalising strategies and the first maternity hospitals – a sociological interpretation'. Unpublished paper (n.d.).
5. Barker-Benfield, G. J. *The Horrors of the Half-known Life*, Harper and Row, New York (1976).
6. Wood, A. D. ' "The fashionable diseases": women's complaints and their treatment in nineteenth century America'. In Hartman, M. and Banner, L. W. (eds) *Clio's Consciousness Raised: New Perspectives in the History of Women*, Harper and Row, New York (1974).
7. Duffin, L. 'The conspicuous consumptive: woman as an invalid'. In Delamont, S. and Duffin, L. (eds) *The Nineteenth Century Woman: Her Cultural and Physical World*, Croom Helm, London (1978).
8. Jordanova, L. 'Medicine, personal morality and public order: an historical case study'. Paper given at British Sociological Association Medical Sociology Conference, York, 22–24 September (1978).
9. Ehrenreich, B. and English, D. *Witches, Midwives and Nurses*, Glass Mountain Pamphlets, The Feminist Press, New York (1975).
10. Swinscow, T. D. V. 'Personal view', *British Medical Journal*, 28 September (1974).

Ann Oakley is Professor of Sociology and Social Policy at the Institute of Education, London. This article is an extract from her book *Women Confined* which was published by Martin Robertson, Oxford (1980).

# 49

# Second Report on Maternity Services (the 'Winterton report')

## HOUSE OF COMMONS HEALTH COMMITTEE

### Introduction

What happens in pregnancy, birth and the early weeks of life is of the utmost importance to all of us.

The Committee was stimulated into conducting this inquiry by its awareness of the fact that it is now over a decade since the last major inquiry into these matters by the then Social Services Committee, and by hearing many voices saying that all is not well with the maternity services and that women have needs which are not being met.

Such discontent may seem paradoxical in view of the continued fall in perinatal mortality, and the very low levels of maternal mortality. However, although avoidance of death is very important, it cannot be the only determinant of satisfactory maternity services. We set out on this inquiry with the belief that it is possible for the outcome of a pregnancy to be a healthy mother with a healthy, normal baby and yet for there to have been other things unsatisfactory in the delivery of the maternity care. Women want a life-enhancing start to their family life, laying the groundwork for caring and confident parenthood, and we set out to discover if this is what they obtain.

Becoming a mother is not an illness. It is not an abnormality. It is a normal process which occurs during the lives of the majority of women and can indeed be seen as a manifestation of health. It is physically very demanding and is a time when women are vulnerable in many ways. They require help and support during the process of being pregnant, giving birth, and postnatally and some of this, though not all, needs professional help. In some circumstances the quality of the professional help is literally vital. But it is the mother who gives birth and it is she who will have the lifelong commitment which motherhood brings. She is the most active participant in the birth process. Her interests are intimately bound up with those of her baby.

For all these reasons we made normal birth of healthy babies to healthy women the starting point and focus of our inquiry. Getting this right is vital for society as a whole and has a fundamental bearing on the quality of life of most women and their families.

Sadly, there are those for whom things go wrong. Nature is not perfect, babies sometimes die, and others are disabled or unhealthy. It is the responsibility of the maternity services to minimise such occurrences and to treat the babies and their parents well and reduce their suffering when possible. Having normality and health as our main focus, we have nevertheless devoted considerable attention to those facing problems or unhappy outcomes.

## Policy developments in the maternity services

We believe that the debate about place of birth, and the triumph of the hospital-centred argument, have led to the imposition of a whole philosophy of maternity care which has tended to regard all pregnancies as potential disasters, and to impose a medical model for their management which has had adverse consequences in the whole way in which we think about maternity care.

Strong views are held on the question of place of birth, and as we have seen, the issue of safety has been used as the primary driving force behind the development of the pattern of normal maternity care for low-risk as well as for high-risk women. However, it is now widely acknowledged that these strong views are not all equally supported by evidence. On the basis of what we have heard, this Committee must draw the conclusion that the policy of encouraging all women to give birth in hospitals cannot be justified on grounds of safety. There is no convincing and compelling evidence that hospitals give a better guarantee of the safety of the majority of mothers and babies. It is possible, but not proven, that the contrary may be the case. Given the absence of conclusive evidence, it is no longer acceptable that the pattern of maternity care provision should be driven by presumptions about the applicability of a medical model of care based on unproven assertions.

## What women want

We conclude that there is a strong desire among women for the provision of continuity of care and carer throughout pregnancy and childbirth, and that the majority of them regard midwives as the group best placed and equipped to provide this.

There is a widespread demand among women for greater choice in the type of maternity care they receive, and that the present structure of the maternity services frustrates, rather than facilitates, those who wish to exercise this choice.

Many women at present feel that they are denied access to information in the antenatal period which would enable them to make truly informed choices about their care, their carer and their place of birth. They are unnecessarily deprived of access to their medical notes. Too often bad news is given in an unsympathetic way. Too often they experience an unwillingness on the part of professionals to treat them as equal partners in making decisions about the birth of their child.

The choices of a home birth or birth in small maternity units are options which have substantially been withdrawn from the majority of women in this country. For most women there is no choice. This does not appear to be in accordance with their wishes.

Until such time as there is more detailed and accurate research about such interventions as epidurals, episiotomies, Caesarian sections, electronic fetal monitoring, instrumental delivery and induction of labour, women need to be given a choice on the basis of existing information rather than having to undergo such interventions as routine.

We conclude that the experience of the hospital environment too often deters women from asserting control over their own bodies and too often leaves them feeling that, in retrospect, they have not had the best labour and delivery they could have hoped for.

## The evidence from the professionals

The discussions we have heard about the case for providing continuity of care and the enabling of women to control their own pregnancies and deliveries have been far too heavily influenced by territorial disputes between the professionals concerned for control of the women whom they are supposed to be helping.

The present system of shared [antenatal] care between hospitals and the community should, by and large, be abandoned. Hospitals are not the appropriate place to care for healthy women.

The desirable development of community-based antenatal care, combined with ready access to specialist assessment, will best be advanced by the general acceptance of the right of midwives to refer women directly to obstetricians or other appropriate specialists. Systems to ensure the prompt notification of GPs of such referrals will be necessary. Continuity of care in these circumstances is likely to be facilitated by encouraging women to hold their own notes.

We recommend that protocols are drawn up in every district health authority and Health Board to ensure the rapid referral of babies becoming ill at home and requiring specialised attention. To facilitate this, the midwife should be able to refer directly to the paediatrician, while also notifying the GP of such referrals.

## The maternity services of the future

### Introduction

The evidence that we have received in the course of this inquiry has persuaded us that the philosophy of approach to maternity care that is most characteristically summarised in the phrase 'no birth is normal except in retrospect' has been and continues to be an impediment to the delivery of a style and pattern of maternity care that will meet the expressed wishes of the majority of women who use these services. The exclusive concentration on this particular aspect of the risks of birth has sometimes been used as a rationalisation for a process whereby women increasingly feel excluded from control over the type of care they receive during pregnancy and childbirth and feel increasingly treated as passive recipients of an imposed and unexplained series of interventions 'on their behalf' and not as active partners in the birth of their own children. These are the predominant themes which emerged from our analysis of the evidence presented to this inquiry by women and their representatives. These problems were widely, though not uniformly, acknowledged by the professionals involved in the delivery of maternity services. There was broad agreement that women need better continuity of care and carer, more choice and control over their pregnancies and the birth of their children, more information about the options available to them, and more support after the birth of their children.

### A new philosophy

Although home births now represent a tiny proportion of confinements in this country, we believe that the prominence of the debate on this issue is a result not of the demands of a vociferous and unrepresentative minority, but of a perception that the home is an ideal setting in which to satisfy the aspirations of women. The debate about home births brings into their sharpest focus the key issues which lie at the heart of the widespread dissatisfaction with what is currently provided by the maternity services. We have no evidence on which to base any reliable assessment of how many women would choose home confinements if their choice was unconstrained, but we are persuaded that it would almost certainly be a substantially higher proportion than at present. Nor does it appear to us that there exists at present a reliable way to measure precisely the impact of any pattern of maternity care on maternal, perinatal and infant mortality and morbidity.

We do not suggest that the admirable record of achievement in these fields should be disregarded, or that the *proven* advantages of advances in medical care during and immediately after pregnancy and childbirth should be abandoned. We must continue to give attention to how to achieve better care for mothers and babies in all contexts. But policy should not be driven by the illusion that we can abolish death. Whether or not PNM [perinatal mortality] rates have reached or are approaching an irreducible minimum we do not presume to judge. We would however point out that a significant improvement in the perinatal mortality rate would be achieved if the lowest social class PNM rate could be improved to the level of the highest social class, and if the worst geographical areas could achieve the figures of the best. These are not related to levels of concentration of births in large district general hospitals, nor to the increased use of high technology in the birth process, since both these are at high levels everywhere. They are far more likely to be susceptible to other forms of social advance and support for mothers. We certainly concur with the Minister of Health that the time has come for a shift in emphasis in the development of policy for the maternity services which gives due weight to other criteria for success additional to the reduction of perinatal mortality . . . Physical morbidity and mental trauma in new mothers have not received sufficient attention, yet they are extremely important for the sake of those women and for the health and well-being of their babies.

We have concluded from the evidence presented to this inquiry that the present pattern of 'shared care' for women is failing to meet their needs. It has developed in such a way as to provide a fragmented, sometimes inefficient and rigid pattern of care often more determined by the needs of the professions, the unimaginativeness of managers and the self-validating arguments drawn from current prejudices about the division of labour than the wishes of women. We recommend a radical reappraisal of the current system of shared care with a presumption in favour of its abandonment. Rather than focusing attention on the providers of care and on the different types of services they provide, it should be the characteristics of the mother herself which should determine the planning of service she is provided with. There is much evidence to support the view that women require their care to be readily accessible and to be provided by a health professional with whom they have been able to form a relationship and who will be with them during the birth of their baby as well as antenatally and postnatally.

An important factor in making this type of care successful is the flexibility of the midwifery input – so that the midwife is able to work in both the hospital and in the community and can be wherever the woman needs her. With this type of care for low-risk pregnancies there will be a minimum amount of involvement from an obstetrician during normal pregnancies, that care being reserved for those women who need specific obstetric input thus giving obstetricians more time to devote their valuable skills to treating such women. We recommend that the development of midwifery-managed maternity units, combined with effective continuity of midwife care between the community and hospital, should be pursued by all DHAs.

*Midwives*

We are persuaded that the key to the development of a pattern of maternity services which is more flexible and responsive to women's needs is a reassessment of the role of midwives. They represent a resource which is inefficiently and inappropriately deployed in the NHS at present, and we believe that there is the potential to unlock very considerable resources to fuel the development of the maternity services at perhaps relatively little cost. What we have seen and heard of the development of genuine team midwifery services persuades us that these represent the most promising way forward towards developing a pattern where women can approach, if not achieve, the ideal of one-to-one care and continuity between antenatal, intrapartum and postnatal care.

When midwives are given the duty to manage their own caseloads, their terms of employment must recognise their professional status and encourage them to make their own judgement about the best use of their time . . . We should no more expect midwives to sit around shuffling paper or twiddling their thumbs in order to fit in with rigid shift patterns than we expect such things to be imposed upon obstetricians. They should work as salaried professionals, not as hourly workers. Midwives' terms of employment must be designed to give priority to the needs of others.

We have received no urgent request for an increase in the number of midwives in this inquiry. We believe this is because midwives recognise that they are forced to use their time inefficiently in the present structure of the maternity services. A great deal more could be done with existing resources to meet the needs of women if midwives were treated as proper professionals. There are some 35,000 practising midwives in the UK and some 650,000 births per year. Even allowing for part-timers, managers and non-working midwives within that total, there must be approximately one working midwife for every 30 births each year. That, with that level of provision, we are still failing to provide women with what they want is a striking demonstration of how inefficient is the present use of midwives by the NHS.

The successful development of team midwifery will demand great energy and commitment from midwives themselves. We have been disturbed by the evidence we have received of demoralisation and deskilling amongst this expensively trained profession. The RCM [Royal College of Midwives] tell us that out of 104 423 qualified midwives in the UK, only 34 629 registered an intention to practise last year. The medical professions have also expressed some doubt as to whether their training currently equips them to take on this enhanced role. To generate that commitment amongst midwives will require the rekindling of pride in their role and the restoration of its status as an independent profession. To this end we recommend:

- that the status of midwives as professionals is acknowledged in their terms and conditions of employment which should be based on the presumption that they have a right to develop and audit their own professional standards;
- that we should move as rapidly as possible towards a situation in which midwives have their own caseload, and take full responsibility for the women who are under their care;
- that midwives should be given the opportunity to establish and run midwife managed maternity units within and outside hospitals;
- that the right of midwives to admit women to NHS hospitals should be made explicit.

In the context of the development of the profession of midwifery, we were disturbed by the anxieties we heard expressed by some witnesses about the Nurses, Midwives and Health Visitors Bill which has been passing through Parliament while we have been conducting this inquiry . . . A profession without its own governing body and its own powers of standard setting and discipline is not a true profession as we understand it. We hope that when the recommendations of this report have been implemented and tested, perhaps by the end of this century, we will have reached a position where midwives will be fully acknowledged as an independent profession deserving the status that goes with such a position, and that this will be acknowledged by statute.

## General Practitioners
We were disturbed by the amount of evidence we received that GPs were obstructing women who wished to choose a different pattern of maternity care from that of shared care with a hospital confinement . . . we recommend that it be a duty placed upon all GP practices to have in place arrangements for women to have a home confinement with GP cover or midwife-only cover if they so desire.

## Obstetricians
We recommend that senior house officers should function as trainees, with principal responsibility for normal labours being taken by midwives. Abnormalities in labour should be dealt with by registrars who should always have the option of direct supervision by trained obstetricians (at senior registrar or consultant level).

The evidence from consumer groups . . . suggests that the small number of women in the specialty of obstetrics has a malign influence on the course of its development, as well as possibly risking depriving of proper medical attention those women who, for cultural or religious reasons, will only accept such care from a woman. Whatever the merits of those particular arguments, we are convinced, like the Minister of Health, that an increase in the proportion of women obstetricians could only be highly desirable. Miss Mellows, herself an obstetrician, told us in oral evidence:

> I do think the staffing problem is very important, and it is not just job satisfaction, it is the quality of life. I am concerned about the number of women who go into our specialty and then leave it and part of the problem is the hours of work. You become a consultant and then you are on call one in two or one in

three, and this is [a] very large commitment and it is something which people . . . should not be expected to do. They cannot run their lives satisfactorily, particularly the women with families.

At present approximately half of all doctors qualifying are women, but . . . only 12 per cent of consultants are women . . . This percentage has not increased over the last 25 years.

The Department [of Health] should encourage the investigation of new working practices, such as shift work, part time working, and job shares, which will make pursuing a career in obstetrics and gynaecology more compatible with a normal family life.

### The way forward

We recommend that midwives should be afforded the same rights as all other professions over the control of their education. Whether in NHS or other institutions, midwifery studies should be afforded independent faculty status. Selection of candidates, curriculum planning, assessment processes and course validation must remain under the control of the midwifery profession. We would expect these principles to be upheld not only in the training establishments but also by the statutory bodies that set overall national standards for training and approve and monitor the courses.

The House of Commons Health Committee report from which these extracts were taken was originally published in 1992 by HMSO, London. It is often referred to as the 'Winterton report' after its Chairman.

# 50
# Normal rubbish: deviant patients in casualty departments

## ROGER JEFFERY

### English casualty departments

Casualty departments have been recognised as one of the most problematic areas of the NHS since about 1958, and several official and semi-official reports were published in the following years. The major criticisms have been that Casualty departments have to operate in old, crowded, and ill-equipped surroundings, and that their unpopularity with doctors has meant that the doctors employed as Casualty Officers are either overworked or of poor quality. 'Poor quality' in this context seems to mean either doctors in their pre-registration year, or doctors from abroad.

The reasons for the unpopularity of Casualty work amongst doctors have usually been couched either in terms of the poor working conditions, or in terms of the absence of a career structure within Casualty work. Most Casualty staff are junior doctors and there are very few full-time consultant appointments. Other reasons which are less frequently put forward, but seem to underlie these objections, relate more to the nature of the work, and in particular to the notion that the Casualty department is an interface between hospital and community. Prestige amongst doctors is, at least in part, related to the distance a doctor can get from the undifferentiated mass of patients, so that teaching hospital consultancies are valued because they are at the end of a series of screening mechanisms. Casualty is one of these screening mechanisms, rather like general practitioners in this respect. However, they are unusual in the hospital setting in the freedom of patients to gain entrance without having seen a GP first; another low prestige area similar in this respect is the VD clinic. Casualty has been unsuited to the processes of differentiation and specialisation which have characterised the recent history of the medical profession, and this helps to explain the low prestige of the work, and the low priority it has received in hospital expenditure.

The material on which this paper is based was gathered at three Casualty departments in an English city. These departments would appear to be above average in terms of the criteria discussed above: all were fully staffed; only two of the seventeen doctors employed during the fieldwork period were immigrant; and the working conditions were reasonable. The data presented came from either fieldwork notes or tape-recorded, open-ended interviews with the doctors.

## Typifications of patients

Moral evaluation of patients seems to be a regular feature of medical settings, not merely amongst medical students or in mental hospitals. In general, two broad categories were used to evaluate patients: good or interesting, and bad or rubbish. They were sometimes used as if they were an exclusive dichotomy, but more generally appeared as opposite ends of a continuum.

> [CO to medical students] If there's anything interesting we'll stop, but there's a lot of rubbish this morning. On nights you get some drunken dross in, but also some good cases.

In most of this paper I shall be discussing the category of rubbish, but I shall first deal with the valued category, the good patients.

## Good patients

Good patients were described almost entirely in terms of their medical characteristics, either in terms of the symptoms or the causes of the injury. Good cases were head injuries, or cardiac arrests, or a stove-in chest; or they were RTAs (Road Traffic Accidents). There were three broad criteria by which patients were seen to be good, and each related to medical considerations.

(i) *If they allowed the CO to practise skills necessary for passing professional examinations.* In order to pass the FRCS examinations doctors need to be able to diagnose and describe unusual conditions and symptoms. Casualty was not a good place to discover these sorts of cases, and if they did turn up a great fuss was made of them.

(ii) *If they allowed staff to practise their chosen speciality.* For the doctors, the specific characteristics of good patients of this sort were fairly closely defined, because most doctors saw themselves as future specialists – predominantly surgeons. They tended to accept, or conform to, the model of the surgeon as a man of action who can achieve fairly rapid results. Patients who provided the opportunity to use and act out this model were welcomed. One CO gave a particularly graphic description of this:

> But I like doing surgical procedures. These are great fun. It just lets your imagination run riot really [laughs] you know, you forget for a moment you are just a very small cog incising a very small abscess, and you pick up your scalpel like anyone else [laughs].

For some COs, Casualty work had some advantages over other jobs because the clientele was basically healthy, and it was possible to carry out procedures which showed quick success in terms of returning people to a healthy state.

*(iii) If they tested the general competence and maturity of the staff.* The patients who were most prized were those who stretched the resources of the department in doing the task they saw themselves designed to carry out – the rapid early treatment of acutely ill patients. Many of the COs saw their Casualty job as the first in which they were expected to make decisions without the safety net of ready advice from more senior staff. The most articulate expression of this was from a CO who said:

> I really do enjoy doing anything where I am a little out of my depth, where I really have to think about what I am doing. Something like a bad road traffic accident, where they ring up and give you a few minutes warning and perhaps give you an idea of what's happening ... And when the guy finally does arrive you've got a rough idea of what you are going to do, and sorting it all out and getting him into the right speciality, this kind of thing is very satisfying.

Good patients, then, make demands which fall squarely within the boundaries of what the staff define as appropriate to their job. It is the medical characteristics of these patients which are most predominant in the discussions, and the typifications are not very well developed. This is in marked contrast to 'rubbish'.

## Rubbish

While the category of the good patient is one I have in part constructed from comments about 'patients I like dealing with' or 'the sort of work I like to do', 'rubbish' is a category generated by the staff themselves. It was commonly used in discussions of the work, as in the following quotes:

> It's a thankless task, seeing all the rubbish, as we call it, coming through.

> I wouldn't be making the same fuss in another job – it's only because it's mostly bloody crumble like women with insect bites.

In an attempt to get a better idea of what patients would be included in the category of rubbish I asked staff what sorts of patients they did not like having to deal with, which sorts of patients made them annoyed, and why. The answers they gave suggested that staff had developed characterisations of 'normal' rubbish – the normal suicide attempt, the normal drunk, and so on – which they were thinking of when they talked about rubbish. In other words, staff felt able to predict a whole range of features related not only to his medical condition but also to his past life, to his likely behaviour inside the Casualty department, and to his future behaviour. These expected features of the patient could thus be used to guide the treatment (both socially and medically) that the staff decided to give the patient. The following were the major categories of rubbish mentioned by the staff.

*(i) Trivia.* The recurring problem of Casualty departments, in the eyes of the doctors, has been the 'casual' attender. For the staff of the Casualty departments I studied, normal trivia banged their heads, their hands or their ankles, carried on working as usual, and several days later looked into Casualty to see if it was all right. Normal trivia treats Casualty like a perfunctory service, on a par with a garage, rather than as an expert emergency service, which is how the staff like to see themselves.

They come in and say 'I did an injury half an hour ago, or half a day ago, or two days ago. I'm perfectly all right, I've just come for a check-up.'

[Trivia] comes up with a pain that he's had for three weeks, and gets you out of bed at 3 in the morning.

*(ii) Drunks.* Normal drunks are abusive and threatening. They come in shouting and singing after a fight and they are sick all over the place, or they are brought in unconscious, having been found in the street. They come in the small hours of the night, and they often have to be kept in until morning because you never know if they have been knocked out in a fight (with the possibility of a head injury) or whether they were just sleeping it off. They come in weekend after weekend with the same injuries, and they are always unpleasant and awkward.

*(iii) Overdoses.* The normal overdose is female, and is seen as a case of self-injury rather than of attempted suicide. She comes because her boyfriend/husband/parents have been unkind, and she is likely to be a regular visitor. She only wants attention, she was not seriously trying to kill herself, but she uses the overdose as moral blackmail. She makes sure she does not succeed by taking a less-than-lethal dose, or by ensuring that she is discovered fairly rapidly.

In the majority of overdoses, you know, these symbolic overdoses, the sort of '5 aspirins and 5 valiums and I'm ill doctor, I've taken an overdose'.

By and large they are people who have done it time and time again, who are up, who have had treatment, who haven't responded to treatment.

*(iv) Tramps.* Normal tramps can be recognised by the many layers of rotten clothing they wear, and by their smell. They are a feature of the cold winter nights and they only come to Casualty to try to wheedle a bed in the warm for the night. Tramps can never be trusted; they will usually sham their symptoms. New COs and young staff nurses should be warned, for if one is let in one night then dozens will turn up the next night.

[Tramps are] nuisance visitors, frequent visitors, who won't go, who refuse to leave when you want them to.

[Tramps are] just trying to get a bed for the night.

These four types covered most of the patients included in rubbish, or described as unpleasant or annoying. There were some other characterisations mentioned less frequently, or which seemed to be generated by individual patients, or which seemed to be specific to particular members of staff. 'Nutcases' were in this uncertain position: there were few 'typical' features of psychiatric patients, and these were very diffuse. 'Smelly', 'dirty' and 'obese' patients were also in this limbo. Patients with these characteristics were objected to, but there was no typical career expected for these patients: apart from the one common characteristic they were expected to be different.

## Rules broken by rubbish

In their elaboration of *why* certain sorts of patients were rubbish, staff organised their answers in terms of a number of unwritten rules which they said rubbish had broken.

These rules were in part consensual, and in part ideological. These rules, then, can be seen as the criteria by which staff judged the legitimacy of claims made by patients for entry into the sick role, or for medical care. These are rules inductively generalised from accounts given by staff.

(a) *Patients must not be responsible, either for their illness or for getting better: medical staff can only be held responsible if, in addition, they were able to treat the illness.*

The first half of this rule was broken by all normal rubbish. Drunks and tramps were responsible for their illnesses, either directly or indirectly. Tramps are responsible for the illnesses like bronchitis which are a direct result of the life the tramp has chosen to lead. Normal overdoses knew what they were doing, and chose to take an overdose for their own purposes. Trivia *chose* to come to Casualty, and could be expected to deal with their illnesses themselves. All normal rubbish had within their own hands the ability to effect a complete cure, and since there was little the Casualty staff could do about it, they could not be held responsible to treat the illnesses of normal rubbish. Comments which reflected this rule included,

> I don't like having to deal with drunks in particular. I find that usually they're quite aggressive. I don't like aggressive people. And I feel that, you know, they've got themselves into this state entirely through their own follies, why the hell should I have to deal with them on the NHS? So I don't like drunks.

> I think they are a bloody nuisance. I don't like overdoses, because I've got very little sympathy with them on the whole, I'm afraid.
> [Q: Why not?]
> mm well you see most of them don't mean it, it's just to draw attention to themselves, you see I mean they take a non-lethal dose and they know it's not lethal.

The staff normally felt uncertain about the existence of an illness if there was no therapy that they, or anyone else, could provide to correct the state, and it would seem that this uncertainty fostered frustration which was vented as hostility towards these patients. One example of this was in the comments on overdoses, and the distinctions made between those who really tried to commit suicide (for whom there is some respect) and the rest (viewed as immature calls for attention). This seems to be behind the following comments:

> It's the same I'm sure in any sphere, that if you're doing something and you're treating it and – say you're a plumber and the thing keeps going wrong because you haven't got the right thing to put it right, you get fed up with it, and in the end you'd much rather hit the thing over the . . . hit the thing with your hammer. Or in this case, to give up rather than go on, you know, making repeated efforts.

(b) *Patients should be restricted in their reasonable activities by the illnesses they report with.*

This rule has particular point in a Casualty department, and trivia who have been able to delay coming to the department most obviously break this rule. This is implicit in the comments already reported about trivia. However, there is another aspect to this rule, the requirement that the activities being followed should be reasonable, and the obvious offenders against this rule are the tramps.

If a man has led a full productive life, he's entitled to good medical attention, because he's put a lot into society.

[Tramps] put nothing in, and are always trying to get something out.

Obviously the Protestant Ethic of work is alive and well in Casualty departments.

*(c) Patients should see illness as an undesirable state.*

The patients who most obviously offend against this rule are the overdoses and the tramps. The overdoses are seen to want to be ill in order to put moral pressure on someone, or to get attention. Tramps want to be ill in order to get the benefits of being a patient – a warm bed and warm meals.

*(d) Patients should cooperate with the competent agencies in trying to get well.*

The major non-cooperative patients were the drunks and the overdoses. Drunks fail to cooperate by refusing to stay still while being sutured or examined, and overdoses fight back when a rubber tube is being forced down their throats so that their stomachs can be washed out. These are both cases where patients *refuse* to cooperate, rather than being unable to cooperate, as would be the case for patients in epileptic or diabetic fits. Similarly, they refuse to cooperate in getting 'well' because they cannot be trusted to live their lives in future in such a way that would avoid the same injuries.

In general, then, patients had a duty to live their lives in order to avoid injury, to remain well, and patients who did not do this were not worth helping. These four rules seemed to cover the criteria by which normal rubbish was faulted. It can be seen that each of them required quite fine judgement about, for example, whether a patient was uncooperative by choice or because of some underlying illness.

## Punishment

Rubbish could be punished by the staff in various ways, the most important being to increase the amount of time that rubbish had to spend in Casualty before completing treatment. In each hospital there were ways of advancing and retarding patients so that they were not seen strictly in the order in which they arrived. Good patients, in general being the more serious, could be seen immediately by being taken directly to the treatment area, either by the receptionist or by the ambulanceman. Less serious cases, including the trivia, would go first to a general waiting area. Patients there were normally left until all serious cases had been dealt with. Sometimes staff employed a deliberate policy of leaving drunks and tramps in the hope that they would get annoyed at the delay and take their own discharge.

The other forms of punishment used were verbal hostility or the vigorous restraint of uncooperative patients. Verbal hostility was in general fairly restrained, at least in my presence, and was usually less forthright than the written comments made in the 'medical' notes, or the comments made in discussions with other staff. Vigorous treatment of patients was most noticeable in the case of overdoses, who would be held down or sat upon while the patient was forced to swallow the rubber tube used. Staff recognised that this procedure had an element of punishment in it, but defended themselves by saying that it was necessary. However, they showed no sympathy for the victim, unlike cases of accidental self-poisoning by children. Drunks and tramps who were uncooperative could be threatened with the police, who were called on a couple of occasions to undress a drunk or to stand around while a tramp was treated.

Punishment was rarely extended to a refusal to see or to treat patients. The staff were very conscious of the adverse publicity raised whenever patients were refused treatment in Casualty departments, and they were also worried by the medico-legal complications to which Casualty departments are prone, and this restrained their hostility and the extent of the delay they were prepared to put patients to. A cautionary tale was told to emphasise the dangers of not treating rubbish properly, concerning a tramp who was seen in a Casualty department and discharged. A little later the porter came in and told the CO that the tramp had collapsed and died outside on the pavement. The porter then calmed the worries of the CO by saying 'It's all right, sir, I've turned him round so that it looks as though he was on his way to Casualty.'

At the time of writing this article, Roger Jeffery was a Lecturer in Sociology in the Department of Sociology, University of Edinburgh. This article is an edited version of one that was originally published in *Sociology of Health and Illness*, 1(1), 90–108 (1979).

# 51
# Food-work: maids in a hospital kitchen

## ELIZABETH PATERSON

## Introduction

Whilst an undergraduate I spent several vacations working as a maid in the kitchens of a fairly large teaching hospital, and became interested in the implications of performing that type of work. As a result the job developed into participant observation and an attempt to examine the setting in a manner which contrasted with many traditional organisational analyses, which often neglected the purposes and definition of the actors concerned and stressed organizational goals.[1]

What follows is an ethnographic account of how the maids did 'food-work' for all practical purposes, given a variety of organisational and architectural constraints. The paper outlines the routines in which they engaged, some of which proved to be dirty, menial and boring; the common sense assumptions they made about the tasks, the materials used to perform them and the people destined to receive the final product; the 'strain' this type of work placed on the maids' conception of self; and finally the strategies utilised to combat these undesirable effects.

## Kitchen maid routine

It was from the daily institutionalised routines that passed as 'maids' work' that the meaning of 'food-work' emerged and description of these processes may lead to some understanding of the everyday assumptions that the maids, and to some extent the other kitchen staff also, made while dealing with the food.

The kitchen provided meals for around 700 patients, for the doctors', sisters' and nurses' dining rooms, the service room in the maternity hospital, the staff of the sterilisation department and for the canteen which catered primarily for technical staff.

During observation the maids' routine consisted of a variety of tasks. They emptied food containers from the heated trolleys returned from the wards and placed them in their appropriate storage areas. They prepared carrots for soup-making by processing sackfuls through 'the machine' (skinner), scraping off the remaining black sections, chopping and mincing them. Similar vegetables had to be processed in an equally tedious manner, including the washing of lettuce for salad. Maids also cleaned, battered and coated large boxes of fish. They pared, cored and sliced apples for puddings and prepared any other fruit which appeared on the menu. They removed from chickens any giblets remaining after factory processing and any excess fat, while generally up to the elbows in tepid, greasy water.

Routinely from eight a.m. onwards food was being cooked for lunch in immense vessels, stirred by wooden 'oars', dished into assorted containers and placed in heated trolleys to wait until noon. In addition each meal necessitated a succession of trolley-emptying, dish-washing and plugging-in, the process being repeated continually throughout the day, although by supper time most of the daily maids had gone off duty and had been replaced by others.

When all the food had been processed for that day, and occasionally even before, ingredients were prepared for the *next* day's dishes. Consequently besides regular accepted routines, the week's menu fleshed out the structure of the day. It indicated not only what had to be prepared or cooked immediately, but what had to be prepared that day for the next or even subsequent days.

## Working assumptions

From the above description of the grinding forward of a routine day it is clear that food is very much work to those within a kitchen, just as death is work to the staff of a hospital and old people are work to the staff of an old people's home. The need to 'get through the day' has an important effect on how they conceive of what they work upon and around.

As a result the typical, common sense ways of thinking about food and its preparation within kitchen walls are different from those outside an area catering for such large numbers and where food is not the object of work. Elsewhere, food is usually considered in small quantities, carefully washed, prepared, cooked to exact times, dished when ready and consumed in small amounts by the person concerned, family or acquaintances. On the other hand, to maids dealing with it in bulk the food became like a factory product and its preparation had meaning in that sense.

As an extension of this type of thinking – food as work – it was categorised in relation to the routines of work and its easy completion. When busy – and during the period of study the maids generally were – foods were typified as 'bad' or 'good', not according to taste but by their relevance for work control.[2]

Washing lettuce for salad was a job which maids tried to avoid. It was a long, boring task and also a back-breaking one, because it necessitated bending over a low sink while holding each leaf under the tap. It had to be performed in such a tedious fashion because lettuce, above most other foods, worried both providers and receivers. Because lettuce is uncooked and tends to lie unadorned on the plate (in the hospital at least), it is patently obvious if it has brown patches, is dirty or is harbouring some wildlife. As a result a maxim about lettuce-washing existed: 'Rather get into trouble for taking a long time than get into trouble for missing slugs'. Hence 'doing lettuce' elicited sympathy from colleagues, a maid was considered brave to tackle it on her own and therefore it was a tactic which led to being classed as a 'good worker'.

On the other hand, 'good' foods were those which required little or no preparation by maids, such as macaroni and cheese, or ones which meant that few boilers or friers had to be washed afterwards. So in this additional way the menu gave meaning to the day's routine, whether it would mean hard work or not, by indicating whether 'good' or 'bad' foods had to be prepared.

### 'Unexpected' practices

From the description of how the food was routinely prepared, cooked and dished, and how maids typically thought about food in the kitchen, practices in that part of the hospital might seem incompatible with typical notions concerning the aims and standards of hospitals in general. One notable example of 'unexpected' practices concerned cooks rather than maids, but it very clearly illustrates the pervading attitude. Even in an area of patient catering to which one would expect careful attention to be given, special diets, the approach to food was similar.

After consultations about the health and choices of patients, dieticians made out diet sheets for specific diseases and conditions. For salt-free, high- and low-protein and sugar-free diets one would expect that the food would be carefully weighed and prepared. Despite this impression of scientific control, science seemed to be abandoned when the diet sheet left the hands of the dietician. She made frequent visits to the diet's cook, but the latter seemed more concerned with the arrangement and control of work routine than with any desire to achieve accuracy. The cook wanted to receive the diet sheet as early as possible in the morning in order to begin preparing dishes for tea. Any late adjustments meant that the cook's routine was upset; dieticians who were late were invariably labelled 'lazy'. In addition, cooks on diet duty often experienced great difficulty in obtaining from the supervisor the foods indicated on the sheet, so they often had to make do with second (or third) best. Many discovered only too late that a certain food did contain the forbidden salt or sugar.

However, such unexpected practices in doing food-work might appear less surprising when we reflect on some earlier points – that food is *work* to maids and others within the kitchen, certain expected routines had to be got through in the day with only limited staff and materials being made available. They 'do what they can' given the circumstances.

### Visibility

In addition to these considerations the concept of visibility is central to any discussion of dirty and careless practices. The hospital kitchen was situated far from the visitors' entrance with few wards beyond it, with the result that there was seldom sufficient reason for outsiders to pass and glance in. Doctors and other non-domestic staff would only be interested in entering the kitchen while 'food-work' was in progress if they had a specific aim, which was unlikely given their preoccupations.

Since control is more likely to be exercised when behaviour is conspicuous and when violation of standards leaves tangible evidence, when it *was* expected that any deviation from expectations would be noticed, a conscious presentation of cleanliness was required by the supervisor. We have seen how much care was taken over lettuce-washing. In sum the kitchen and its staff were presented as clean and savoury in line with the 'front' that the rest of the hospital maintained, and any discrepant information and 'dirty work' concealed.

## 'Staff' and 'patients'

Up to this point the discussion appears to indicate that the 'unexpected' standards of food production were similar for all categories served by the kitchen. However this was not the case. Standards differed for doctors and sisters, who were considered of high social worth, for nurses and technical staff who were lower in the hierarchy, for private patients who were considered almost as worthy as staff, and for 'ordinary' patients, whose status was considered lowest of all. This was related to the power of the respective categories; their power to demand accounts for food that was deemed unsatisfactory; the power resting in the fact that all groups except 'ordinary' patients could be said to pay for their meals.

Staff also got priority with containers, i.e. they received shiny new ones, or plates and glass dishes as opposed to metal trays, whereas any bashed object that could conceivably hold food was placed in the patients' trolleys. Different maids and cooks prepared staff and patients' meals, the staff side being allocated a larger quota than the patients' side, perhaps indicating the desire to perform staff preparation more thoroughly.

Ward C contained private patients and they often received the same food as staff, except for those patients on special diets. Patients on this ward got personalised extras, such as individual moulds for jelly, parsley in a small container which could be sprinkled on food if desired, sole instead of haddock and so on. They were also likely to receive 'treats' such as strawberry tarts, while these delights were never offered to other patients. However, it must not be overlooked that much of this personalised treatment may have stemmed from the fact that the food was being served for much smaller numbers. So decisions about the worth and financial contributions of clientele in this instance had a quite dramatic effect, especially for bored patients for whom food could have become the only highlight in the day's dull routine.

## Implications for maids

Although the impression may have been given that maids performed 'food-work' routines and engaged in dirty and discriminatory practices with equanimity this was not invariably the case. Although much had become taken for granted they frequently reacted unfavourably towards the job and how it affected them as human beings in general and as women in particular. In a large variety of ways the work had implications for their self conception and their general well-being.

Behaviour in the role of bulk food-producer often conflicted with that of food-producer in the home, and this 'role strain'[3] was felt particularly acutely among newcomers or those whose relatives or friends were also patients. A further element of the maids' problem was that since their products seldom reached the consumer direct, there was no one to praise them. They produced only transient things like cleanness and scraped carrots. In addition the maids saw the work as very hard and the allocation of duties as unfair. The job was also dangerous because of the likelihood of falling on the greasy floors, being burned on the multitude of hotplates and ovens, or being cut by knives or other dangerous equipment. Furthermore maids were subordinate to all others in the kitchen hierarchy, low in power and in status.

It was considered a tough and demeaning job even in comparison with being a maid in other sections of the hospital; other maids did not have to wear the unbecoming caps and aprons in addition to their overalls; they were allowed a greater degree of autonomy in organising their work; and they could increase their status by contact with nursing staff. How lowly kitchen maids were considered in hospital eyes was illustrated by the fact that not only had they to queue silently on Friday lunchtime to be handed their pay abruptly 'like a food ration', but kitchen maids received theirs after all other maids and cooks; consequently they had to stand around longer and their half-hour lunch break was reduced considerably.

Finally, it has been extensively documented that a large portion of kitchen maid work was physically unpleasant. In most occupations there are elements of this dirty work, disgusting, degrading or immoral tasks which the incumbents try to avoid or regulate – for example, by allocating this sort of work to others. In the kitchen cooks' dirty work was allocated to maids.

In sum there were few maids who did not resent the implications of their work for their conception of themselves as clean, attractive, concerned and fairly independent women.


## Maids' strategies

As a result of the problems outlined maids utilised a variety of tactics to negate the undesirable effects of the organisational setting, of the dirty, strenuous, repetitive, demeaning and unsatisfying work.

### Making adjustments

Maids tried to 'distance themselves' from their position within the kitchen in an attempt to control the definition of themselves in the situation. To indicate that they did not wish to be classed as a 'skivvy', most expressed the forced nature of their work, i.e. 'this is not the *real* me'. To distance themselves from their subordinate position maids attempted to develop a joking relationship with those cooks considered amenable to this approach. A maid might jokingly blame someone else for a mistake or make mock apologies to superiors. For they found that they could be disrespectful to authority if what they said was heavily disguised as a joke. However, such comments were not always accepted as a joke, and negotiation often occurred over whether or not the initial remark or 'insubordination' was merely some fun or whether a message of more serious consequence was intended. As a result, maids had to handle joking carefully in order to avoid disrupting working relationships completely.

Distance from their position as 'skivvy' was also expressed by sullen replies, biting comments after the superior had departed, or, as happened repeatedly in the kitchen because the facilities were available, by loud banging of containers and equipment. Maids often symbolically rejected being ordered around by appearing aloof, walking slowly and taking an extremely long time to perform a task.

Conversational topics were also part of this comprehensive fabric of behaviour which disassociated their role in menial and dirty tasks from their 'real' selves, the good housewives, the interesting people. Talk not only passed time but gave evidence of the lives these women took part in outside work.

Regulating appearance was yet another method used to negate the role. All kitchen maids were forced to wear unattractive nylon caps. The older women with short hair objected to the cap spoiling the style, so they crumpled it into a ball and pinned it at the back. Many of the older maids had their hair styled regularly, and maids and cooks tended to wear a great deal of perfume as if to combat any clinging odours of 'food-work'.

Furthermore, in addition to these distancing tactics, maids worked the system.[4] They would take things from the kitchen as if in compensation for being employed there. They consumed pieces of cooked meat that were lying around; they carefully chose the nicest tomatoes to eat with their toast. Maids would be annoyed if there was nothing for them to pinch; if, for example, all the tomatoes had been used up before breakfast for patients' meals, and not enough remained to take for their own break, an extra box would appear from the larder, with claims that they were bound to need them later.

Taking food out of the premises was far less common, although it would be fair to say that no kitchen maid's family went short of tomatoes; large turnover and ease of handling made them a popular prey. And although there were continual complaints about the shortage of [cleaning] cloths, most of the married women ensured that they had a constant supply of the better ones for private use. They got the most out of the kitchen as if to compensate for being engaged in a rather demeaning job.

*Combating monotony*

It has been shown that work was not only subordinate and dirty but that several of its aspects were extremely boring, a factor in many low-status occupations. Hence methods of overcoming the tedium were important for doing 'food-work'.

Most maids took a variety of 'smoke-breaks', generally before breakfast, before lunch and before leaving in the afternoon. These were enjoyed in the toilet due to the scarcity of other 'back regions' or 'free places'.[4] The toilet was one of the few areas almost accepted by senior staff as a place of escape from work routines for short periods of time. Unfortunately outside the actual cubicles – in the cloakroom – there were only two chairs, so maids were often found sitting on the cupboards, on the sinks or even on the floor. So the day would be routinely broken up; at about nine o'clock each morning maids asked each other, 'Are you going to the toilet?'; at around nine fifteen the signal was 'It's toilet time'.

'Floor time', the period when respective 'sides' washed the areas of the kitchen allotted to them, also broke the monotony of work like scraping carrots all morning. In addition they had the more illicit 'tea time', taken apart from the regular breaks, and occurring in the vegetable room, another quite secluded region. In addition the older women went to the refectory each Saturday lunch time for a drink (although the break only lasted half an hour) and on Sunday, when the refectory was closed, they drove to a hotel nearby. For these trips they had to remove their working overalls, and in this way they could step out of their role as maids for a short time at least.

## Conclusions

This necessarily truncated description of how maids engaged in some aspects of 'food-work' has outlined the dirty, menial and boring routines which came to be accepted as 'maids' work', and the assumptions they made about that work, the materials involved and the recipients of the final product. This occupation had several undesirable, demeaning effects on the maids' conception of self and led to a variety of strategies or adjustments on their part, many of them tolerated by supervision.

What has been described may disturb those who organise catering in medical (and other) institutions, and is highly relevant to debates concerning the generally poor state of hospital meals and the periodic outbreaks of food-poisoning among patients. But it has been made clear throughout the discussion that there were numerous practical factors involved in the behaviour displayed; there would be many 'good' organisational reasons for 'bad' hospital food.

## Notes and references

1. For a detailed critique of organisational analyses, see David Silverman, *The Theory of Organisations: A Sociological Framework*, Heinemann, London (1971).
2. This 'good'/'bad' categorisation is common in other sorts of occupation. The workers' clientele is often typified in such a manner. See Raymond Gold, 'Janitors versus tenants: a status-income dilemma', *The American Journal of Sociology*, 57, No. 5, pp. 487–493 (March, 1952) and Raymond Gold, 'In the basement: the apartment-building janitor', in Peter Berger (ed.), *The Human Shape of Work*, Macmillan, New York (1964) for discussion of 'good' and 'bad' tenants.
3. William J. Goode, 'A theory of role strain', *American Sociological Review*, 25, No. 4, pp. 483–496 (August 1960).
4. See Erving Goffman, *Asylums: Essays on the social situation of mental patients*, Penguin, Harmondsworth (1970).

At the time of writing this article, Elizabeth Paterson was a Research Fellow and sociologist at the MRC Medical Sociology Unit, Institute of Medical Sociology, Aberdeen. This is an edited version of an article originally published in Atkinson, P. and Heath, C. (eds) *Medical Work: Realities and Routines*, Gower, Farnborough, pp. 152–169 (1981).

# Part 7
# Prospects and speculations

## INTRODUCTION

The final part of this Reader illustrates the extraordinary diversity of published material written about the future prospects for health, disease and health care in western industrialized societies. The editors have chosen eleven articles to represent this rich territory, ranging from a systematic analysis of epidemiological trends extrapolated into the near future, to contrasting visions of a fictional twenty-first century which seem at least plausible evolutionary developments from present-day circumstances. The styles of writing and the predictions are more varied here than in earlier parts of this book, as you might expect from an authorship which includes three biologists, a journalist, several doctors of different persuasions and a social worker who writes science fiction.

The selection begins in the distant future with J. D. Bernal's vision of 'The flesh' as an increasingly troublesome encumbrance, which will ultimately be dispensed with, freeing the 'cerebral mechanism' to commune with others like itself. The individual ceases to exist and is subsumed in a compound mind, transcending concepts of health, disease, life and death. This view of the body as a flawed machine, liable to go wrong at any moment and requiring constant maintenance from skilled technicians, is a prevalent one in modern culture. But speculation about a biological 'fix' for the ills of human flesh generally goes hand-in-hand with anxieties about the products of biological wizardry running amok and escaping from social control. Several articles in this part of the book address this issue, but before the biologists get another chance to predict the future, we return briefly to the present-day.

When health policy analysts Margaret Whitehead and Göran Dahlgren ask 'What can be done about inequalities in health?' they are not looking for a magic-bullet to cure manual workers of their tendency to die before the professional classes. No biological tinkering with nature will remedy the persistent poverty and social disadvantage experienced by a substantial minority of people in many European societies, including the United Kingdom, which – as J. N. Morris pointed out in his article in Part 3 – underlies the growing inequalities in health. Whitehead and Dahlgren's prescription for reversing this trend is to break the frozen inactivity and face these complex issues by prioritizing four areas for concerted attention: infant health, working conditions, equitable distribution of services, and an audit of the health impact of European Community policies on health inequalities. The authors believe there are 'grounds for modest optimism' that European nations can begin to tackle the problems.

One strand, among many, in strategies to raise standards of health is described by Lester Breslow, an American public health doctor, who offers 'A health promotion primer for the 1990s'. He advocates a community approach that enables all citizens to collaborate in constructing a health-promoting social and physical environment, in preference to the traditional medical model of making individuals the sole custodians of their own health and blaming them if they adopt unhealthy lifestyles. The likelihood that such an approach will be promoted by public health doctors in the United Kingdom seems remote to Paula Whitty and Ian Jones. In 'Public health heresy: a challenge to the purchasing orthodoxy', they accuse their profession of reneging on their traditional commitment to public health measures as the prime means to improving the nation's health and selling out in return for a role in the new purchasing authorities. They warn that decades of evidence that hospital medicine cannot redress deep-seated inequalities in health are in danger of being side-lined as public health doctors are seduced into 'getting their hands back on the purse strings of clinical health services'. Whitty and Jones foresee the possible collapse of public health medicine as a specialty when the purchasing bubble bursts and the profession has nowhere to go.

The custodians of the community approach to health promotion in the future will be environmentally-aware GPs, according to Patrick Pietroni in 'The greening of medicine'. Whitty and Jones recognize the competition posed by fund-holding GPs, who can determine what forms of primary care will be available in a district and already meet a number of health promotion targets. In Pietroni's vision of the future, GPs will be sensitive to the wishes of the consumer/patient, including the desire for orthodox and alternative health care to be integrated within the same primary care team, as it is in his Marylebone practice. The GP will reclaim his traditional role as spiritual healer as well as dispenser of remedies, at the same time stepping down from the pedestal of the expert to engage in a negotiation between equals about treatment. Pietroni points to the need for *sustainable* growth in social structures that impact on health, together with a new realism that disease cannot be eradicated by throwing more health care at it.

This theme is taken up by Alexander Leaf, another public health doctor, who catalogues the 'Potential health effects of global climatic and environmental changes'. Unless the developed and developing nations adopt sustainable industrial policies and curb population growth, Leaf warns of a bleak future in which plankton in the oceans die from excess radiation, crops fail to thrive and the global food web collapses. An equally stark future emerges from 'The welfare man', part of a short story by Chris Beckett, whose daytime job as a social worker must have informed his prediction that, sometime in the next century, most of the population will live in a competitive world of market forces and the welfare state will exist only for the 'dreggies', the no-hopers at the bottom of the social heap.

It seems a giant step from Beckett's dreggie housing estates inside their electrified fences to the long-stay geriatric ward visited by journalist Sally Vincent in 'Exits'. But

Vincent was virtually the only visitor to this isolated outpost of society, whose inhabitants are the subject of a growing debate about how vigorously the welfare state should strive to keep death at bay. When medical technology and the pharmaceutical industry can prolong life to the point of total dependency on others, should we pre-arrange while in our full senses, for medical assistance to vacate our lives and our hospital beds at the 'proper time'? Or is this another manifestation of youth viewing old age as a life not worth living (as Peter Laslett's article in Part 3 suggests)? This question also raises fears that some means will be devised of identifying the 'undeserving' for despatch. Benno Müller-Hill recognizes the threat of discrimination against the 'genetically disadvantaged' as well as the potential for health gains resulting from rapid scientific progress in his own discipline, medical genetics. The Human Genome Project aims to identify each of the one-hundred thousand genes that encode the biological basis of human anatomy, physical function and (to a disputed degree) mental abilities. Müller-Hill foresees 'The shadow of genetic injustice' in a future society where everyone carries their individual genetic 'print-out' on a smart card and employers calculate your chance of staying productive before giving you the job.

Another geneticist, Steve Jones, takes a different view. In 'The evolution of Utopia', he predicts that genetically-based diseases will become less prevalent as a result of social processes rather than medical advances. As intermarriage increases between previously isolated social groups, genetic deficiencies in one partner are masked by genetic strengths in the other; for example, the child of a white Briton and a black Briton will not develop either cystic fibrosis (which only affects whites) or sickle cell disease (which only affects blacks). He does not expect to see mass genetic screening for the pragmatic reason that a personal genetic print-out for everyone would be exceedingly expensive; but individuals might be helped to avoid environmental hazards to which their genes make them unusually susceptible. However, the proliferation of information about variations in personal biology could lead to a future in which no-one considers themselves to be in good health. In 'The last well person' another doctor, Clifton Meador, predicts that in nations rich enough to afford the diagnostic tests everyone will become so knowledgable and so paranoid about their health that every little blip in the daily assessment of health status will lead to a trip to the doctor.

So which future will it be? In this collection you can choose from a sensitive, caring, sustainable world engaged in collaborative promotion of collective good health; or a brutal meritocracy where everyone is judged not only on their social acceptibility but also on their genetic resilience to environmental pollution and radiation damage; or a stratified society where health is inequitably distributed along old familiar lines and the health service undergoes radical reconstruction once every five years.

# 52
# The flesh

## J. DESMOND BERNAL

In the alteration of himself man has a great deal further to go than in the alteration of his inorganic environment. Man has altered himself in the evolutionary process, he has lost a good deal of hair, his wisdom teeth are failing to pierce, and his nasal passages are becoming more and more degenerate. But the processes of natural evolution are so much slower than the development of man's control over environment that we might, in such a developing world, still consider man's body as constant and unchanging. If it is not to be so then man himself must actively interfere in his own making and interfere in a highly unnatural manner. Biologists are apt, even if they are not vitalists, to consider [evolution] as almost divine; but after all it is only nature's way of achieving a shifting equilibrium with an environment; and if we can find a more direct way by the use of intelligence, that way is bound to supersede the unconscious mechanism of growth and reproduction.

In a civilized worker the limbs are mere parasites, demanding nine-tenths of the energy of the food and even a kind of blackmail in the exercise they need to prevent disease, while the body organs wear themselves out in supplying their requirements. On the other hand, the increasing complexity of man's existence, particularly the mental capacity required to deal with its mechanical and physical complications, gives rise to the need for a much more complex sensory and motor organization, and even more fundamentally for a better organized cerebral mechanism. Sooner or later the useless parts of the body must be given more modern functions or dispensed with altogether, and in their place we must incorporate in the effective body the mechanisms of the new functions. Surgery and biochemistry are sciences still too young to predict exactly how this will happen. The account I am about to give must be taken rather as a fable.

Take, as a starting point, the perfect man such as the doctors, the eugenists and the public health officers between them hope to make of humanity: a man living perhaps an average of a hundred and twenty years but still mortal, and increasingly feeling the burden of this mortality. Sooner or later some eminent physiologist will have his neck broken in a super-civilized accident or find his body cells worn beyond capacity for repair. He will then be forced to decide whether to abandon his body or his life. After all it is brain that counts, and to have a brain suffused by fresh and correctly prescribed blood is to be alive – to think. The experiment is not impossible; it has already been performed on a dog and that is three-quarters of the way towards achieving it with a human subject. But only a Brahmin philosopher would care to exist as an isolated brain, perpetually centred on its own meditations. Permanently to break off all communications with the world is as good as to be dead. However, the channels of communication are ready to hand. Already we know the essential electrical nature of nerve impulses; it is a matter of delicate surgery to attach nerves permanently to apparatus which will either send messages to the nerves or receive them. And the brain thus connected up continues an existence, purely mental and with very different delights from those of the body, but even now perhaps preferable to complete extinction. The example may have been too far-fetched; perhaps the same result may be achieved much more gradually by using of the many superfluous nerves with which our body is endowed for various auxiliary and motor services. We badly need a small sense organ for detecting wireless frequencies, eyes for infra-red, ultraviolet and X-rays, ears for supersonics, detectors of high and low temperatures, of electrical potential and current, and chemical organs of many kinds. We may perhaps be able to train a great number of hot and cold and pain receiving nerves to take over these functions; on the motor side we shall soon be, if we are not already, obliged to control mechanisms for which two hands and feet are an entirely inadequate number; and, apart from that, the direction of mechanism by pure volition would enormously simplify its operation. Where the motor mechanism is not primarily electrical, it might be simpler and more effective to use nerve-muscle preparations instead of direct nerve connections. Even the pain nerves may be pressed into service to report any failure in the associated mechanism. A mechanical stage, utilizing some or all of these alterations of the bodily frame might, if the initial experiments were successful in the sense of leading to a tolerable existence, become the regular culmination to ordinary life.

But this is by no means the end of [man's] development, although it marks his last great metamorphosis. Apart from such mental development as his increased faculties will demand from him, he will be physically plastic in a way quite transcending the capacities of untransformed humanity. Should he need a new sense organ or have a new mechanism to operate, he will have undifferentiated nerve connections to attach to them, and will be able to extend indefinitely his possible sensations and actions by using successively different end-organs.

The carrying out of these complicated surgical and physiological operations would be in the hands of a medical profession which would be bound to come rapidly under the control of transformed men. The operations themselves would probably be conducted by mechanisms controlled by the transformed heads of the profession, though in the earlier and experimental stages, of course, it would still be done by human surgeons and physiologists.

It is much more difficult to form a picture of the final state, partly because this final state would be so fluid and so liable to improve, and partly because there would be no reason whatever why all people should transform in the same way. Probably a great number of typical forms would be developed, each specialized in certain directions. If we confine ourselves to what might be called the first stage of mechanized humanity and to a person mechanized for scientific rather than aesthetic purposes –

for to predict even the shapes that men would adopt if they would make of *themselves* a harmony of form and sensation must be beyond imagination – then the description might run roughly as follows.

Instead of the present body structure we should have the whole framework of some very rigid material, probably not metal but one of the new fibrous substances. In shape it might well be rather a short cylinder. Inside the cylinder, and supported very carefully to prevent shock, is the brain with its nerve connections, immersed in a liquid of the nature of cerebro-spinal fluid, kept circulating over it at a uniform temperature. The brain and nerve cells are kept supplied with fresh oxygenated blood and drained of de-oxygenated blood through their arteries and veins which connect outside the cylinder to the artificial heart–lung digestive system.

The brain thus guaranteed continuous awareness, is connected in the anterior of the case with its immediate sense organs, the eye and the ear – which will probably retain this connection for a long time. The eyes will look into a kind of optical box which will enable them alternatively to look into periscopes projecting from the case, telescopes, microscopes and a whole range of televisual apparatus. The ear would have the corresponding microphone attachments and would still be the chief organ for wireless reception. Smell and taste organs, on the other hand, would be prolonged into connections outside the case and would be changed into chemical testing organs, achieving a more conscious and less primitively emotional role than they have at present. The remaining sensory nerves, those of touch, temperature, muscular position and visceral functioning, would go to the corresponding part of the exterior machinery or to the blood supplying organs. Attached to the brain cylinder would be its immediate motor organs, corresponding to but much more complex than, our mouth, tongue and hands. This appendage system would probably be built up like that of a crustacean which uses the same general type of arm for antenna, jaw and limb; and they would range from delicate micro-manipulators to levers capable of exerting considerable forces, all controlled by the appropriate motor nerves. Closely associated with the brain-case would also be sound, colour and wireless producing organs. In addition to these there would be certain organs of a type we do not possess at present – the self-repairing organs – which under the control of the brain would be able to manipulate the other organs, particularly the visceral blood supply organs, and to keep them in effective working order. Serious derangements, such as those involving loss of consciousness would still, of course, call for outside assistance, but with proper care these would be in the nature of rare accidents.

The remaining organs would have a more temporary connection with the brain-case. There would be locomotor apparatus of different kinds, which could be used alternatively for slow movement, equivalent to walking, for rapid transit and for flight. On the whole, however, the locomotor organs would not be much used because the extension of the sense organs would tend to take their place. Most of these would be mere mechanisms quite apart from the body; there would be the sending parts of the television apparatus, tele-acoustic and tele-chemical organs, and tele-sensory organs of the nature of touch for determining all forms of texture. Besides these there would be various tele-motor organs for manipulating materials at great distances from the controlling mind. These extended organs would only belong in a loose sense to any particular person, or rather, they would belong only temporarily to the person who was using them and could equivalently be operated by other people. This capacity for indefinite extension might in the end lead to the relative fixity of the different brains; and this would, in itself, be an advantage from the point of view of security and uniformity of conditions, only some of the more active considering it necessary to be on the spot to observe and do things.

The new man must appear to those who have not contemplated him before as a strange, monstrous and inhuman creature, but he is only the logical outcome of the type of humanity that exists at present. Although it is possible that man has far to go before his inherent physiological and psychological make-up becomes the limiting factor to his development, this must happen sooner or later, and it is then that the mechanized man will begin to show a definite advantage. Normal man is an evolutionary dead end; mechanical man, apparently a break in organic evolution, is actually more in the true tradition of a further evolution.

A much more fundamental break is implicit in the means of his development. If a method has been found of connecting a nerve ending in a brain directly with an electrical reactor, then the way is open for connecting it with a brain-cell of another person. Such a connection being, of course, essentially electrical, could be effected just as well through the ether as along wires. At first this would limit itself to the more perfect and economic transference of thought which would be necessary in the co-operative thinking of the future. But it cannot stop here. Connections between two or more minds would tend to become a more and more permanent condition until they functioned as dual or multiple organisms. The minds would always preserve a certain individuality, the network of cells inside a single brain being more dense than that existing between brains, each brain being chiefly occupied with its individual mental development and only communicating with the others for some common purpose. Once the more or less permanent compound brain came into existence two of the ineluctable limitations of present existence would be surmounted. In the first place death would take on a different and far less terrible aspect. Death would still exist for the mentally directed mechanism we have just described; it would merely be postponed for three hundred or perhaps a thousand years, as long as the brain cells could be persuaded to live in the most favourable environment, but not for ever. But the multiple individual would be, barring cataclysmic accidents, immortal, the older components as they died being replaced by newer ones without losing the continuity of the self, the memories and feeling of the older members transferring themselves almost completely to the common stock before its death. And if this seems only a way of cheating death, we must realize that the individual brain will feel itself part of the whole in a way that completely transcends the devotion of the most fanatical adherent of a religious sect. It is admittedly difficult to imagine this state of affairs effectively. It would be a state of ecstasy in the literal sense, and this is the second great alteration that the compound mind makes possible. Whatever the intensity of our feeling, however much we may strive to reach beyond ourselves or into another's mind, we are always barred by the limitations of our individuality. Here at least those barriers would be down: feeling would truly communicate itself, memories would be held in common, and yet in all this, identity and continuity of individual development would not be lost. It is possible, even probable, that the different individuals of a compound mind would not all have similar functions or even be of the same rank of importance. Division of labour would soon set in: to some minds might be delegated the task of ensuring the proper functioning of the others, some might specialize in sense reception and so on. Thus would grow up a hierarchy of minds that would be more truly a complex than a compound mind.

The complex minds could, with their lease of life, extend their perceptions and understanding and their actions far beyond those of the individual. Time senses could be altered: the events that moved with the slowness of geological ages would be apprehended as movement, and at the same time the most rapid vibrations of the physical world could be separated. As we have seen, sense organs would tend to be less and less attached to bodies, and the host of subsidiary, purely mechanical agents and perceptors would be capable of penetrating those regions where organic bodies cannot enter or hope to survive. The interior of the earth and the stars, the inmost cells of living things themselves, would be open to consciousness through these angels, and through these angels also the motions of stars and living things could be directed.

The new life would be more plastic, more directly controllable and at the same time more variable and more permanent than that produced by the triumphant opportunism of nature. Bit by bit the heritage in the direct line of mankind – the heritage of the original life emerging on the face of the world – would dwindle, and in the end disappear effectively, being preserved perhaps as some curious relic, while the new life which conserves none of the substance and all the spirit of the old would take its place and continue its development. Such a change would be as important as that in which life first appeared on the earth's surface and might be as gradual and imperceptible. Finally, consciousness itself may end or vanish in a humanity that has become completely etherialized, losing the close-knit organism, becoming masses of atoms in space communicating by radiation, and ultimately perhaps resolving itself entirely into light. That may be an end or a beginning, but from here it is out of sight.

J. Desmond Bernal was a writer, physicist and communist. He was involved, until his death in 1971, in the politics of science. The extract 'The Flesh' included here is drawn from *The World, the Flesh and the Devil: An Enquiry into the Future of the Three Enemies of the Rational Soul*, first published in 1929 by Cape, London, and republished by Indiana University Press, Bloomington.

# 53
# What can be done about inequalities in health?

## MARGARET WHITEHEAD AND GÖRAN DAHLGREN

A mountain of evidence has accumulated on the issue of inequalities in health. The existence and the extensive nature of the problem have been described in several European countries,[1-7] including lately those in the centre and east of the region.[8] This widespread evidence shows systematic and avoidable differences among social, ethnic, and geographic groups in the population in terms of both health status and access to, uptake of, and quality of health care. Many of these differences are also unjust and unfair.[9]

The debate is no longer about whether inequalities in health exist, but what can be done about them. This is the question asked by many policy-makers and practitioners when faced with the facts. But the solutions may seem so complex that people can easily become frozen into inaction. This is the impression gained from the 1991 draft health strategy for England,[10] as well as other policy documents in Europe.

Is this pessimism justified, or can the knowledge and experience gained from around Europe be used to make a start on tackling the issue? Background research carried out for a World Health Organisation discussion paper on the subject[11] has convinced us that there are grounds for modest optimism.

### Changing climate

Three general observations can be made on the various responses from different parts of Europe. First, in some places inequality in health has changed from a political non-issue in the 1960s and 1970s to one occupying centre stage·in the past few years; in several countries it has become politically feasible and timely to take action. In some places, the medical profession has taken a leading role in raising awareness of the issue and campaigning for action, whereas in others it has been conspicuously silent.

Second, where action has taken place it tends to start with small, manageable problems rather than tackling the whole subject in a comprehensive, coordinated plan. Particular issues have been addressed when a cause of public concern is seized upon and used to gain support for a policy initiative. Specific health targets to improve health status among disadvantaged groups can be found in programmes concerned with health care, social services, and working conditions. Curiously, the impact that wider programmes aimed at improvement of economic or social conditions will have on health is rarely acknowledged explicitly, though undoubtedly it will be substantial.

Third, initiatives have been taken at different levels, from national governments to small neighbourhood groups or individual health professionals working through their daily contacts. Successful initiatives often entail cooperative action across sectors on the living and working conditions of socioeconomic groups at high risk of poor health.

Such responses show that something can be done about inequalities in health, but there is no universal blueprint for success. On the contrary, effective policy to tackle inequalities in health has to be tailored to suit the systems operating in a specific country or district. However, there are some common factors and much is to be learnt from the varied experiences of other countries.

## Options for change

Several starting points could be considered. Here, we propose four types of action to illustrate some of the options.

### A focus on infant health
One approach to choosing priorities for action is to start with a particular health problem or disease that shows disparities between social groups and to tackle the determinants of the health problem either singly or in combination. Since social inequalities in health are evident for most diseases and from birth to old age, there is a wide choice of starting points. We have chosen infant health as an example, because inequalities in infancy are striking and regarded as unacceptable by the public. Attention to infant health also represents an investment in the future health of the nation, and it is an issue on which health services can take an active lead.

Disparities in health are evident in perinatal and infant mortality and morbidity, in birthweight, in infectious diseases and accidents, in height (an indicator of nutrition in childhood), and in dental health. The pattern continues throughout childhood. If all children in the United Kingdom enjoyed the same survival chances as the children of professionals and managers, over 3,000 child deaths a year might be prevented.[12]

A national strategy to tackle these differences comprehensively would recognise first the need for an adequate income for parents, as well as improvements in child care and housing. But more specific actions can be taken, particularly within health service policy. It has been estimated, for instance, that perinatal mortality in the UK could be reduced by 20 per cent if all antenatal screening tests of proven value were fully implemented.[13] Several of the tests seek disorders with strong social gradients, and uptake of antenatal care is lower in less advantaged social groups; action to improve implementation, access, and uptake would therefore have a positive effect not only on the overall perinatal mortality but also on the gap between social groups.

The same could be said for other maternal and child health services: if we ensured that all sections of the community had access to contraception and abortion services, for instance, the prevalence of undesirable factors such as early and unwanted pregnancies, high parity, and insufficient spacing between births would decline. Similarly, if immunisation services reached every child, death and disability from infectious diseases, which at present are commonest in infants living in the poorest circumstances, would be reduced. The Netherlands health authorities have improved immunisation rates among babies of Moroccan and Turkish immigrants through changes in clinic times and schedules to take account of cultural barriers to services use.[14] Inequalities in the dental health of children have been decreased by local measures such as fluoridation of the water supply.[15] Also, there are individual doctors and nurses who make sure that the pregnant women and mothers with small babies in their care receive all their social security entitlements and nutritional supplements.

Enhanced social and psychological support from caregivers is also important, since it can affect the health of mothers and babies on a range of morbidity and quality-of-care indicators.[16,17] Since there is strong evidence that maternal smoking reduces average birthweight, there is a place for sensitive support and advice on quitting smoking in pregnancy; such action would have an effect on inequalities in those countries where there is a social gradient in maternal smoking. However, education is likely to be effective in this context only if offered with some understanding of the way some women use smoking as a means of coping with difficult social conditions.[18] In successful schemes sponsored by statutory and voluntary agencies women from disadvantaged communities have given each other support to recover from depression, to overcome social isolation, and to reduce child behaviour problems.[19]

The point is that, if the health sector made a concerted effort to ensure universal access to the essential services under its control, it could make a valuable contribution to reducing inequalities in infant and child health. Health professionals would then be in a much stronger position to press for the necessary improvements outside the health care sector.

The approach of choosing a disease or health problem as a starting point has the advantage that effort is concentrated on a single issue. The World Health Organisation's programme on immunisation, for example, has very effectively mobilised effort to reduce or even eradicate specific infectious diseases in Europe. However, a drawback of the disease-oriented approach is the risk that there will be a predominantly medical response when wider strategies are also needed.

*Improvement of working conditions*
Another approach is to choose one or more of the health-damaging factors related to the conditions in which people live and work. Conditions that restrict opportunities for people to achieve their full health potential include poverty, unemployment, inadequate or unsafe housing, stressful or dangerous working conditions, and restricted access to a nutritious diet. Richard Smith has set out wide-ranging proposals on what the medical profession could do in relation to unemployment and health.[20] There have been several calls lately for a response from public health professionals to the problems of housing and homelessness.[21–23] In this article, we focus on working conditions to illustrate that a range of possibilities is available at different levels of organization.

In addition to accidents at work and designated occupational diseases, common work-related disorders include musculoskeletal disorders and stress-related illness linked to the workplace. Working conditions play an important role in inequalities in health

– the lower the occupational class the more likely are people to experience poor working conditions, including physical strain, serious injury, greater noise and air pollution, shift-work, a monotonous job, and a forced pace of work with fewer voluntary pauses.[1] In Sweden, poor working conditions were judged to be the main determinant of inequalities in somatic diseases among occupational groups.[24] Since work-related migration has escalated across Europe, some appalling conditions have arisen for migrant and other low-paid workers, and there are instances of international companies applying different standards in different countries and of children working in unprotected conditions.

So what can be done? Despite achievements made over centuries to improve working conditions and reduce risks of serious accidents, there is obviously a need for further countermeasures. There have been some promising initiatives that point to several types of action. Firstly, governments could experiment with incentive schemes in addition to traditional safety legislation, though this will always be important. In Sweden, for example, a special fund was created by the Government by means of a short-term tax on business from September to December, 1990. The substantial sum of money raised is being paid back over 5 years in grants to companies that put forward good proposals for improvement of working conditions. Such a fund can be raised in other ways – the state of Victoria in Australia uses a levy on tobacco products to create a substantial health promotion fund each year.

Secondly, people in the workforce could become more active in investigating and putting forward ideas for improvements in their own immediate surroundings with encouragement and help from researchers and occupational health personnel. When the Swedish Labour Organisation (LO; the national confederation representing over two million manual workers in the country) realised that its members had an above-average risk of ill health, it initiated a 5-year programme to improve health and narrow the gap between the members and other groups. Although the programme was centrally funded and coordinated, people in each separate branch decided their own priorities for action. The workers of one company near Stockholm, for instance, chose to focus on the reduction of heart disease, but to include not only changes in personal behaviour but also negotiated improvements in the factory canteen, better provision for shift-workers, changes in working hours, and more appropriate training for safety delegates.[25] There is also scope for much more cooperation between researchers and people in the workforce, so that workers survey their own working conditions and health problems and put forward ideas for improvements, based on their experience of the job.[26-27]

Thirdly, environmental and public health professionals could become more skilled at identifying work-related illness and could press harder for improvements in the workplace. In the UK, four projects have been initiated to identify work-related illnesses more effectively in primary health care settings. Occupational health workers are employed jointly by family health services authorities and general practitioners to build up occupational histories in patients' notes. Patients are interviewed at the doctor's surgery and hearing and lung function are tested. Individual patients are then advised on their right to compensation and social security benefits and put in touch with self-help support groups. In addition, the database on patients is used to look at patterns of illness and to relate diseases to specific industries or hazards.[28]

The approach of choosing a risk factor in the environment has the advantage that some of the clearly inequitable root causes of ill health are tackled. Several diseases could be affected by action on one risk factor. On the other hand, health is rarely a prime consideration in decisions on housing, employment, and trade and industry policy. Trade-offs over priorities have to be made which mean that rapid progress is unlikely.

### Adding equity to the equation

A third approach is to make sure that in any health policy more attention is paid to how health status, health hazards, and health services are distributed within a population. All too often at present, policies rely solely on overall rates of health indices and risk factors and the distribution is overlooked.

Perhaps this point is easiest to illustrate in the context of preventive services, such as cervical cytology. Many schemes aim to achieve uptake rates of 90 per cent or more and thus the prevention of a substantial number of deaths. However, if no attention is paid to the fact that cervical cancer is more prevalent in certain social groups, which also tend to have low uptake of preventive services, an uptake rate of 90 per cent may not secure the predicted saving of life – the people at highest risk of the disorder are likely to be within the 10 per cent of the population who do not take up the service. Here is what we propose in this case: that targets are set to reach all sections of the population; that use of services by social groups and geographic area is monitored; and that additional plans are made to increase use in low-uptake areas (for example, by means of mobile screening clinics, by active case-finding and opportunistic screening in general practice, or by employing extra nurses for home visits).

These general principles could be applied to most of the priority targets in national health strategies around Europe – the reduction of smoking-related diseases, accident prevention, improvements in nutrition and rates of physical activity, pollution control, and so on. Action on smoking-related diseases, for example, should recognise the heavier burden of such illness among less privileged groups and their poorer survival chances.[1,29] Action to reduce such inequalities could include: tobacco pricing policy, known to have the strongest influence on consumption in low-income and younger age groups;[30] restrictions on tobacco advertising and sponsorship, particularly those forms aimed at groups at high risk; the use of educational techniques, which are most effective in the less educated groups;[31] more sensitive advice and support for those living in stressful, disadvantaged conditions;[18] and action on inequalities in referral and specialist investigations by different groups of doctors – oncologists, cardiologists, public health specialists, and general practitioners, for example – auditing their referral and treatment procedures.

This approach has been adopted by Finland, which has set national health goals on both the level and the distribution of health and health care.[32] In Sweden, a parliamentary bill adopted in June, 1991, requires all national public agencies and authorities to report to Parliament on specific goals to reduce inequalities in health in different social and occupational groups and to analyse the health impact of all national policies. An Institute of Population Health has been set up to develop policies to improve health-related conditions for disadvantaged groups and to make sure these are scientifically sound. Thus, formal mechanisms are now in place for monitoring of, reporting on, and planning action on inequalities in health across Government departments in Sweden. In the Netherlands, a national research and policy development committee on inequalities in health has also been set up to inform policy decisions.[33]

Evidence from the committee was available when a new health insurance system was being discussed and the possible effects of the proposed changes on equity were fully aired.

The efficiency and effectiveness of health strategies in general would improve as the problems of those at greatest risk were taken into account, and also the health gap would decline in the long term as improvements raised the level of health of the most disadvantaged groups.

### Auditing European policy

The dramatic changes happening in Europe provide unique opportunities to address the issue of inequalities in health, not only within countries but also between them. The increasing health divide between the east and west of Germany is now one nation's problem, impossible to ignore.

For countries already in the European Community and the many that may join, decisions made in Brussels will have an increasingly important effect on living and working conditions around the region. Policy decided at the Community level has a strong influence in each member state on, for example: price, availability, and quality of food; production, pricing, and promotion of tobacco; availability and price of alcohol; water safety standards; working conditions; pollution control; and transfer of health personnel between countries.

Furthermore, the economic policy of the European Community aims to even out the differences between countries; large amounts of money are redistributed towards less developed regions to foster development. The Social Fund also concentrates effort in the most disadvantaged areas, giving priority to unemployed people, people with disabilities who wish to join the labour market, and migrant workers and their families. The European Commission is working on common policies for immigration and refugee asylum, and looking at the different benefits obtainable from health and social services.

Although there is great potential for these policies to affect health in general and health inequalities in particular, health impact is not explicitly taken into consideration in any of these decisions and there are many anomalies – the funding of tobacco growing in one part of Europe and restriction of tobacco promotion in the rest, for example.

What is needed at the Community level is a health impact approach to assess as far as possible the effect on health inequalities of European policy decisions. In the long term, the aim would be to have explicit health objectives for all policies affecting the health status of the population.

Although the European Community level has no official remit on health matters, people interested in public health in each member state can press for action on such issues through several channels – for example, by lobbying the health-related committees of the European Parliament; by briefing each member state during its six-month term holding the presidency of the Community; and by liaising with the umbrella organisations that represent non-governmental agencies from different countries.

After the revision of the Treaty of Rome in December, 1991, the Community may have a little more authority to take action on major health issues. In the long term, however, the power of the Community to reduce inequalities in health could be enhanced by the appointment of a senior member of the Commission to coordinate the actions of the ten departments that currently cover health-related matters.

Alternatively, a separate public health directorate could be created with a major focus on equity in health.

Within the context of European action, it would also be logical to implement the resolution unanimously adopted by the World Health Assembly in 1986 which called on all member states of the World Health Organisation 'to use the health status of the population and in particular its changes over time among disadvantaged groups as an indicator for assessing the quality of development'. Acceptance of this recommendation would mean the introduction of an indicator of social development alongside the gross-national-product index of economic development. The use of social inequalities in health as an indicator for social progress and quality of development would also reinforce the understanding of the economic and social roots of the health divide. To change European policy in this way is obviously a long-term challenge, but it has the potential for great influence on inequalities.

## Conclusion

These are just some of the available ways in which to start taking action on inequalities in health. We argue that national and local health strategies would be more efficient and more likely to achieve their targets if more attention were paid to the issue of equity. The gains could be even greater if efforts at different levels and in different sectors were coordinated into soundly based national and European policies. But the strongest arguments of all for doing something about inequalities are still those concerned with fairness and basic human rights.[9] Substantial sections of the community are prevented from achieving their full health potential, which is surely unacceptable for Europe in the 1990s.

## References

1. Fox, J. (ed.) *Health Inequalities in European countries*, Gower, Aldershot (1989).
2. Illsley, R. and Svensson, P-G. (eds) *The Health Burden of Social Inequities*, WHO Regional Office for Europe, Copenhagen (1986).
3. Kohler, L. and Martin, J. (eds) *Inequalities in Health and Health Care*, WHO/Nordic School of Public Health, Gothenberg (1985).
4. Department of Health and Social Security, *Inequalities in Health: Report of a Research Working Group* (The Black Report), DHSS, London (1980).
5. Whitehead, M. *The Health Divide*, Penguin, London (1988).
6. Gunning-Schepers, L. J., Spruit, I. P. and Krijnen, J. H. (eds) *Socio-Economic Inequalities in Health: Questions on Trends and Explanations*, Ministry of Welfare, Health, and Cultural Affairs, The Hague (1989).
7. Vogel, J., Andersson, L-G., Davidsson, U. and Häll, L. (eds) *Inequality in Sweden*, report no. 58, Statistics Sweden, Stockholm (1988).
8. Wnuk-Lipinski, E. and Illsley, R. (eds) 'Social equity and health in non-market economies', *Social Science and Medicine*, **31**, 833–889 (1990).
9. Whitehead, M. *The Concepts and Principles of Equity and Health*, WHO Regional Office for Europe, Copenhagen (1990).
10. Department of Health, *The Health of the Nation: a Consultative Document for Health in England*, London, HMSO (1991).
11. Dahlgren, G. and Whitehead, M. *Policies and Strategies to Promote Equity and Health*, WHO Regional Office for Europe, Copenhagen (in press).

12. Whitehead, M. 'Deaths foretold', *Guardian* (7 Dec 1988).
13. Wald, M. J. (ed) *Antenatal and Neonatal Screening*, Oxford University Press, Oxford (1984).
14. Gunning-Schepers, L. A. *A Policy Response to Socio-Economic Differences in Health*, Paper presented to the meeting of the European Community project on socio-economic factors in health and health care, Lisbon (May 1991).
15. Carmichael, C. L., French, A. D., Rugg-Gun, A. J. and Furness, A. J. 'The relationship between social class and caries experience in five year old children in Newcastle and Northumberland after 12 years of fluoridation', *Community Dental Health*, 1, 47–54 (1984).
16. Oakley, A., Rajan, L. and Grant, A. 'Social support and pregnancy outcome', *British Journal of Obstetrics and Gynaecology*, 97, 155–162 (1990).
17. Enkin, M., Keirse, M. and Chalmers, I. *Guide to Effective Care in Pregnancy and Childbirth*, Oxford University Press, Oxford (1990).
18. Graham, H. 'Women and smoking in the United Kingdom: the implications for health promotion', *Health Promotion*, 3, 371–382 (1989).
19. Pound, A. 'Newpin and child abuse', *Child Abuse Review*, 5, 7–10 (1991).
20. Smith, R. *Unemployment and Health*, Oxford University Press, Oxford (1987).
21. Morris, J. N. 'Inequalities in health: ten years and little further on', *Lancet*, 336, 491–493 (1990).
22. Acheson, E. D. 'Edwin Chadwick and the world we live in', *Lancet*, 336, 1482–1485 (1990).
23. Roderick, P., Victor, C. and Connelly, J. 'Is housing a public health issue? A survey of directors of public health', *British Medical Journal*, 302, 157–160 (1991).
24. Lundberg, O. 'Den ojämlika ohälsan. Om klass – och könsskillnader i sjuklighet' (*Inequities in Health – Differences in Class and Gender Morbidity*), Almqvist and Wiksell International, Stockholm (1990).
25. Lundberg, B. *The LO Health Project: Trade Union Health Promotion in Sweden*. Paper presented to the European Conference on Health Promotion in the Workplace, Barcelona (April 1991).
26. Reich, M. and Goldman, R. 'Italian occupational health: concepts, conflicts and implications', *American Journal of Public Health*, 74, 1031–1041 (1984).
27. Lundberg, B. and Starrin, B. *Fighting Health Hazards at Work: Experiences from Participatory Research on Workplace-related Health Issues*, Research report No. 1., Centre for Public Health Research, Karlstad, Sweden (1990).
28. Sheffield Occupational Health Project, *Occupational Health Workers in Primary Health Care*, Sheffield Occupational Health Project, Sheffield (1989).
29. Kogevinas, M., Marmot, M. G., Fox, A. J. and Goldblatt, P. O. 'Socio-economic differences in cancer survival', *Journal of Epidemiology and Community Health*, 45, 216–219 (1991).
30. Townsend, J. 'Cigarette tax, economic welfare and social class patterns of smoking', *Applied Economics*, 19, 355–369 (1987).
31. Jamrozik, K., Vessey, M., Fowler, G., Wald, N., Parker, G., and Van Vunakis, H. 'Controlled trials of three different anti-smoking interventions in general practice', *British Medical Journal*, 288, 1499–1503 (1984).
32. Ministry of Social Affairs and Health, *Health for all by the Year 2000: The Finnish National Strategy*, Ministry of Social Affairs and Health, Helsinki (1987).
33. Gunning-Schepers, L. 'How to put equity in health on the political agenda', *Health Promotion*, 4, 149–150 (1989).

Margaret Whitehead is an independent health policy analyst and Visiting Fellow at the King's Fund Institute in London, who can be contacted at The Old School, Ash Magna, Whitchurch, Shropshire, SY13 4DR. She has published widely on the subjects of inequalities in health and the implementation of health promotion strategies. Göran Dahlgren is an economist and Senior Advisor to the Director General of the Swedish International Development Authority. His work on the health implications of macro-economic policy has been influential in developing Sweden's health policy. He has also worked in several Third World countries. This article, which is reproduced in its entirety, was first published in *The Lancet*, 338, 26 October, 1059–1063 (1991).

# 54

# A health promotion primer for the 1990s

## LESTER BRESLOW

### Individual versus community focus

One important question for those concerned with improving health is whether to emphasize identifying and treating individuals at high risk or to tackle the problem at the community level. Almost any effort to advance health may focus on the individual or on the community. One may seek to detect persons with blood cholesterol levels above 250 mg [per 100 ml of blood] and follow up to reduce their levels to 200 mg, or one may attempt to lower average levels in a community from 220 mg to 210 mg [per 100 ml of blood]. Both would be substantially effective. There is nothing inherently good or bad about either approach; it is merely a question of which lens to use and how to achieve the corresponding purpose.

Medical practitioners tend to focus on individual patients and specific aspects of their health. That approach enables physicians, ideally in partnership with the patient, to assess the patient's health and to follow a path toward maintaining or improving health.

In contrast, the public health mode seeks improvement in the conditions of life for all people in the community. That course is based on favourable experience in assuring safe water supplies and otherwise creating a sanitary environment in which to reduce communicable diseases. Public health practitioners continue to concentrate on the conditions of life that lead to disease. For example, they seek to change the circumstances that favour tobacco use, rather than trying to persuade individuals not to use tobacco. Public health action thus attempts to establish community conditions that facilitate healthful choices for all people. Recently, the Institute of Medicine (IOM) reaffirmed the mission of public health as

> ...fulfilling society's interest in assuring conditions in which people can be healthy.[1]

Milton Terris emphasized that promoting health means social assurance of a decent standard of living, including adequate nutrition, working conditions, and education.[2]

On the other hand, John Knowles pleaded for the responsibility of the individual, stating that

> ... over 99 per cent of us are born healthy and are made sick as a result of personal misbehaviour and environmental conditions. The solution to the problem of ill health in modern American society involves individual responsibility, in the first instance, and social responsibility through public legislation and private voluntary efforts, in the second instance.[3]

## Health promotion: some concepts and issues

Probably the most widely cited definition of health promotion comes from the Ottawa Charter for Health Promotion (1987):

> Health promotion is the process of enabling people to increase control over, and to improve, their health. To reach a state of complete physical, mental and social well-being, an individual or group must be able to identify and to realize aspirations, to satisfy needs, and to change or cope with the environment. Health is, therefore, seen as a resource for everyday life, not the objective of living. Health is a positive concept emphasizing social and personal resources, as well as physical capabilities. Therefore, health promotion is not just the responsibility of the health sector, but goes beyond healthy lifestyles to well-being.[4]

This concept integrates ideas of community and personal effort in health promotion by focusing on the process of enabling individuals, through social action, to 'take control' of their own health. Another formulation that combines purpose and modality is that health promotion consists of

> ... the advancement of well-being and the avoidance of health risks by achieving the optimal levels of the behavioural, societal, environmental and biomedical determinants of health.[5]

As consensus on the meaning of health promotion evolves, the concept clearly will emphasize social action to strengthen members of society and will go beyond disease prevention by

1. regarding health as more than the absence of disease;
2. aiming to change conditions and institutions.

A fundamental issue is the definition of health itself. What is to be promoted? Beyond disease control, how shall health be delineated? What are the fundamental aims and objectives of health promotion? To what extent is it a task for each individual, for physicians (in roles beyond traditional medical service), or for the community as a whole? Also, what ethical and political considerations surround health promotion? Finally, how may the endeavour best be evaluated? The following sections expand on each of these issues.

### Definition of health

Whether health consists of something more than freedom from disease is an important issue for health promotion. The question goes to the heart of what shall be promoted. If our focus is exclusively on avoiding disease and injury, then the term *disease prevention* is appropriate, and the term *health promotion* may be restricted to social efforts to minimize disease and impairment, such as assuring good housing, adequate income, and safe working conditions. If, on the other hand, health is conceived as a state of 'physical, mental, and social well-being' as proposed by WHO, then it is necessary to define health as more than 'the absence of disease and infirmity'.

While WHO's statement is still not universally accepted as a working definition, the evolution of health increasingly evokes the notion that it includes well-being. Health can be regarded as a state toward the positive end of a spectrum as well as escape from the negative end, manifested by disease and ultimately death. It is certainly not something to be obtained by 'consumers' from 'providers'. That formulation, so common nowadays, grossly distorts the role of medicine in assisting people to regain, preserve, or improve health as an asset for achieving a full, enjoyable life.

A recent publication by the international Epidemiological Association and WHO describes two aspects of health: *health balance* and *health potential*.[6] Health balance is essentially the Hippocratic notion of dynamic equilibrium between the human organism and its environment. In the constant interaction between the two, the organism does not collapse or deteriorate but maintains a basically stable relationship with the world outside. A vigorous person even strives to change the environment, making it more amenable to life for oneself and others. In this positive view, health is not merely defensive.

Health potential consists of reserves – the capacity of an individual to cope with environmental influences and thus keep in balance. This concept is related to but goes further than the idea of resistance to microbiologic agents that can harm the organism. Health reserves also include the capacity to withstand the adverse effects of noise, factors causing atherosclerosis, ionizing radiation, loss of a loved one, and the myriad other hazardous circumstances of living. Psychological reserves, though in less well delineated categories, also help to maintain balance with one's environment. Ideally, of course, optimal levels of these reserves are desirable, not just those that border upon or indicate pathology.

It is possible now in health endeavours to focus on achieving maximal health in the sense of staying in equilibrium with one's physical and psychosocial environment, and not limit health efforts to avoiding or minimizing pathology. We must seek both maximum longevity and maximum health throughout life. Good health is, of course, not the aim of life, but it does constitute a major resource for life. It means more than freedom from physical and mental disturbances, such as those listed in disease nomenclature; it includes with equal importance the energy and reserves of health that permit one to lead a buoyant life, full of zest, competent to meet challenges. Indeed, one could enjoy considerable health of this kind even while having some handicapping conditions.

## Aims and objectives of health promotion

Accepting that health means both the current state of a human organism's equilibrium with the environment and the potential to maintain that balance, health promotion aims

... to maintain and expand function generally and to build reserves against forces adverse to health.[7]

The relationship between health promotion and disease prevention may best be portrayed as a continuum ranging from extreme infirmity to bounding health. Every person's degree of health may be found somewhere on the continuum. Promotion of health means facilitating at least the maintenance of a person's current position on the continuum relative to age and, ideally, advancing toward its positive end. Disease prevention, on the other hand, means avoiding specific diseases that carry one toward the negative end.

In some important respects, health promotion and disease prevention are two sides of the same coin. Many of the same actions – for example, obtaining adequate exercise and appropriate nutrition – that are aimed at accomplishing one also achieve the other. To the extent that such measures are directed against a particular disease, such as cessation of smoking to minimize the risk of lung cancer, they must be regarded as disease prevention. To the extent that the same measures are aimed at advancing health generally, for example, preserving optimum respiratory and cardio-vascular systems, they may be regarded as health promotion. To limit the term *health promotion* to health-supportive measures avoids grappling with the issue of what constitutes health – an issue that seems ripe for consideration.

## Means and responsibility for health promotion

A subtle but important difference has occurred between the time when *exposure* to hazardous agents such as contaminated water posed the main health problem and the present time, when *access* to hazardous agents such as alcohol and tobacco consti-tutes the main problem. Nowadays, personal choice enters substantially into the process. It has become the final segment of the exposure pathway. The choices made by individuals, however, do not occur in a vacuum. They reflect not only availability of whatever is involved but also, to a considerable extent, the social milieu in which the choices are made. Health promotion thus embraces both improving the health aspects of the physical and social environment in which people live and improving personal health practices.

Conceptually, individual action as a factor in determining disease and health (one's place on the health continuum) is clear enough. Responsibility for such action is, however, by no means so clear. Since the action is ultimately taken by each person, and since individuals in advanced industrial societies confront so many choices that can affect their health, many observers have pointed out that personal choices con-cerning food, exercise, use of alcohol, tobacco, and the like largely determine indi-vidual health. This emphasis on ultimate personal choice, without reference to other factors in the decision-making process, often implies that the individual is totally responsible for his or her health. Some have objected that such imputation results in 'blaming the victim' and takes no account of another decisive element: the social context in which decisions about drugs and the like are made. For example, cocaine is used for the most part when it is socially available and when one's peers are using it; asserting that the person who uses cocaine has 'free choice' actually obscures the reality. The decision takes place in a system in which the individual is the final, but only one, element in the process.

Thus, understanding the interrelationships between individual health-related actions and their social context becomes critical in attempting to deal with individual actions. Strong moral feelings often confound rationality in approaching such relationships.

Biological factors are also involved. Biological capacity is a fundamental limiting factor in actions affecting health, as it is to all human action. Infants do not make decisions about health, except to withdraw from pain. Two-year-olds given beer or snuff (as sometimes happens) do not have much 'choice' in the matter. Invalids may exercise their personalities, but their physical incapacity often restricts their freedom of choice. People addicted to opiates, nicotine, and other drugs also experience biological influences on health-related decisions, particularly the pain of withdrawal.

Influence of the social milieu on health-related individual actions to promote health, however, usually far exceeds biological factors. This can be seen in the dramatic changes that occur from one generation to the next, or even within a single generation. Prohibition greatly reduced cirrhosis due to alcohol toxicity among American males during the early part of the twentieth century, but that approach to the alcohol problem proved socially untenable, and cirrhosis mortality rose again.

Thus, essential to understanding individual action to promote health is a systems view of the phenomenon. That view takes into account biological, that is, suborganismic, factors on the one hand, and social factors that extend beyond the individual on the other. Although some would focus on individual behaviour, the social context is the dominating influence, within biological limits.

Health professionals also carry special responsibility for health promotion. Their role is to delineate the prospects for preserving life and extending health for most persons at least into the ninth decade of life; to ascertain the barriers to achieving that potential; and to advocate the social and personal actions that are indicated. Although medical services are now largely directed toward overcoming poor health by treating disease, to the extent that medical services are aimed at health promotion, they are certainly part of the total effort.

## Ethical and political concerns

Philosophically, the community approach is consistent with the principle of the collective good, that we are 'our brother's keeper'. Dan Beauchamp recently [1985] outlined what he calls the 'second language of community' in America. The first language of community health was to protect the individual against hazards; a recent example is safety-belt legislation. The second language goes beyond preventing harm to particular people, which is still political individualism. It includes

> ... encouraging citizens to share in reasonable and practicable group schemes to promote a wider welfare, of which their own welfare is only a part.[8]

Instead of 'The life you save may be your own', which represents our tradition of individualism, the public health slogan might become 'The lives we save together might include your own'.

A second, more pragmatic strength of the community approach to health lies in its avoiding dependence on efforts to influence thousands or millions of individuals in their personal behaviour. Two examples of this approach include fluoridation and tobacco advertising. Rather than persuading individuals to take fluoride with their toothpaste or to resist tobacco advertising, the public health approach is to optimize the fluoride content in community water supplies and to stop tobacco advertising on television and radio. A community environmental policy that protects essentially all people is obviously more efficient and effective than seeking protective behaviour by each person. But many such 'protective' measures related to health behaviour are regarded by some as paternalistic and intrusive, if not a violation of rights.

Finally, a great strength of the community approach is its relative permanence. Customarily, it deals with a situation 'once and for all'. Public decisions concerning health can, of course, be changed, but when healthful life conditions are established, it is no longer necessary to deal with an endless chain of individuals whose health may be impaired by the same bad conditions.

The community approach to health, however, often encounters two serious difficulties. First, health promotion typically involves multiple sectors in a society. For example, advocating a policy to curtail cigarette consumption usually brings the health official up against officials of agriculture, industry, and finance. The health issue must be of paramount social importance to prevail over interests of other sectors in a society. Second, the community approach to health must confront the ideology of individual freedom. Cherished by democratic societies throughout the world, freedom in certain of its forms may be threatened by collective action for health. Licensing individuals to operate motor vehicles is widely practised; restricting such license upon conviction for driving while intoxicated is also increasingly accepted. A further step, the systematic sample checking of drivers for intoxication, however, is being legally challenged by civil liberties groups as an infringement on individual freedom.

## Measurement and evaluation

As yet, measurement of health on the positive end of the continuum remains quite primitive, and thus, unsatisfactory. It is important, therefore, to carry WHO's definition forward conceptually and operationally to quantify health, for both the individual and the community. In the meantime, some current although admittedly limited notions and tools can be used to measure progress in health promotion.

### Individual goals

While setting health objectives at national or community levels is now feasible and apparently useful from a public health standpoint, what can be said about a comparable approach to individuals? Perhaps the first target for individuals in advanced industrial nations should be awareness of their health situation. Many people already seem eager for appraisal of their own 'health risk'. Knowledge about one's health situation, derived from a health risk appraisal, together with related attitudes and beliefs, comprises the ground on which to project health goals. Data concerning weight, nutrition, and exercise typify items involved in formulating what one sees as desirable and achievable in health.

A second important step toward personal health consists of obtaining access to medical and other health services as needed, particularly including periodic health maintenance examinations. One difficulty here is that physicians generally have been trained and practise in a complaint/response system. The physician's role in that system is to receive and evaluate the patient's complaint, diagnose the condition, and offer treatment – an excellent way to deal with manifest disease, but not sufficient to help individuals toward health. Within medical service, however, practices in two fields indicate increasing orientation to health as the basic medical service goal. In obstetrics and pediatrics, the focus is preserving and improving, if possible, health during pregnancy, infancy, and childhood. Regimes in those times of life include periodic visits for specific health maintenance procedures, not just responses to disease.

*Specific recommendations*
This kind of health monitoring can now be extended throughout life. For each age period, it is possible to define sets of goals and professional services directed toward health maintenance upon which health monitoring and action can be based. For example, for middle-adult life, ages forty to fifty-nine, health goals might be established as:

1. to prolong the period of maximum physical energy and optimum mental and social activity, including menopausal adjustment;
2. to detect as early as possible any of the major chronic diseases, including hypertension, heart disease, diabetes, and cancer, as well as vision, hearing, and dental impairments. Professional services might include:
   (i)   four professional visits with the healthy person, once every five years, with complete physical examination and medical history; tests for specific chronic conditions; appropriate immunizations; and counselling on changing nutritional needs and physical activities; occupational, sex, marital, and parental problems; and use of cigarettes, alcohol, and drugs;
   (ii)  for those over age fifty, annual tests for hypertension, obesity, and certain cancers;
   (iii) annual dental prophylaxis.

Access to lifetime health monitoring by a physician should therefore be added to health awareness as a basis for establishing and pursuing individual health maintenance objectives.

# A future for health promotion

By the year 2000, chronic disease control should be well under way, at least in the United States. Cardiovascular disease has been declining steadily for more than two decades, and cancer mortality is now declining, having declined first among younger people and now reaching persons aged fifty-four. A heavy disability burden will, of course, unfortunately continue for some years among older persons already affected by the precursors of chronic disease. The diseases themselves, however, will impair people's lives less frequently just as communicable diseases have relinquished their grip on health.

Further 'epidemiologic transition' will increasingly clear the way for attention to health promotion, beyond disease prevention. Pressures for achieving optimal health will rise, along with understanding of how to move in that direction as individuals and as communities. Guidelines for better nutrition, cessation of tobacco use, control of alcohol use, improved patterns of physical activity, and the like are taking hold among increasingly larger segments of the population – with a view toward health, not just disease prevention. As longevity increases due to these and other factors, people will seek to preserve health as a resource for living in the later years rather than merely to avoid disease.

As health promotion becomes more prominent on the health agenda, care must be taken to reach people most in need. Prominent in this category are those in our nation who have been historically neglected in health matters: the poor, racial/ethnic minority groups, and the elderly. Health promotion activities in schools, small as well as large worksites, the medical care system, and neighbourhood gathering places are the way to extend benefits to all persons. Indicators of the conditions that foster health in the whole population should replace GNP [Gross National Product] as the indicator of national well-being. Health indicators would more closely approximate progress toward securing the well-being of people than do the current gross economic indices. The well-being of people – physical, mental, and social – is the ultimate goal of society.

## References

1. Institute of Medicine Committee for the Study of the Future of Public Health (1988), *The Future of Public Health*, National Academy Press, Washington D.C.
2. Terris, M. 'Public health policy for the 1990s', *Annual Review of Public Health* (forthcoming).
3. Knowles, J. H. (1977), 'The responsibility of the individual', *Daedalus*, 106, pp. 57–80.
4. Ottawa Charter for Health Promotion (1987), *Health Promotion*, 1(4), iii.
5. Long-Range Planning Committee (1984), School of Public Health, University of California, Los Angeles.
6. Noack, H. (1987), 'Concepts of health and health promotion', in T. Abelin, Z. J. Brzezinski and V. D. L. Carstairs (eds) *Measurement in Health Promotion and Protection*, WHO Regional Publications, European Series, 22, World Health Organization and the International Epidemiological Association, Copenhagen.
7. Breslow, L. (1983), 'The potential of health promotion', in D. Mechanic (ed.) *Handbook of Health, Health Care, and the Health Professions*, Free Press, New York.
8. Beauchamp, D. E. (1985), *Community: The Neglected Tradition of Public Health*, Hastings Center Report (December), The Hastings Center, New York.

Lester Breslow is a professor of public health and Dean Emeritus of the School of Public Health, at the University of California, Los Angeles. This article, which has been edited, was first published in the USA, in the journal *Health Affairs*, Summer 1990; we have altered some words to conform to English spelling.

# 55

# Public health heresy: a challenge to the purchasing orthodoxy

## PAULA WHITTY AND IAN JONES

The purchaser–provider split introduced by the NHS reforms has been enthusiastically embraced by public health physicians. This reaction was in marked contrast to that of the rest of the medical profession and was exploited by the former Secretary of State for Health as support for the changes. Directors of public health argue that the reforms fully embody the recommendations of the Acheson report on the future of the public health function.[1] Public health's role in purchasing has since attained the status of a new orthodoxy, without there being reason to believe that the necessary investment of its resources will have any impact on the public's health. This paper questions the acceptability of such a role, thereby raising considerable doubts about the future of public health medicine.

### Purchasing and the Acheson report: indistinguishable?

The essential components of the public health function as laid down in the Acheson report are tripartite: to survey the health of the population; to promote and maintain health; and to ensure that the means are available to evaluate exisiting health services. The enthusiasm of public health physicians stems from the belief that purchasing clarifies and fulfils the role given to public health in the Acheson report and moreover anchors the public health specialty firmly within the NHS management structure.

But the assessment of health care needs is already dominating the assessment of the health status of the population. Although this situation is difficult to avoid in the face of purchasing pressure, it represents a profoundly regressive shift for public health physicians.

Quality monitoring has focused on the 'humanity' dimensions of care, such as the improvement of hospital surroundings. Only rarely has a health authority tackled the monitoring of formal patient outcome; therefore public health skills are presently redundant in this aspect of the public health role.

As for Acheson's third component, 'promoting and maintaining health', there is a growing misconception that 'purchasing for health gain' is the process by which this will be achieved. This assumption completely disregards the evidence that the state of the population's health is fundamentally determined by social and economic factors, as has been emphasised in the recent past by the widening of social inequalities; therefore the impact of purchasing health services on the population's health would be expected to be minimal. Rather, the promotion of the population's health requires governmental and societal action.[2] The public health professional has a hope of improving health by appraising and lobbying on relevant economic and social policy issues; coordinating local intersectoral action on health related issues; and, in a more limited way, by organising disease prevention programmes, such as immunisation and screening.

The confusion over purchasing and health gain has been fed by the government's most recent green paper, *The Health of the Nation*.[3] The tacit aim of this document is to improve the health of the population, but the failure to acknowledge poverty as a major health determinant and the focus on approaches advocating change in individual lifestyle as the means of preventing disease show a misunderstanding of effective health promotion strategies. The emphasis on indicators of health service utilisation as targets gives credibility to the belief that purchasing can influence health. Surprisingly, the paper has met with only limited criticism from public health professionals. The generally enthusiastic response can only support the impression of complicity, willing or otherwise, with the myth that purchasing health services will improve the health of the population.

No one would of course argue that the maximisation of benefit in individual patients should not be the legitimate goal of purchasing authorities. Public health medicine has an accepted role in evaluating that service benefit. It cannot be over-emphasised, however, that the most important of the three public health functions, to promote and maintain the health of the population, can never be achieved through purchasing.

## Direct conflicts between the new role and legitimate public health concerns

The corporate responsibility resulting from executive membership of directors of public health in the new style health authorities has been accepted as a necessary trade off of independence for influence. However, inadequate thought has been given to the implications, in particular for the independence of the annual report. Admittedly, this tension has always been present to a degree, but the right of health authorities to gag their members has never before been so clearly enshrined. Such constraints are the more worrying should the health service continue to be subject to strong political direction from the government – remember the fate of the Black report? The freedom for a director of public health to comment on policies affecting his or her local population is paramount, and this freedom should not be traded for influence over the organisation of clinical health services.

## Motives: selfless or self seeking?

The contrasting response to the reforms from the remainder of the medical profession can be partly explained by the threat of curtailed clinical autonomy. Conversely, there may be perceived gains in professional terms for public health physicians, and professional rivalry cannot be discounted as a factor in the response of public health professionals.

### Can we learn from the past?

There are some historical parallels between the new purchasing role and the status of the specialty in the interwar years (1918–40). Many public health physicians perceive this period as one in which they had considerable power.[4] During this time they had administrative control of local government hospitals and were increasingly involved in the running of personal health services. The impact on public health of the medical officers of health during this era was minimal: they had 'wearied of their traditional public health activities and . . . had progressively been seduced into hospital administration.'[5] Allowing for the very different social and political backgrounds of the periods under comparison, it would be foolhardy to ignore the implications of this historical precedent. Directors of public health are clearly enjoying the opportunity to get their hands back on the purse strings of the clinical health services, but this opens them up to the danger of being 'seduced' into over-involvement in administration, to the detriment of broader public health activities.

## The specialty's future under the new regime: naive optimism?

The goals of public health are, as we have seen, in danger of being displaced from promoting the public's health to ensuring the availability of health services. But there are other dangers inherent in public health medicine's advocacy of the purchasing role.

In districts where public health has become dominated by 'needs assessment' public health physicians are in danger of becoming 'technical assistants' to purchasing teams. Thanks to the persistent rhetoric, expectations of needs assessment are unrealistically high, whereas progress has been extremely slow, and the inevitable failure of public health to deliver the goods is bound to result in bitter disappointment. Already there are instances where this sacred cow of purchasing has been taken over by exasperated providers. If needs assessment does not lose favour altogether it is likely to become a more limited activity that could just as easily be contracted out to academic departments, at much reduced costs. In addition, when and if purchasing teams get around to evaluating health care outcomes, the urgent requirement is for original research and development, making contracting out to academic departments the most appropriate option. Where would the specialist public health contribution to purchasing be then?

### The fate of purchasing

The potential impact of fundholding general practitioners on district health authorities is enormous and could negate the district's role altogether. Public health is in danger of being isolated from 'bottom up' initiatives. For example, fundholding general practitioners have the potential to work with case managers in producing integrated primary care. In addition, purchasing authorities are now even less democratic than many trust boards, and therefore providers may prove better able to work with local populations.

## Conclusions

This paper has examined the relation between the NHS reforms, the Acheson report, and the government's most recent green paper, *The Health of the Nation*. We have shown that the enthusiasm for purchasing among public health physicians is excessive, considering that purchasing is likely to be ineffective in improving the population's health and may even be in direct conflict with this goal.

Time and time again the specialty of public health medicine has been unable to control its future, a scenario that will be fully deserved if repeated because of apathy, naivety, or the pursuit of professional power. In this case, the specialty could prove as expendable as its commitment to the public's health.

## References

1. Department of Health and Social Services, *Public Health in England: the Report of the Committee of Inquiry into the Future Development of the Public Health Function*, Cmd 289, Acheson report, HMSO, London (1988).
2. European Office of the World Health Organisation, *Targets in Support of Health for All by the Year 2000 in the European Region*, WHOEURO, Copenhagen (1985).
3. Secretary of State for Health, *The Health of the Nation*, HMSO, London (1991).
4. Godber, G. E. 'Medical officers of health and health services', *Community Medicine*, 8, 1–14 (1986).
5. Webster, C. 'Medical officers of health – for the record', *Radical Community Medicine*, 3 (Autumn), 10–4 (1986).

Paula Whitty is Honorary Lecturer in Public Health Medicine at the Health Services Research Unit, Department of Public Health and Policy, London School of Hygiene and Tropical Medicine. Ian Jones is a Research Fellow at the Health Services Research Unit, Department of Geography, Queen Mary and Westfield College, London. This article, which has been edited, appeared originally in the *British Medical Journal*, 304, 1039–1041, 18 April (1992).

# 56
# The Greening of medicine

## PATRICK C. PIETRONI

Originally the Green revolution was a phrase used to describe new high-yield wheat strains that had been developed in Mexico and were subsequently exported to India to help solve the sub-continent's chronic food shortages. Since then, the 'Greening process' has affected many of our social organisations as well as our individual beliefs and has come to mean much more. We can identify five major areas where change has taken place and how they have or have not affected the practice of medicine.

### The consumerist element

The consumer movement is second only to the concern for the environment as a principal feature of the Greening process. It can be understood in terms of power-relationships between consumer and supplier or, in medicine, between patient and doctor. We now see evidence of this in changing attitudes amongst both doctor and patient. The 'doctor knows best' approach has had to alter as it has become clear to some patients that we don't always know best. How much to tell a patient about his diagnosis and/or prognosis? How much to involve a patient in the decision-making regarding treatment are now questions we must ask ourselves and indeed have a legal obligation to do so. The vexed question of informed consent in complex operations and research studies will not go away.

The growth of the self-care movement – and alternative medicine – are probably the two most obvious examples of the consumer/patient wanting more power. In the first group the patient wants to be an active participant both in the treatment and prevention of his condition – (the explosion in health clubs, jogging, yoga groups, keep-fit, etc., are an expression of that), and the alternative medicine movement is in part an expression of the consumer/patient voting with his feet. The consumerist element in health care is seen in the various campaigns often mounted successfully by patients themselves, either against a particular medical attitude, e.g. the natural birth movement, or for 'breast is best'.

## The environmental element

The need to care for the environment is the one overriding and unifying belief that binds the Green movement together. Petitioning for the abolition of a planned by-pass or the preservation of a wild-life sanctuary are quintessential Green issues. Concern over the pollution of rivers, the ozone layer, the emission of CFCs, the dumping of nuclear waste, etc. is now at the forefront of public debate and is no longer merely a fringe or counter-culture activity. How can we live on our planet and not destroy it or so affect the quality of our lives that we do not make ourselves sick?

The major arena for concern has been over food and water. Interest in nutrition is one of the hallmarks of Green medicine – the level of additives, the question of preservation and irradiation, the use of antibiotics and hormones in meat production. The question of salmonella in eggs and the purification of water are only two recent glaring examples of how, all of a sudden, doctors have had to wake up to the real concern there is amongst patients regarding these aspects of our environment.

The concern for the environment is linked to the 'back to nature' movement. For a section of the population the doctors' insistence on drugs as the only intervention for treatment is unacceptable.

It is increasingly clear that if we are to understand the relationship between ill-health and ecological destabilisation, the medical profession will need to involve itself more directly in matters regarding the environment. Not only are many of the modern epidemics (heart disease, arthritis, cancer) partly related to environmental factors, but political reactions stimulated by the rise of the Green movement will ensure that no government will be able to ignore the validity of public concern. The specialities of community health, environmental health and occupational health have all been relegated to Cinderella status in the medical profession. The next two decades may see these areas of medicine requiring more government research than the 'high status' specialties of heart surgery, transplantation and genetic engineering.

## The inter-personal element

Like the consumer movement and the environmental movement, the feminist movement has been one of those broad sea-changes against which we can both understand and make sense of many of the changes we see in our society and in the practice of medicine. The emergence of the feminist movement has not only had a profound impact on, say, the number of women who now become doctors, but on our understanding of the psychological processes of diseases and treatments that heretofore have been described through masculine eyes using masculine language.

Not withstanding the presence of white witches, midwives and nurses, healing and health care has always been a masculine-dominated preserve. The gods of medicine, Apollo, Aesculapius, Chiron, were all male and equally important were warrior gods. We still talk of 'fighting the disease', 'the war against cancer', 'the magic bullet', 'stamping out infection'.

Menopause is described as a 'process of failure', the 'ovaries are shrunken', 'breasts and genitals atrophy', and it is not too difficult to comprehend why there is a widely accepted view that the menopause is a pathological process. It is in highlighting the words and phrases found in medical text-books, both past and present, that the male bias towards women can be identified. This bias ensured that women's role in medicine was limited to that of the comforting healer. Female practitioners were few and far between and almost always attracted the opprobrium and disapproval of their male colleagues.

We can see more clearly the masculine bias in medicine when we look at those conditions and disorders which affect women in particular – child birth, menstruation, menopause, breast feeding, contraception, cervical smear, breast cancer, obesity, anorexia and bulimia, sexual dysfunction. One does not have to be an ardent feminist to recognise that much of medicine, with its male bias, has ensured that the exchange between a male doctor and a female patient results in women feeling less in control and more at the mercy of the doctor.

Another feature of the Greening process is the move towards more gentle nurturing interventions and therapies. If we categorise drugs, surgery and radiotherapy as the active, interventionist, masculine therapies, then we can see the emergence of listening, counselling, massage, relaxation and meditation as more nurturing, containing, feminine therapies.


## The spiritual element


Up until very recently, scientific Western medicine has been content to view man and his diseases from a perspective which is primarily a form of mechanistic materialism. Since the Renaissance and Descartes, we have separated the physical from the metaphysical. Descartes saw the body as a clock. The pursuit of reason and reductionist science enabled us, as Francis Bacon said, to put the body on the rack and make it reveal its secrets. Nowhere is this move away from the spiritual to the material more evident than in our approach to terminal illness and death. There is no greater factor which determines the nature of our health care systems than our attitudes towards death. Much of medicine is organised and devoted to do battle with death. This has now been extended to the ageing process as well. We have developed an impressive array of procedures, clinical agents, multivitamins, mineral preparations and reconstructive surgical procedures, transplants, etc. whose aim is to prolong life. There is clearly a legitimate task for medicine, but we need to begin to ask ourselves the question 'why?' What is it that we are afraid of and is this attitude towards ageing and death healthy? Certainly within ecological texts, the relationship between life and death and the survival of one species at the expense of another, form a very central part of their study.

Once we begin to ask questions about death, we inevitably have to ponder on the question of the spirit/the soul. Following the Age of Reason, the cure of the soul was given to the priests, whilst medicine concentrated on the body and latterly, on the mind. This, of course, is a fairly recent separation for medicine has always been closely linked to the spirits and the gods. Many of the earliest healers were indeed priests. Jesus was known as the great healer. Plato, the father of Western philosophy wrote:

The cure of the part should not be attempted without treatment of the whole. No attempt should be made to cure the body without the soul and if the head and body are to be healthy you must begin by curing the mind, for this is the greatest error of our day in the treatment of the human body that physicians first separate the soul from the body.

What we are now witnessing in our society and what forms an essential part of many Green groups is the return of the spirit. The recognition that man cannot live by bread alone, that to be whole and healthy implies an integration of that part of ourselves that medical science discarded 300 years ago. Its modern expression in health care takes several forms. First, the vast majority of alternative practitioners are spiritual healers. Over 40,000 are registered with one or other organisation in this country – more than the number of GPs. The number of patients seeking 'laying on of hands' or some spiritual intervention, grows each month. Another manifestation of the return of the spirit has been in the use of the concepts of energy or life-force that underpins many of the alternative therapies. Patients seek these practitioners because they will be asked about their energy flow, their sense of harmony and balance. Acupuncture, homœopathy, reflexology, spiritual healing, all operate on the understanding that ill health occurs as the result of some 'energy block'. Many patients understand this language and respond to it. It is the language of the spirit. Science has rejected this model and regards it as an outdated concept.

## The sustainable element

The final characteristic of the Greening process in society is the most difficult to describe but is probably the most important to grasp. It is much less tangible than the other four so far outlined. For Greens, one of the factors that cause many of the problems they describe – pollution, over-population, resource scarcity – is over-consumption or the pursuit of growth, in the economic sense, that typifies many Western economies. In the sixties, when concern regarding the world's resources seemed to reach a peak, many of the prophecies outlined in the books, reports and conferences were doom-laden, and the solutions proposed had a 'hair shirt' air about them. No growth and negative growth were phrases that were often used. Today, the accepted wisdom is that to address many of the problems that beset us, we need to adopt a policy of *sustainable* growth.

If it is to be pursued, how then does this principle apply to medicine and health care? The pursuit of health and positive health has become a major industry, much of it taking place within the alternative health movement. The health food industry and the 'look well–feel well' approach has overwhelmed the public and the medical profession alike. It is in danger of creating a tyranny of its own in the same way as we have created an expectation that all disease will eventually be eradicated if we were given enough research grants, developed the right instrumentation and discovered the appropriate drugs. Gene therapy is now held up as the latest saviour in the way steroids were in the 60's, Interferon in the 70's, antibiotics in the 50's. At the other end of the pole, the public is told if you eat the right lentils, meditate in the right way and exercise, you will be healthy. Both of these approaches, in my view, are misguided. We can no more eradicate disease than we can rid the sea of storms.

If we are to develop the notion of sustainable health, we need first to acknowledge the limitations of what is possible, recognise that ageing and death are normal and moderate our drive for perfection with a pursuit of the ordinary.

## Conclusions

What impact, if any, have these 'Green' ideas had on the practice of medicine today?

The Government reforms in the UK such as the NHS & Community Care Act, 1990, appear to address the need to 'put the patient first'. The rhetoric underpinning the reforms – 'the user-centred seamless service' – all suggest that the power relationship between patient and doctor is being addressed at policy level. It is still unclear whether this will provide for a better service or whether the adversarial relationship between patient and doctor will result in a deterioration of care at all levels.

With regard to health, the environmental concerns have, as yet, to influence the training of doctors in any substantial way and medicine remains a personal service profession, where the community and global issues are rarely addressed. We may need to develop and train a new form of 'planetary doctor' if the issues are to be tackled with any seriousness. The feminist influence on medical care is making inroads, not only into research areas but also into the training of future doctors. Many of the more feminine modes of healing – counselling, massage, hydrotherapy – are beginning to find a legitimate place within many General Practices and hospital outpatient departments.

The hospice movement and the debates around euthanasia suggest that the taboo regarding our approach to death and dying are gradually being eroded. Many more people are making living wills and doctors are more openly discussing the conflict they encounter when caring for someone who is terminally ill.

It would appear from the above conclusions that one could be reasonably optimistic regarding the future in health care. Unfortunately it is the case that most Western economies and cultures have not addressed the last of the 'Green ideas' – that of sustainability. Medicine is still striving to find the 'magic bullet' for cancer. Gene therapy, embryo research and transplant surgery are all seen as the next phase in medical care. No doubt miracle cures will occur, but these approaches to health care are not sustainable and we continue to neglect the 'simple needs of the many in order to concentrate on the complex and costly conditions of the few.'[1]

## Reference

1. De Kadt, E. *Inequality & Health*, University of Sussex, Brighton (1975).

Patrick C. Pietroni is a general practitioner who was instrumental in setting up the Marylebone Health Centre in London, which opened in 1987 and combines orthodox medical approaches to primary health care with complementary therapies. He is also the Director of the Centre for Community Care and Primary Health at the University of Westminster. This article, which has not been previously published in this form, presents some of the ideas that he discusses fully in his book, *The Greening of Medicine*, published by Victor Gollancz Ltd., London (1990).

# 57
# Potential health effects of global climatic and environmental changes

## ALEXANDER LEAF

The subject of climatic and environmental changes that result from human activity has been much in the news recently. Discussions of the greenhouse effect, thinning of the ozone layer, rising levels of carbon dioxide, global warming, chlorofluorocarbons, and acid rain have made the terms common in print. Atmospheric physicists and other scientists have examined the physical consequences of these effects, but the impact of environmental change on the health and survival of humans has received relatively little direct attention, with some notable exceptions.[1] Although the direction of environmental change seems clear, much uncertainty remains about its magnitude and tempo. When we hear that the mean temperature at the earth's surface may rise 2 to 5°C in the next 100 years, or that the oceans may rise by 1 metre in the next 50 to 100 years, should we be alarmed? How will such climatic and environmental changes influence human health? Can we predict their consequences with sufficient accuracy to take action to curb them, or is the uncertainty so great that action would be foolhardy given other urgent problems that need solutions today? Can we put action on the back burner while we wait and see?

This essay examines the impact global environmental and climatic changes may have on human health so that it can be kept in focus as we decide whether action or inaction is our best course. I begin with a brief summary of what climatologists have discovered about our climate and atmosphere.

### Environmental effects of global climatic changes

The term 'greenhouse effect' refers to the effect that the accumulation of carbon dioxide and other gases in the earth's atmosphere has on the balance between the energy the earth receives from solar radiation and the energy it loses by radiation from its surface back to space. Since the Industrial Revolution, the combustion of fossil fuels has added carbon dioxide, the predominant greenhouse gas, to the atmosphere at an accelerating rate. Carbon dioxide and other greenhouse gases – methane, nitrous oxide, and chlorofluorocarbons – are largely transparent to the visible light and ultraviolet waves that warm the earth's surface with solar energy. Like water vapor, however, they absorb the longer infrared waves emitted from the earth, trapping energy in the atmosphere and warming the earth's surface. If there were no gases in the atmosphere capable of absorbing infrared radiation, the surface temperature of the earth would be about 40 kelvins colder, the oceans would freeze over, and life as we know it would not be possible.[2]

Carbon dioxide is our society's single largest waste product – the estimated world production in 1988 was 5 billion metric tons[2] – and its changing level in the atmosphere has been well documented for the past 30 years. The concentration of carbon dioxide has increased from 315 parts per million in 1958 to 352 parts per million in 1988, substantially higher than at any time in the past 160 000 years.[1] Half the carbon dioxide produced since the start of the Industrial Revolution remains in the atmosphere today. The rest has been incorporated into living matter or sequestered more definitively in the oceans. Our increasing dependence on fossil fuels makes a continuing rise in the carbon dioxide level inevitable.

The increase in the carbon dioxide level has caused the mean surface temperature of the earth to rise 0.6°C in the past 100 years, and increases of 2 to 5°C in the next 50 to 100 years have been predicted.[3] Chlorofluorocarbons (especially efficient absorbers of infrared radiation) in aerosols and refrigerants and methane from decaying organic matter and cattle flatus also accumulate in the atmosphere and contribute to the greenhouse effect.

That industrial processes cause carbon dioxide and other greenhouse gases to accumulate in the atmosphere is little disputed, but the magnitude and timing of the predicted rise in temperatures are controversial, and its consequences are even more uncertain. Although a mean increase of 2 to 5°C may sound trivial, it equals the change since the last ice age. Its distribution and timing could cause drought and desertification in areas that are now fertile and more arable areas into the higher latitudes. It could change the patterns of tropical and monsoon rains that are so important to vegetation and agriculture in Africa, Asia, and South America. It could melt the polar icecaps. If the West Antarctic ice sheet were to melt, sea levels would rise by about 6 m (20 ft).[3]

Even the expected rise of 1 m due to thermal expansion and the melting of glaciers and icecaps[4,5] will inundate large population centers and much fertile land. The expected rise may create 50 million environmental refugees worldwide, more than triple the number of all refugees today.[1] Mainland coastal regions as well as low islands will be in danger. Cities built on barrier islands and the fertile plains that typically surround river deltas are in jeopardy. A substantial part (18 to 34 percent) of Bangladesh (the classic case, with its impoverished millions) could disappear, displacing 15 to 35 per cent of the country's population. In addition, land will be rendered unfit for agriculture by the rising salinity of water tables. Large areas of the wetlands that nourish the world's fisheries will also be destroyed. Displaced people and less arable land would compound the problem of feeding the world's increasing population.

Another consequence of global warming is increased precipitation; warmer air increases the evaporation of sea water, creating more clouds and more rain and snow.

But the precipitation will not be evenly distributed. Climatic modeling does not yet allow sufficient spatial resolution to permit the predictions of changes in areas less than hundreds of kilometers square. Nevertheless, gross predictions have been made. In the United States, the southwestern desert will shift north to cover the midwestern grain belt, which will move into Canada. Temperatures favorable for growing grain will move from mid-Europe and the middle United States to Canada and Siberia, but whether fertile soils, adequate rainfall, and the other essentials of growth will exist in the higher latitudes is uncertain. California will be hard hit by drought. Southern California will have a drier winter, the season when most precipitation falls. Even if total precipitation levels remain unchanged, the warmer temperatures will cause more of the winter's precipitation to fall as rain, which will mean quick runoffs, winter flooding, and less melting snow to support water needs in the summer.

The condition of water supplies, already a major problem, is likely to deteriorate further: the intrusion of salt into surface water as sea levels rise, increased flooding, and runoffs contaminated with pesticides, salts, garbage, excreta, sewage, and eroded soil are all likely.

The rise in the level of atmospheric carbon dioxide may increase photosynthesis and the growth of plants under some circumstances, but not always. With increased temperatures and dryness, it may even curtail plant growth. Its effect on weeds and agricultural pests is largely speculative. Other air pollutants, such as sulfur dioxide and nitrogen oxides (the chief contributors to acid rain), ammonia, hydrogen sulfide, and dimethyl sulfide, are also toxic to vegetation. Industrial nitrogen oxides and both natural and industrial hydrocarbons are thought to be responsible for toxic levels of tropospheric ozone, which contributes to smog. Levels of ozone over the eastern United States during the summer are high enough to cause damage to crops and vegetation.[2,6] A similar phenomenon may be responsible, together with acid rain, for the deterioration of forests in Germany and eastern Europe.

Another environmental disturbance with widespread potential health consequences is the depletion of the ozone layer in the stratosphere. Only in the past few years have scientists understood that gases liberated in industrial processes reduce the ozone layer in the stratosphere, which forms a shield protecting us and other living things from the damaging effects of the sun's ultraviolet radiation. Our understanding of global climatic changes is clearly limited.

Ultraviolet light is the portion of the electromagnetic spectrum between 200 and 400 nm [nanometres], which is arbitrarily divided into the subregions' ultraviolet-A, ultraviolet-B, and ultraviolet-C. DNA and the aromatic amino acids absorb maximal amounts of ultraviolet-C, substantial amounts of ultraviolet-B, and minimal amounts of ultraviolet-A radiation. The pathological consequences of ultraviolet radiation seem chiefly attributable to its disruption of DNA and proteins.

Chlorofluorocarbons, which are used in aerosols, refrigerants, and other industrial products, rise to the stratosphere, where they become highly reactive and destroy ozone in photolytic reactions. Nitrous oxide, a byproduct of internal-combustion engines, industrial processes, and microbial activity, also rises to the stratosphere, where it also destroys ozone. Ozone is formed slowly by the action of sunlight on the rare molecules of oxygen in the stratosphere, some 20 to 50 km above the earth.[7] The half-time for the recovery of ozone levels in the stratosphere is three to four years.[8,9] Any process that accelerates the decomposition of ozone will interfere with its steadystate levels, and once depleted, the ozone layer may require 8 to 10 years for reconstitution.[9] In spring 1985 a hole in the ozone layer over Antarctica was discovered, and it thereafter grew to continental dimensions. In March 1988 thinning of the ozone layer over the North Pole was also noted. Seasonal ozone depletion in these regions is dependent on the slow circulation of the atmosphere and the presence of chlorofluorocarbons and nitrogen oxides at high altitudes. Atmospheric scientists are monitoring these processes and measuring the increased incidence with which harder ultraviolet-B waves reach the earth's surface under the ozone holes.[10] Although human populations are small in these parts of the globe, their oceans are rich in phytoplankton, which are the beginning of the food chain for all aquatic creatures. Ultraviolet-B radiation can penetrate several meters below the ocean's surface, where phytoplankton obtain the sunlight essential for photosynthesis. Phytoplankton are highly vulnerable to damage by ultraviolet-B radiation, so the potential for ecologic disaster is uncertain but considerable.

Biological diversity, which is already being reduced by human activities, may be one of the chief casualties of environmental changes. 'In one sense,' says E. O. Wilson,[11] 'the loss of diversity is the most important process of environmental change, because it is the only process that is wholly irreversible. Its consequences are also the least predictable, because the value of the earth's biota (the fauna and flora collectively) remains largely unstudied and unappreciated.'

## Health consequences of global climatic change

The health consequences of global warming are potentially great but are currently speculative. A mean rise of 2 to 5°C in the next 50 to 100 years will increase the number of days with temperatures over 38°C (100°F). Washington, D.C., which now averages 1 day a year with temperatures over 38°C, will average 12 such days by the middle of the next century.[12] Increased mortality from heat stress can be expected if ambient temperatures exceed 32°C (90°F) on a substantial number of days per year. This will chiefly affect elderly people, whose numbers are increasing rapidly, chronically ill and debilitated persons, and perhaps infants. The magnitude of the increase in mortality is not yet clear. Air conditioning could reduce the number of sufferers, but air conditioning expends energy and increases the consumption of fossil fuels that create the greenhouse warming. The increase in mortality may also be offset to some extent by a decreased number of deaths from hypothermia and cold.

It has been predicted that with global warming, respiratory irritants will further pollute the air, causing increased morbidity and mortality from lung diseases such as bronchitis, bronchiectasis, asthma, and chronic obstructive pulmonary disease. Air pollution is also likely to be exacerbated by industrial activities, which will increase as the world's population grows and more nations strive for a higher standard of living.

The thinning of the stratospheric ozone shield and the increase in ultraviolet-B radiation reaching the earth are expected to have direct health effects. The incidence of all kinds of skin cancer among white populations will increase with more exposure to ultraviolet-B. The incidence of melanoma has already increased; in the United States, it has risen 83 per cent over the past seven years. Unlike basal-cell and squamous-cell carcinoma, which seem to increase in proportion to total exposure to ultraviolet radiation, melanoma appears to be associated with acute exposure, as in the case of severe sunburns. How much public education will offset this increase by encouraging reduced exposure to solar radiation and the use of sunscreen lotions is unpredictable.

An increased incidence of cataracts may be a more widespread health effect of ultraviolet-B radiation than cancer because it will affect all populations. To a considerable extent, the loss of vision due to cataracts is correctable today with surgery and the implantation of prosthetic lenses, but the occurrence of a large increase in the number of cataracts in younger people would nevertheless create problems. Cataracts are currently the third largest cause of preventable blindness in the United States.

The effects of ultraviolet-B radiation on the skin have been studied intensively in recent years. The composite effect of these changes in the skin is a systemic reduction in the immune response. The depression of the immune system by ultraviolet-B radiation may have special importance when sanitation is poor and infectious diseases are prevalent. In countries whose health care systems are deficient, an increased incidence of infectious diseases is likely. Sanitary facilities will be further taxed by population increases and crowding; the incidence of waterborne infections will increase. The incidence of airborne diseases is also likely to increase because the air will be more polluted with respiratory irritants and population density will grow. If rising sea levels and regional droughts cause large population shifts, people with infections and unimmunized people are likely to appear in countries with developed health care systems, with a resulting increase in the incidence of diseases such as measles, pertussis, and poliomyelitis, as well as that of tuberculosis, leprosy, and other chronic illnesses. Malnutrition is also known to impair the immune system and to increase the frequency and gravity of infections. Food shortages that primarily affect the underdeveloped world are almost certain, and infectious diseases will be even more devastating than they are now. Whether the transfer of tropical diseases into the United States and other industrialized countries will increase is unclear. Global warming will change the habitats of insect vectors, and increases in the incidence of insect-borne diseases are possible. Contaminated water supplies will contribute to the spread of infectious diseases.

Probably the most widespread and devastating consequences of global environment changes are likely to result from their effects on agriculture and food supplies for the world's burgeoning population. In Africa, the people who are 'food insecure' (defined by the World Bank as not having enough food for normal health and physical activity) now number more than 100 million.[13] Clearly, many of the anticipated climatic effects will harm agricultural productivity: drought will decrease yields, the number of pests will increase, arable coastal land will be submerged, soils will become more saline, desertification and the amount of arid land will grow, soil erosion will increase, and larger amounts of ultraviolet-B radiation and air pollutants will interfere with photosynthesis. Shrinking food supplies will cause further hunger, malnutrition, and starvation, especially in poor countries that are already only marginally self-sufficient with respect to food. Food production in the oceans may be reduced by the effects of ultraviolet-B radiation on phytoplankton and by the warming of the ocean water.

A reduced land mass and the large projected increases in population in the coming decades are likely to result in heightened rates of environmental destruction; forests will be demolished to provide fuel, as in Nepal, or farmland and pasture, as in Brazil, with the attendant soil erosion and potential desertification. Each year 6 million hectares (14.8 million acres) of productive land turn into worthless desert, creating in three decades an area roughly the size of Saudi Arabia. More than 11 million hectares (27.2 million acres) of forest are destroyed yearly – in three decades, an area roughly the size of India.[14] As more people strive for higher standards of living, with all that implies in further energy needs and accelerated consumption of the world's natural resources, all these problems will be amplified.

## The present

Some or all of these possibilities will probably come to pass. The pace at which change occurs is a very important determinant of the consequences for the environment and health. Given sufficient time, nature is highly adaptable, and in theory society is also adaptable. In the past, the pace of climatic change has been measured in tens or hundreds of thousands of years; today we talk in terms of decades. Genetic changes do not occur so rapidly. But before shrugging off possible changes in the future, we need to examine the present, which may be even more unsettling. The root cause of the climatic and atmospheric changes stems from the pressure of the current population explosion and the desire of people everywhere to improve their standards of living. [Note] the exponential rate of growth of the world's population. The 5 billion mark was reached in July 1986, and the population will stabilize at between 8 and 14 billion people in the next century, according to United Nations projections. More than 90 per cent of the increase will occur in the poorest countries, and of that, 90 per cent in the world's already bursting cities.[14]

Industrial production has grown more than 50-fold over the past century, with four-fifths of this growth since 1950. The world manufactures seven times more goods today than it did as recently as 1950. A further 5- to 10-fold increase in output will be needed just to raise the level of consumption in the developing world to that in the industrialized world by the time population growth stabilizes in the next century.[14] The industries most heavily reliant on environmental resources and most heavily polluting are growing fastest in the developing world, where growth is urgent and the capacity to minimize damaging side effects is smaller. Industrialization, agricultural development, and rapidly growing populations in developing countries will need much more energy. Today the average person in an industrialized country uses more than 80 times as much energy as someone in sub-Saharan Africa.[14] Thus, any realistic global energy program must provide for the substantially increased use of energy by developing countries. Such a program has not been created. A fivefold increase in energy use would be required to bring consumption in the developing countries up to the level in industrialized countries by 2025.[14] Our planetary ecosystems cannot sustain such an increase, especially if it is based on non-renewable fossil fuels. Global warming and the other polluting effects of increased consumption probably rule out even doubling the use of energy from current sources. The impact on the biosphere will be profound, as economic growth extracts raw material from forests, soils, seas, and lands. Today every country seems to be rushing to promote economic growth.

The report of the World Commission on Environment and Development of the United Nations,[14] which I have cited in this section, summarized the present situation eloquently.

When the century began, neither human numbers nor technology had the power radically to alter planetary systems. As the century closes, not only do vastly

increased human numbers and their activities have that power, but major, unintended changes are occurring in the atmosphere, in soils, in waters, among plants
and animals, and in the relationships among all of these. The rate of change is
outstripping the ability of scientific disciplines and our capabilities to assess and
advise. It is frustrating the attempts of political and economic institutions, which
evolved in a different, more fragmented world, to adapt and cope.

# References

1. Brown, L. R. (ed.) *State of the World, 1989: a Worldwatch Institute Report on Progress Towards a Sustainable Society*, W. W. Norton, New York (1989).
2. McElroy, M. B. 'The challenge of global change', *Bull. Am. Acad. Arts. Sci.*, **42**, 24–38 (1989).
3. Hansen, J., Fung, I. and Lacis, A. *et al.* 'Predictions of near term climate evolution: what can we tell decision-makers now?' in, *Preparing for Climate Change: Proceedings of the First North American Conference on Preparing for Climate Change: A Cooperative Approach, October 27–29, 1987*, Government Institutes, Washington D.C./Rockville, Md., 35–47 (1988).
4. Emanuel, K. A. 'The dependence of hurricane intensity on climate', *Nature*, **326**, 483–5 (1987).
5. Schneider, S. H. 'The greenhouse effect: science and policy', *Science*, **243**, 771–81 (1989).
6. Seinfield, J. H. 'Urban air pollution: state of the science', *Science*, **243**, 745–52 (1989).
7. McElroy, M. B. and Salwitch, R. J. 'Changing composition of the global stratosphere', *Science*, **243**, 763–70 (1989).
8. National Research Council, Committee on the Atmospheric Effects of Nuclear Explosions, *The Effects on the Atmosphere of a Major Nuclear Exchange*, National Academy Press, Washington D.C. (1985).
9. Pittock, A. B., Ackerman, T. P., Crutzen, P. J., MacCracken, M. C., Shapiro, C. S. and Turco, R. P. *Environmental Consequences of Nuclear War*, 1, John Wiley, Chichester (1985).
10. Roberts, L. 'Does the ozone hole threaten Antarctic life?' *Science*, **244**, 288–9 (1989).
11. Wilson, E. O. 'Threats to biodiversity', *Sci. Am.*, **261**(3), 108 (1989).
12. Revkin, A. C. 'Endless summer: living with the greenhouse effect', *Discover*, **October**, 50–61 (1988).
13. World Bank, *Report of the Task Force on Food Security in Africa*, World Bank, Washington, D.C. (1988).
14. World Commission on Environment and Development, *Our Common Future*, Oxford University Press, Oxford (1987).

Alexander Leaf, M.D. works at the Department of Preventative Medicine, Harvard Medical School and the Massachusetts General Hospital, Boston, USA. This is an edited extract from a longer text which was originally published in 1989 in the *New England Journal of Medicine*, **321** (23), 1577–1583.

# 58
# The welfare man

**CHRIS BECKETT**

Special Category. Anyone in Europe would have instantly recognized what kind of place this was: the concrete buildings, the trampled parks, the graffiti, the ubiquitous Dreamer Shops renting out software with names like 'WARM GORE', 'SEX HEAVEN', 'BARBARIAN RAIDER' . . . It was a dreg estate and the people who inhabited it were *dreggies*. Their ID cards were different to other people's, they were subject to different laws, they spoke differently, smelled differently, they wore tattoos and shaved bald patches on their heads for the ingestion of electronic dreams . . .

Here were a chippie, two dreamer places, a grocery, a sweetshop. There were four boys mixing glue and homegrown tobacco on the steps of the long-defunct fountain. There were shaven-headed young mums pushing buggies. There was a block of offices with bars over the windows and a three-metre-high wire fence. The office had a large blue sign with a logo that depicted one hand reaching down protectively to another. DEPARTMENT OF SPECIAL CATEGORY ADMINISTRATION it said. 'Fort Apache' the Knowle South DeSCA office was called by the staff who worked within its walls.

'Well, colleagues. It's 9.25, so perhaps we had better make a start. For those of you that don't know me, my name is Cyril Burkett and I am the Assistant Regional Registration Officer. This is a Contested Initial Registration Conference within the meaning of the 2003 Act, concerning Stacey Blows of 34 Lilac Flats. Miss Blows herself has been invited to attend at ten o'clock. Let's start with a round of introductions . . .'

Jovial Charlie Blossom, with his sports jacket and his Scout tie, explained he was the Registration Liaison Officer from the Housing Section.

'Joy Frost, Headmistress, Virginia Bottomley Memorial School,' barked out the dapper woman to Charlie's left. 'Stacey Blows' daughter, Ulrike, is our pupil.'

Cyril smiled. Joy was a tough old boot. You had to be to teach in a Special Category School – and face the abuse not only of the children but of the rest of your profession. Teachers in the last remnant of the state sector were seen as no-hopers unable to cope with the fiercely competitive world that was education outside the Estates.

Dr Rajman introduced himself irritably. (Why should he attend meetings at the DeSCA if they couldn't pay his fees?)

A very young and pretty WPC called Fran Stimbling explained that she was on temporary secondment to the DeSCA Constabulary from Avon & Somerset Police and that she had come in the absence of Sergeant Walker and had no personal knowledge of Stacey Blows.

'Welcome, Fran,' said Cyril.

Then a small, thin, frightened woman introduced herself as Christine Wothersmere, a Welfare Investigator in the Community Hygiene Team (as the Child Protection Unit had been renamed since accepting sponsorship from the manufacturers of TCP). She was, in other words, a kind of social worker, a member of Cyril's own former profession – though it was very different nowadays, an almost entirely clerical function, feeding statistics into data-processing systems, reporting to computers and lawyers for instructions.

And a very elegant, large person beside her explained that she was Harriet Vere-Richards and was a voluntary Lay Representative appointed by Bristol City Council. There were letters of apology from the Probation Service and from the Benefits Section.

'Good,' said Cyril, 'welcome, everybody. Stacey Blows, who was born on 6th September 1995, holds *de facto* Special Category citizenship as a result of having grown up in this Estate and having a Special Category parent. Now that she is approaching 21, it is our task to determine whether she ought to be registered as a Special Category citizen in her own right. Stacey, as is her legal right, has indicated that she would oppose registration, and she will be here to put her views to us in person after we have had a preliminary discussion among ourselves. A transcript of the meeting will be made available to her and she will be entitled to take the matter to court under section 8 of the Act if she does not agree with our decision.'

He tapped the keyboard of the speech processor, which proceeded to read out the background report.

'Stacey Blows' mother is Jennifer Pendant, White British, of 65 Rose Corner. Her father is Roger Blows, Mixed Race British, of 105 John Major Way, Artcliffe North. She attended South Knowle Secondary School and left without any formal qualifications, though she possesses basic literacy and numeracy skills up to Age Ten Standard. She has never worked and now lives on National Basic Benefit. From the ages of 14 to 16 she was Accommodated under the 2005 Children Act at one of the Child Protection Service's Group Homes. She then moved into a flat at 58c Japonica Gardens where her first child, Ulrike, was born on May 1st, 2011. Stacey Blows indicates that she is not sure who Ulrike's father is and has named two different possible men when asked. Her second child, Wolfgang, was born in 2012. His father was allegedly one Archduke Wayne Delphonse Delaney, now serving a prison sentence for armed robbery and Line offences. Following the birth of Wolfgang, she moved to her present address where Kazuo was born in 2014.'

The conference – or those members of it who were listening – smiled at the German and Japanese names. It was a fashion that had swept the British Estates because of the dominance of the Dreamer market by the two superpowers. (In the case of the Germans, who increasingly did not bother to dub their Dreamware in English, not only the names but the language itself was starting to penetrate the Dreamer-fed *argot* of the Estates.)

'Kazuo's father was allegedly one Benjamin Tonsil, whose present whereabouts Stacey does not know. Stacey has several offences for shoplifting and two minor Line violations. The Community Hygiene Team have also been involved in investigating various allegations of child neglect, which Mrs Wothersmere will fill us in on.'

Cyril cleared his throat. 'Yes . . . Now . . . Before going any further, I need to remind the conference of the criteria for registration laid down under section 5 of the Act. If you remember we have firstly to be able to agree that Stacey demonstrates what is called in the legal jargon *"substantial fecklessness"* in two or more of the *"core areas"*: Financial Affairs, Family Relationships, Basic Citizenship, Health and Hygiene. Secondly, as this is a contested case, we have to demonstrate that non-registration would be, in the words of the Act *"contrary to the public interest."* Now, if we can start with the first core area, which is Financial Affairs. Any comments here?'

Charlie Blossom immediately launched into the long and (to him) hilarious story of Stacey Blows' repeatedly vandalized electricity meter, enthusiastically supported by WPC Stimbling who read out a long list of criminal offences against Western Electricity in a shocked breathless voice. Cyril's mind wandered. He doodled on his pad, underlining random words. Stacey. *Stacey.* STACEY. Those old American names: Jason, Stacey, Wayne . . . Stacey's parents must have been among the last to use them. Strange to remember there was a time when America was associated with style and freedom and fun . . .

'I am growing old,' thought Cyril. He was dreading a lonely retirement. He was dreading having time to look back over his life: so many compromises, so many decisions ducked as he climbed his little career-ladder through all the reorganizations and restructuring and rationalizations. Each step had somehow seemed reasonable and justifiable at the time, the best he could do. But all the time the old public welfare system was being slowly dismantled around him – leaving only a rump service in which the remnants of all the agencies were gradually amalgamated together: Housing and Social Services, Social Services with Health, Health with Social Security . . . He had started out wanting to help people; he had become the administrator of an Underclass. Well, that's society's choice not mine, he had always told himself, and at least it pays the mortgage and has a decent pension scheme.

Stacey had her hair shaven in stripes, so as to allow easy contact to the scalp for the electrodes of Dreamer sets, which supplemented sensory stimulation with low-voltage jolts to the brainstem and hypothalamus. Her arms were covered in tattoos of Teutonic warriors, and cross-hatched with self-inflicted scars. Her ears were riddled with holes from which bones, hearts, swastikas, dice, St Christophers and miniature Suzuki motorcycles were suspended. She wore a long tee-shirt with Japanese characters and a picture of a burning Zero fighter – and a short black skirt that left her thin, pale legs quite bare. On her forehead was a deathshead 'Liebe–Hass' hologram, on her hip a little scabrous feral child with its face smeared with something sticky and cheap and red.

Everyone went quiet, as they always did in these moments when they had finished picking over a person's life and were confronted with the real human being. Only Joy and Cyril looked Stacey in the eye.

'Welcome, Stacey,' he said, 'do have a seat. Let's start by checking you know everyone here . . .'

The child – little Kazuo – reached out across the table for one of the carafes of water that stood there. Stacey smacked him hard and everybody winced.

'Well, I knows 'im, ja,' she said, looking at Dr Rajman, who blushed. 'I knows 'im. 'E gives I me 'scriptions for me fags.'

She suddenly treated them all to a smile of dazzling and utterly unexpected sweetness.

'Ja, und I knows 'er,' she went on, in the strange slow Germanized West country burr that was the *patois* of the Bristol Estates. 'She gets I Kaz's milch and that and tells I I ain't feedin' 'im prarper. Und Mister Blarssom und Miss Frarst, I know them . . .'

WPC Stimbling was introduced.

'And I'm Harriet Vere-Richards,' gabbled the Lay Representative, sensing that her moment had come. 'You don't know me, Stacey, but I'm here to look after your interests. I'm not a professional person like the other people here, you see. I'm just an ordinary Bristol person like yourself . . .'

There was a moment of silence in which this preposterous statement was allowed to quietly fade into the air.

'Now Stacey,' said Cyril after a decent interval, 'we understand that you don't want to be registered as a Special Category Citizen. I wonder if you could tell us a bit about why?'

'Well, it's just I thought I'd like to be an or'nary person with a white card, you know, und not be a dreggie any more, und feel people's laughing at I and that . . .'

'I'm sure we all understand that, but I wonder where you would live if you weren't Special Category any more? Because of course, you'd have to give up your tenancy here within six months.'

Cyril was courteous, but his mind was far away. He had been here so very many times before.

'Well, o'course, I 'adn't really thought yet, but I'd look in the papers and that . . .'

'What about money, Stacey? You know, don't you, that only Special Category citizens can apply for National Basic Benefit? You don't get benefits outside unless you've subscribed to a private scheme.'

Kazuo started reaching out for the water again. Stacey distracted him by giving him a packet of sweets, which he devoured three or four at a time.

'I could get a jarb,' she said, without much conviction.

'Good for you, but of course then there'd be the care arrangements for the children . . .'

'Wolfie's in the nursery now und ich bin trying to get a place for Kaz . . .'

'But you mustn't forget, Stacey, that you only get free nurseries in the Estates. Outside you have to pay the market rate which is about two thousand Units per week I believe.'

Stacey looked flustered. The deathshead on her forehead glowed red. (It was made to respond to changes in skin temperature, and was supposed to give outward expression to Love and Hate – Liebe und hass – those powerful forces in the crude, elemental, violent life of every Estate.)

'I 'ates meetings,' she muttered.

'You see, Stacey,' Cyril explained, 'we've been talking a bit about your circumstances, and we really do think that it isn't the right moment for you to drop your Special Category status. Of course you are entitled to your say, and you're entitled under the Act to go to court if you don't agree with our decision, but I'd like you to think carefully about what is really right for you and see if we can't come to some agreement. Will you do that?'

He paused and Stacey nodded humbly, as people usually did at this point. (Only a few of them erupted into rage as they saw the net closing around them.)

Joy Frost, the headmistress, stepped in. 'Stacey, I think you and I get on pretty well don't we?' Stacey nodded. 'Well, listen. You used that silly word "dreggie," and there are a lot of other silly words that are used about Special Category citizens. But what I always tell people to remember is this: Special Category means what it says. You are *special*. I for one happen to believe you *need* special help, and I believe you deserve it. By keeping you Special Category we are making sure that you get a whole range of services that you couldn't otherwise get. A time may come, Stacey, when you don't need those things – and when that day comes, you get back to us and we'll be the *first* to say "Hooray! Well done! Let's get you off that register at once!" – but we do think you need those services now.'

Cyril smiled. Joy was one of the few DeSCA employees he knew who really and sincerely believed that the Department's whole purpose was to better the lives of its customers. It was a belief she lived out every day of her life.

'So what do you say, Stacey,' said Joy. 'Be honest, doesn't it make sense?'

Stacey nodded reluctantly. Kazuo emptied the carafe across the table. There was a pause while Charlie fetched some paper towels and Dr Rajman dabbed angrily at his sodden personal organizer.

'But before you finally make up your mind,' said Cyril, 'there are some obligations attached to registration as well as benefits. It's part of my job to spell them out for you.'

Although he know this section of the Act off by heart, Cyril had the habit of opening the copy of the Act that lay in front of him, and smoothing down the relevant page. The rules were made by society as a whole and not by him. Only by reminding himself and them of this fact could he look the customers in the face.

'First of all, there are some rules about your movements outside the Estate. As you know, the general rule is that you can go where you like when you like. The only thing is: you are obliged to show the duty officer your ID when you cross the Line, and to tell him where you're going and when you're coming back. It is an offence not to co-operate with the duty officer on the Line. And of course, your movement can be restricted by Exit Restriction orders if you commit offences.'

'It's only when people are silly that the court orders come into it,' said Joy Frost.

Stacey nodded. You got caught shop-lifting down in Broadmead and you got a one-month Exit Restriction. You got caught burgling a house in Clifton and you got Restriction for six months or a year. Everyone knew that!

Joy turned to Mrs Vere-Richards: 'It always sound so awful, but you've got to remember that in the old days, you were just sent to prison!'

'Absolutely!' agreed the Lay Representative. She was an activist in the *Forward with Europe* party. She knew quite well that one of the benefits of the Compromise was a reduction in the prison population.

'Secondly,' Cyril went on, 'there are some rules about credit. You can't get a credit card if you are on the Special Category register, you can't get a bank loan and you can't enter into a hire-purchase agreement. If you really need a loan, you have to sort it out with our own Benefit Section here at the DeSCA.'

Charlie Blossom chuckled: 'I wish I could get those rules applied to my wife!'

'I wish someone could apply them to me,' piped in WPC Stimbling.

'*Absolutely!*' said Mrs Vere-Richards.

'But seriously, Stacey,' said Joy Frost, 'the credit rules are purely and simply for your own benefit: to save you all the worry and trouble of getting in debt.'

Stacey smiled: 'Ja, I'd 'ate it if they gave I one of them cards.'

'Sensible girl!' said Charlie.

'The only other restriction,' Cyril went on, 'is about voting in elections . . .'

'Oh, I ain't bothered about that!'

'All as bad as each other, eh, Stacey?!' chuckled Charlie.

'Absolutely!' laughed Mrs Vere–Richards.

The skull on Stacey's forehead had returned to its normal lurid green.

Chris Beckett is a social worker who has published several science fiction stories, including one in the 1993 edition of *The Years Best SF* anthology. This extract from a story with the same title appeared in the science fiction magazine *Interzone*, **August**, 48–56 (1993).

# 59
# Exits

## SALLY VINCENT

Dying is our most catastrophic expectation. Not death itself, we hasten to add, but dying. People who have witnessed an agonised and protracted death tend not to develop their experience into a conversation piece. Like a generation of first-world-war soldiers, they maintain their trauma in a kind of shamed and unbelieving silence. To have observed a calm and painless passing, however, is often described as a privilege and an honour, as though something undeserved but immeasurably enriching has been bestowed upon us. At such times a sense of grief seems to be both ameliorated and suspended by the stark relief of knowing that the dreadful has happened and, hey, it wasn't that dreadful. The dying was easy. There is nothing to fear. If we could only be sure that we, too, could glide as smoothly from the terminal of our choice, how much better (in a curious way) life would be.

As quantum leaps go, it is only a small step to conclude that if we could have some measure of control over the manner of our dying we would also, by way of a handy bonus, have our lives in control. Dignity is the word that springs to mind. We would have dignity. If our existence was not punctuated at either end by the twin parentheses of pain, bewilderment, helplessness and incontinence, what we leave behind in the memory banks of those we sought to impress would never bear the taint of indignity. In contemplation of the desirability of an easy, self-controlled death, we have moved inexorably into the field of the possibility of voluntary euthanasia as a universal rite of passage.

For two and a half thousand years, the moral rectitude of the medical profession was adequately served by the Hippocratic Oath. The old Greek was unequivocal on the issue of voluntary euthanasia. 'I will give no deadly medicine to anyone if asked, nor suggest any such counsel', was what he wrote and what physicians have been content to avoid thereafter, or at any rate up until 1947. It was then that the World Medical Association was formed and the Hippocratic Oath retranslated into the modern idiom of the Declaration of Geneva, which entirely omits the no-deadly-medicine line along with various archaic references to Apollo, Aesculapius and

All-Heal. Subsequent re-editings of the Declaration have moved further from the Hippocratic emphasis on the sanctity of life and towards a more trade union approach where a doctor's consecration of his life to the service of humanity becomes nicely balanced by a code of conduct designed to protect and preserve the sanctity of a doctor's professional security.

The English text of the International Code of Medical Ethics innocuously embraces the ethic of voluntary euthanasia in its 'easy death' connotation when it states, '[when] a physician provides medical care which might have the effect of weakening the physical and mental condition of the patient, he must do so only in the patient's interest'. By 1977, voluntary euthanasia no longer meant 'easy death'. In full recognition of common usage and its erosion of 'easy death' into 'mercy killing', the BMA was moved to affirm that, 'Practitioners who are in conscience opposed to euthanasia must be fully protected in future legislation'. In other words, over the past 47 years, the British medical ethos has abandoned the Hippocratic condemnation of euthanasia and taken up arms to protect conscientious objectors from the obligation of killing people. No matter how they beg and plead.

However they may advise the Government, [the House of Lords Select Committee on Medical Ethics] will be less concerned with the minutiae of moral philosophy attending the issue of voluntary euthanasia than they are with the anomalies of a legal system that comes down like a ton of bricks on doctors who conscientiously do not object. The most likely outcome will be to decriminalise the practice of voluntary euthanasia along the lines of the system operating in the Netherlands.

'If asked', a Dutch physician – or at any rate 78 per cent of Dutch physicians – will give his 'deadly medicine' and, assuming he has sought another's 'counsel', filled in a lot of forms and notified the coroner, he will not have to waste his time justifying his action in a court of law. It is hoped – or feared – that a similar exemption from prosecution will swell the ranks of British doctors currently amenable to the role of mercy killer, from a mere 48 per cent to better resemble the Dutch model. Thereafter, British citizens diagnosing their lives as not worth living, will have little trouble finding a doctor with the know-how and wherewithal to take them literally, and a consultant rheumatologist called Dr Nigel Cox will take his place in medical history as the very last martyr to the cause of voluntary euthanasia.

It is the Cox case upon which our present deliberations are based. There was never any argument about what happened. Mrs Lillian Boyes had been Dr Cox's patient for three years. They knew each other well. By all accounts, Mrs Boyes's rheumatoid arthritis had her on her knees. As her condition worsened, she was reported to have suffered the agonies of the damned, 'howling like a dog' and pleading to be released from her misery. Dr Cox prescribed morphine-based drugs in increasing doses until it became clear that the pain from the disease and from the bone-deep bed sores resulting from years in hospital had become intractable. The lady made it clear to all concerned that she wished to die. It was in direct response to her awareness of her own best interests that, in 1991, Dr Cox injected potassium chloride into the vein of Mrs Lillian Boyes, as a result of which she very quickly died. Dr Cox's choice of potassium chloride – a poison with no therapeutic qualities – over the conventional anaesthetic cocktail which hastens death as a secondary effect, gave unequivocal evidence of his primary intention.

The charge was attempted murder. Had Mrs Boyes's body not been swiftly cremated, the charge would have been murder, but since it was not possible for anyone to ascertain whether or not she would have died without the lethal injection, the lesser crime was nominated.

Several members of the jury shed tears when they brought in a guilty verdict. Dr Cox was given a suspended sentence of one year's imprisonment, reprimanded by the Disciplinary Committee of the General Medical Council for failing to observe established practices and went back to work, accompanied by the sympathy, good wishes and admiration of his peers. Public support of voluntary euthanasia reached an all-time high.

The popularity of the leniency of the Cox decision was predicated largely upon public imagination, bounded by our desire to abolish pain and to have the ultimate say in our own fate. It was clear to everyone that in the spirit, if not the letter of the law, Mrs Boyes was the best judge of her own predicament and her own salvation. We can comprehend that somebody with a terminal illness and unremitting pain would long for oblivion, if they had reason to believe there was no alternative. And since Mrs Boyes had that reason, the responsibility for her death was her own. Dr Cox was merely the merciful operative.

Which of us would not hope to be similarly merciful, given the opportunity to load the needle, hold the cup, crush the pills, do the decent thing? But what if the recipient of our best attentions is less helpful with his prognosis? What if he has no opinion on the matter whatsoever?

Anthony Bland was nineteen and a half years old when, like Mrs Boyes, he inadvertently became a test case for the legalisation of euthanasia. A victim of the Hillsborough Stadium disaster, Anthony was diagnosed as clinically brain dead and lay in a permanent vegetative state for two and a half years, with no prospect of a reversal for his lamentable condition. He could, however, breathe unaided, and presumably would have done so indefinitely if artificially fed and regularly medicated for the various infections that beset the unconscious body. It is inarguable that Anthony's life had no discernible meaning to himself and was the cause of considerable sadness and grief to those who loved him. Mr and Mrs Bland decided that 30 months of living death was probably enough for any one family and in common with thousands of grieving relatives before them, they felt that in the absence of their son's opinion as to what was best for him, they must make the decision for him.

Had we never heard of Anthony Bland, there would have been no further debate about his fate. But we did know about him. And we cared. The media saw to that.

This happened a month ago: the father of a friend – I'll call her Margaret – suffered a massive stroke and was admitted to a London hospital. There he was carefully examined and it was discovered that while he was otherwise in fine fettle for a man of his age, he was now effectively brain dead. Only two things distinguished Margaret's father from Anthony Bland. One, he was 92 years old, and two, the incident of his brain damage was not a matter of public record. Margaret sat at her father's bed-side and held his hand. Then she was called to the consultant physician's office, where it was given to her straight. The doctor explained that her father's case was irreversible. In the tones of one who knows of what he speaks, he gave Margaret the benefit of his best advice. He suggested that if, with her permission, the hospital were to refrain from feeding and medicating her father, he would be physically as well as mentally dead within 19 days.

Margaret went back to her father and took his hand. She knew what was involved. She thought of the bed shortage. She knew that in all probability a younger, worthier candidate for the care and resources that might be lavished upon her father was worsening in the wings. She knew that she wouldn't want to lie there, lingering on. She knew her father was never a chap to relish that kind of prospect either. She pressed his freckly old hand and strained every nerve to imagine a response from him. All that happened was that he sneezed. And then she said no. No, she did not want her father to starve to death, nor did she want him to drown in his own lung fluid. She knew she was being bolshie, but dammit all, what was the rush? Her father was a good citizen. He'd paid his dues.

Margaret felt the disapproval. There was nothing she could put her finger on, of course, just a general air of impatience, mainly exemplified by the consultant's swift and brisk departure from her sight.

The old man died seven days later, just 12 days short of the date predicted by the starving method. Those decisions are taken every day in our hospitals. Passive euthanasia – the withdrawal of life-sustaining systems, up to and including food, when those systems clearly have no therapeutic purpose – is not illegal. It was by virtue of the public nature of Anthony Bland's tragedy that his parents' decision on his behalf was considered insufficient. The decision had to be made by the President of the Family Division of the High Court, affirmed by the Court of Appeal and thereafter upheld by the Appellate Committee of the House of Lords. Anthony starved to death, or to put it more accurately, Anthony was starved to death. The moral stance taken by the learned Lords who doubtless debated long and hard over the Bland case, was no different to the one taken by Dr Cox. In both cases the patient was intended to die. Whether the execution is technically 'active' or 'passive', the end and the motive are identical.

Dame Cecily [Saunders] is synonymous with the hospice movement, with Macmillan nurses and the complete obviation of all further contemplation of euthanasia. Anyone who has ever visited a hospice comes away marvelling at the atmosphere of peace and dignity they found there. Terminal cancer, once the euthanatist's prime target, literally lost its sting. You'd think we'd leave it there.

But the euthanatists have moved their goal-posts. Leave cancer to the hospices, from now on the maximum dread buzz-word is mental incapacity. Senility. Confusion. Alzheimer's disease. Terminal ga-ga-ness. Ending up like a prize marrow in some obsessive gardener's plot. And since these conditions render us incapable of knowing what is good for us, we must foresee their possibility and second-guess ourselves with the compilation of a Living Will. In these documents, properly witnessed and with the soundness of our minds attested to, we may make it abundantly clear that when we cease to be of use to ourselves or to others, we would wish to be bumped off as soon as possible. It is the decent, citizenly thing to do.

Dr Herbert Cohen, a Dutch euthanatist who confines himself to one act of euthanasia per month on the grounds that he finds it emotionally burdensome work, has been at pains to point out that old people who wish to die in order to relinquish their hospital beds to worthier patients should be treated as national heroes, like soldiers who die for their country and mothers who give their last crust to their starving children.

The hidden agenda of the great euthanasia debate is precisely this. It places us at the vanguard of a demographic catastrophe. We are living too long. In the past 50 years, the section of the population with the temerity to survive beyond 65 has increased from 10 to 15 per cent. If something is not done about it, 25 years into the next millennium this unacceptable and unprecedented drain on our resources will have swelled to 19 per cent. A direct link between available resources and what we are prepared to afford for the general good is a vital aspect of the social contract of all primitive cultures. It is not necessarily admirable in its implementation. Today, if we choose not to afford to support the elderly, we must urge them to loose their hold on life. Not because they are ill, but because they no longer contribute to our own survival. The bear eats grannie, we eat the bear. Our modern social contract suggests an equivalent cycle of regeneration. Grannie volunteers for euthanasia, her savings are not frittered away in nursing home fees but go directly to her descendants.

Simple practicalities don't enter the equation. In fact only one in 20 pensioners is entirely dependent on the state benefits to which their contributions entitle them. And, according to an Age Concern survey, people of 65 and over consult doctors less frequently than any other age group.

With touching doctorly elitism, the medical profession takes full responsibility for its part in creating a society progressively impoverished by its elderly. Theirs was the initial miracle, with their spare parts and pacemakers, of life prolongation. Theirs must now be the duty to do something about it! In an article published by the journal of the Royal College of GPs, Dr Mary Bliss, consultant geriatrician and member of the Voluntary Euthanasia Society, has written, 'We cannot expect to enjoy unnatural life unless we are also prepared to accept unnatural death.'

Dr Bliss was more than happy to take me round her geriatric ward. 'It's about time,' she said, 'someone looked at it.' They call it the long-stay ward, because people who come here tend to stay a long time. Three, four, oh anything up to eight years. It's not like a hospice. Nobody stays in a hospice for longer than three weeks. That's one of the differences. People are dying of something to be in a hospice. Here people aren't dying. They've nothing to die from. By virtue of iron constitutions and, in some cases, the officious striving of a medical practitioner in the distant past, they have merely failed to pass away at what they and their relatives might consider a reasonable age. Now they must wait, at great expense, for their frail and decrepit bodies to go the same way as their youth and vigour.

The ward is long and semi-compartmentalised. As you move out of earshot of one television set, you walk into the orbit of another one. Health workers – nurses are too expensive to be wasted on geriatric care – watch Princess Diana announce to the nation her preference for privacy. Dr Bliss tells me that hardly anyone here gets any visitors. The gentleman over there has a daughter, but she doesn't come any more. She said there was no point since he doesn't really recognise her any more. The lady there, the one who seems to be sleeping, has a husband who reckons she should have been dead years ago. Dr Bliss thinks he was right.

Elizabeth, same age as the Queen Mother, sits in solitary silence upon her commode; her eyes bright with humour, she waves to us with the close-fingered economy for which her namesake is famed. Elizabeth tumbles from this position in the course of her stay. They've lost count of the arms and legs she's broken. Elizabeth is saying something. She whispers and we cannot hear. Dr Bliss catches one word. 'She says she's lonely,' says Dr Bliss. Elizabeth's case-notes are two inches thick. Nobody minds me looking through them. From time to time someone has written in tipsy capitals across the page NTBR. Not To Be Resuscitated. They've tried to persuade her to go into a nursing home, but she won't have it. Her only complaint seems to be something to do with a hearing aid. When she came here, three-and-a-half years ago, she seems to have mislaid it. She accepts everything. She accepts her legs won't hold her any more. She is content to be kept safe and warm in this awful place. All she wants, all she's ever asked, is for somebody to find her bloody hearing-aid.

This article is an edited extract from a much longer article with the same title, written by journalist Sally Vincent and published in *The Guardian Weekend*, 19 February, 6–10 and 52 (1994).

# 60
# The shadow of genetic injustice

## BENNO MÜLLER-HILL

The effects of the inevitable discoveries emerging from the Human Genome Project will be catastrophic for some. Now is the time for preventative action to be taken.

Many knowledgeable people have a deep dislike of the Human Genome Project. If you ask them why, some may say that the money would be better spent on different, smaller projects. A few fear that the outcome could be harmful: they foresee a new underclass, unable to get jobs or insurance. These pessimists of course overlook that this underclass already exists: 37 million people have no health insurance of any kind in the United States. Could things become worse?

Proponents of the Human Genome Project imagine great progress in diagnosis of diseases and in their therapy. Some predict that eventually everyone will carry all the sequences of his genes on a compact disk. Others even claim that the present knowledge of man and his mind is nil and that real culture will arise only out of the knowledge of the sequence of human DNA. This, I think, is unlikely.

As pure scientists, these enthusiasts often do not imagine the consequences for society as a whole. My own view is that the project will be truly enlightening about the molecular structure of the human body and brain, and that this knowledge alone is exciting enough to justify the programme. Little is known in molecular biology and many unsuspected medical applications may emerge from this endeavour. As a molecular geneticist I have always defended the Human Genome Project as scientifically sound and important, and I continue to do so. But I have also tried to spread the knowledge of the past criminal misuse of human genetics in Nazi Germany. Until now I have abstained from commenting on the possible effects of the Human Genome Project on society in the future. But science after all consists of making, and testing, predictions. So I have decided to stick my neck out and to make some predictions for the next 30 years.

There is no doubt that the main medical progress will be in diagnostics. Therapeutics may lag behind, possibly for decades, so I will abstain from discussing these aspects here. What will be the main diagnostic results of the Human Genome Project that are relevant to society? I think there are two different areas: genetic ailments of the body and those of the mind.

There are many severe ailments of the body for which there are genetic predispositions. Most of these conditions are extremely rare: only a very few are as frequent as one per cent. At the moment it is in most cases just about possible to say that, according to a family history, a certain risk exists. The Human Genome Project, however, will lead to the identification of DNA defects in the relevant genes. Then, accurate predictions can be made from the blood (DNA): for example, one will be able to predict that a healthy child will die in his or her forties from Huntington's [disease] or from familial Alzheimer's disease. In Huntington's [disease], the time-point of the outbreak of the first symptoms will vary considerably. In other diseases it may vary even more. The predictions will thus not be accurate in the sense that the severeness of the symptoms can be predicted for a particular time, but they will be statistically accurate. This concept is difficult to explain to patients and clients.

There are some similarities between this situation and that in the late nineteenth century, when infections were random and where no treatment was available. Then, many had the bad luck to be infected whereas here we are talking about only a few people. But the late nineteenth century was the time that general health insurance was introduced in countries like Germany. Bismarck's reform in that country had the effect of increasing the industrial output of Germany. Perhaps the time of molecular revelation of rare diseases would be the proper time to introduce general health insurance in the United States?

To continue my predictions for the future. Imagine four potential cases of genetic disablement. (1) When a haemophiliac wants to become a butcher it makes sense to discourage him. (2) When a colour-blind man wants to become a truck driver, he fails at a colour test: his DNA does not need to be tested. (3) When a healthy young man asks for employment and his employer wants to know whether his genotype indicates that he may die in his thirties or forties from Huntington's disease, this is unfair. (4) When a healthy black person seeks employment and is tested for sickle-cell anaemia gene, then is refused employment because there may be an extra risk under certain conditions, this is unfair.

Thus, in my view, practical ability tests are acceptable, but genetic tests for disabilities which may turn up later in life should not be made available to employers. Moreover, DNA testing for employment purposes should not be performed if a large ethnic group would suffer. But it goes without saying that a person presenting a potential employer or insurance company with unsolicited evidence that he does not carry the genes predisposing for various ailments will have a definite advantage.

One can imagine the development of protest movements among those who have decided not to reveal their genetic identity, and there will be fundamentalists who will never have themselves tested because they themselves do not want to know. All these groups will suffer grave social disadvantages. One can also imagine clubs for the 'healthy' that will demand proof of 'genetic fitness'. The turning point may come when the US supreme court decides that genetic injustice is so immense that it is within the law to show an employer or the insurance company falsified genetic identity. (In Germany the supreme court has just decided that pregnant women may lie about the pregnancy to an employer.) From then on, the interest of employers and insurance companies in the genetic identity of their employees or clients will wane.

I think all these developments will be painful but could come to a good end: the genetic bad luck of a very few may, eventually, be helped by many in that general health insurance and tough anti-discrimination laws could become reality. It is, of course, also possible that the genetically handicapped will be simply too few ever to influence the majority to come to their help.

The situation will be different with the genetic ailments of the mind, which I shall now discuss. Here, the percentage of the population involved is much larger and cannot easily be overlooked. Any current textbook of human genetics will contain the assertion that most differences of the human mind and soul (to use an old-fashioned word) are inherited. But in almost all these cases the respective genes have not been located or isolated, and the DNA defects are thus totally unknown. It is claimed that psychiatric diseases such as manic depression or schizophrenia, and also psychological disablements such as low intelligence, are somehow inherited. But the truth is that the extent of family influence or other environmental factors is unclear. Proof that these ailments are essentially genetically determined can come only through the knowledge of the DNA sequences of these genes and their variants. Knowledge of the DNA sequences of a person will then allow one to make statistically accurate predictions about that person's intelligence and mental stability, and thus about their possible fate.

In earlier times, such predictions were the business of charlatans. But belief increases the likelihood of a predicted outcome: placebos against psychic ailments work astonishingly well. The scientific prediction of a person's limitations, and thus his possible fate, has a very dangerous component in that it may lead the individual to inaction and despair. It may also lead the population at large to believe that, as there is no real chance, money should not be wasted to counteract genetic limitations. It could be forgotten that these limitations are also set by environmental factors.

Many medical scientists would like the fame of having isolated one of these genes. Some succumb to the pressure and claim they have obtained evidence where in fact there is little or none. The 'discovery' of genes determining alcoholism, schizophrenia, manic depression and Alzheimer's disease have been peer-reviewed and published in leading scientific journals. They were hailed in the media as breakthroughs – and then they were·shown to be wrong either by their own authors or by others. These errors do not mean that the main qualities of the mind and the soul are not biologically inherited: they show simply that scientists are ordinary people. One can predict safely that many more such non-discoveries will be made. This will be confusing for scientists and painful for the particular patients involved. But eventually the truth will emerge in areas where now we can only make guesses.

Finally, I would like to imagine what may happen if it does turn out that mental health can be shown to have a genetic basis. Let us assume as an example that a gene is isolated which in several mutated forms predisposes for schizophrenia. It will take by then a matter of weeks to determine the complete DNA sequence of such a gene. Will the sequence reveal anything about schizophrenia? For a molecular biologist, knowledge of a sequence means that the function of the protein specified by that sequence is known – for example the protein may form an ion channel or be an enzyme metabolizing a particular molecule. Does this mean that we will understand schizophrenia if we know that it often occurs in people when a certain ion channel or a certain enzyme is damaged?

Many scientists or doctors would answer in the affirmative, but I would like to say, emphatically, that the answer is no. Understanding a biochemical defect brings us no nearer to understanding the thoughts and actions of the schizophrenic. Those opposed to my view would argue that knowledge of the gene will allow us to identify which lifestyles are dangerous for such a person. But we do not need any knowledge of the gene or its product to do this. Pharmacologists, on the other hand, will point out that they now can design rational drugs which may influence precisely the functioning of the relevant gene product. But it is not true that if we know which drug to prescribe, we know all that is necessary to know about schizophrenia. Although the molecular–genetic approach will certainly lead to a frenzy of new drugs on the market, in the end the suffering patients will be helped only partially. It is so much easier to pre-scribe a pill than to change the social conditions that may be responsible for the severity of the symptoms.

I have little faith in the notion that treatment of mental diseases will truly benefit from knowledge of the culprit genes and gene products. But I have no doubt that diagnosis will flourish. Cheap tests will be developed which will allow everyone to be tested for the variants of genes determining psychiatric ailments or psychic qualities outside the doctor's office. Those carrying the disabling genes of schizophrenia, manic depression and low intelligence may constitute ten or more per cent of the US or European population. Medical scientists will test anonymously all possible ethnic and social groups for these genes, and doubtless some ethnic differences will be found. Suddenly, genetic racial injustice will be a fact.

The isolation of the first gene involved in determining 'intelligence' (whatever that is) will be a turning point in human history. Will governments endorse the view of the eugenicists of the 1930s that the carriers of such genes are 'bad and inferior' and that they and their followers are 'good and superior'? Or will they stress privacy and cleverly leave the necessary selection to market forces? Or will they resort to legal measures to speed up the process of the 'physical·disappearance of the unwanted'? And what will the geneticists themselves say? Perhaps they will simply be relieved to find that their own mental genotypes are 'healthy'. But will some of them propose ways to eliminate the 'bad' genes from others?

Anticipating such conflicts, many may conclude that we do not need or want this genetic knowledge. I disagree. The knowledge will simply unveil reality, emphasizing the injustice of the world. It is certainly not enough to face reality bluntly if the future develops as I describe it. It is not enough simply that the right of privacy is ac-knowledged. If those who have this right have no education, health insurance or jobs, the right is not enough. Laws are necessary to protect the genetically disadvantaged. Social justice has to recompense genetic injustice. The details of such legislation can be spelled out only when the genetic facts are known. Deep changes in attitudes are also required. All we can do now is to be prepared. Progress may be painfully fast or slow, and will be full of contradictions. To master it demands firm values. At the extremes, people will have to choose between the values of the Nazis and those of Moses – that is, racism or an appreciation of equal human rights. The choice for politicians of the world's governments will be between international fascism or, if science and justice are combined, a fundamentally improved social structure throughout the world.

I would like to conclude by citing a sentence from *Science and the Future*, pub-lished in 1924, written by the optimist J. B. S. Haldane, 'I think that the tendency of applied science is to magnify injustices until they become too intolerable to be borne, and the average man whom all the prophets and poets could not move, turns at last and extinguishes the evil at its source'.

Benno Müller-Hill is a molecular geneticist working at the Institute for Genetics, University of Cologne, Germany. This article was originally published in *Nature*, 362, 8 April (1993) pp. 491–492.

# 61
# The evolution of Utopia

## STEVE JONES

Most Utopian novels of the future ignore one of the few predictable things about evolution, which is its unpredictability. No dinosaur could have guessed that descendants of the shrew-like creatures playing at its feet would soon replace it: and the chimpanzees who outnumbered humans a hundred thousand years ago would be depressed to see that their relatives are now so abundant while their descendants are an endangered species.

Evolution always builds on its weaknesses, rather than making a fresh start. The lack of a grand plan is what makes life so adaptable and humans – the greatest opportunists of all – so successful. Life's utilitarian approach also means that speculating about the future of evolution is a risky thing to do as it is difficult to guess what a pragmatist will do next. In this [article], I will take the risk.

Humanity evolved by the same rules as those which propel less pretentious creatures. Humans are, of course, more than just apes writ large. We have two unique attributes: knowing the past and planning the future. Both talents guarantee that the outlook for humankind will depend on a lot more than genes. Nevertheless, it should be possible to make some guesses from the biological past as to what the evolutionary forecast might be. One pessimistic but probably accurate prediction is that it means extinction. Although about one person in twenty who has ever lived is alive today, only about one in a thousand of the different kinds of animal and plant has survived. Our species is in its adolescence, at about a hundred and fifty thousand years old (compared to several times this for those of our relatives whose fossil record is good enough to guess their age). Its demise is, one hopes, a long way away; and we can at least reflect about what might happen before then.

The rules which drive evolution are simple and are unlikely to change. They involve the appearance of new genes by mutation, natural selection, and random changes as some genes, by chance, fail to be passed on. To speculate about what will happen to each of these processes is to make predictions about human evolution. Will this biological Utopia be anything like its fictional equivalents (as I hope it will not); will we continue to evolve as rapidly as we have since our beginnings, or is human evolution at an end?

Human beings have interfered quite unknowingly with their biological heritage since they first appeared on earth. Stone tools, agriculture and private property all had an effect on society and in turn on evolution. Many people are concerned that the next phase of human history will be one in which genetics makes deliberate plans for the biological future. This is expecting too much of science. Inadvertent change – evolution by mistake – is much more likely to be important than is any conscious attempt to modify biology.

Even the most determined efforts of doctors, genetic counsellors or gene therapists will have only a small effect on future generations. About one British child in two thousand five hundred is born with cystic fibrosis – but a hundred times as many carry the gene without knowing it. Molecular biology makes it possible to advise people of their condition and perhaps, one day, will provide a cure. Even today's imperfect treatment means that the number of affected children surviving to reproductive age will double in the next thirty years. Nobody knows what the balance will be; whether the fact that more of those with cystic fibrosis pass on the gene will be outweighed by a decrease in the number of sufferers as genetical advice allows parents to plan their reproduction. Many people with phenylketonuria have had children. There was once strong social pressure against those with inborn disease marrying. In the 1950s only a minority of achondroplastic dwarves found a spouse, but in the United States more than eighty per cent of them are now married, often to another dwarf. No doubt, many genes which once disappeared quickly as their carriers died or remained single will now persist.

This is unlikely to have much influence on the biological future. Most inborn diseases which are susceptible to treatment or to pre-natal diagnosis are recessive, so that there are hundreds of times as many copies of the gene in healthy people as in sufferers. As everyone carries several hidden recessive mutations there is little prospect that medicine will pollute a once pure human gene pool by allowing a few more copies to survive.

Many inherited diseases appear anew each generation by mutation. Is the evolutionary future in danger because of an increase in the mutation rate? There are real concerns that modern civilisation – with its dubious benefits of nuclear radiation and poisonous chemicals – will lead to a dramatic increase in the number of mutations. In many science fiction worlds this is, in a few short generations, enough to degrade the human race. The obvious threats, including man-made radiation and chemicals, have a smaller effect than do natural mutagens such as radon gas leaking from granite. The Sellafield nuclear power station in the North of England is the most polluting in the western world and the North Sea the most radioactive body of water. Yet, compared to other sources of radiation, its effects are minor. Avid consumers of shellfish collected near the discharge pipe receive about as much excess radiation as do those who fly from London to Los Angeles and back four times a year and are exposed to cosmic radiation as a result.

The rate of mutation goes up greatly with age. The control of infection means that most people now live for far longer than in earlier times. Mutation can hence take its toll on a much higher proportion of the population. This is very obvious when looking at such changes in body cells, including those which give rise to cancer. The cancer epidemic in the modern world is largely confined to older people. A shift in the pattern of survival has had effects on genes as they reside in body cells.

A more subtle transformation is having a dramatic effect on the mutation rate. In the western world at least, a change in the age at which people have children means that the number of new mutations will probably drop.

Cells which give rise to sperm or eggs are also exposed to the destructive effects of old age. Older parents are more likely to have genetically damaged children than are those who reproduce early. Any change in the age of reproduction will hence have an effect on the mutation rate. If the average age of reproduction goes up, there will be more mutations; if it decreases, there will be fewer. Social progress has led to just such a shift. The general picture, world-wide – a picture which applies to most of the Third World as much as to Britain and the United States – is simple and a little surprising.

Before the improvements in public health over the past few centuries most children died young. Mothers started having babies when they were themselves youthful and continued to have them until they were biologically unable to do so, perhaps twenty-five years later. As infant mortality drops there is less pressure to have children as an insurance against one's own old age. People prefer to have smaller families. The availability of contraception means that parents can choose to delay their first child – sometimes, as in middle-class Britain, until their mid-twenties – but then complete their families quickly. This means that most people stop having children soon after they have started. As a result, the average age of reproduction for both males and females goes down as social conditions improve.

All this means that mothers are younger on the average than they have been for much of the evolutionary past. Fathers, too, are getting more youthful. At the moment, at least, it looks as if the human mutation rate is on the way down. Whether this trend will continue is not known, but it does put fears about a new race of mutated monsters into context.

If mutation is the fuel of evolution, natural selection is its engine. As selection is a more elusive process than mutation it is more difficult to forecast what its future might be. Nature is always liable to come up – as it has so often before – with a nasty surprise with which natural selection must cope. The emergence of the AIDS virus shows that there is an eternal risk of this happening again. However, in the western world at least some of the greatest selective challenges have gone, because of the control of infectious disease.

Once a disease has disappeared (as so many have) the fate of the genes involved in combating it will change. Cypriots carry the inherited anaemia [*thalassaemia*] because the gene once defended their ancestors against malaria. Malaria has now disappeared from Cyprus – as, in time, will thalassaemia, with the incidence of carriers likely to drop by as much as one per cent per generation from its present level of seventeen per cent. In time, and given success – still far distant – in the fight against malaria, the same will happen to the dozens of other genes involved in resisting it elsewhere in the world. Perhaps such genes will, in time, remain only as mute witnesses to their evolutionary past.

There are more subtle ways of looking at the future of selection. Natural selection can only act on differences. If everyone survived to adulthood, found a partner and had the same number of children there would be almost no chance for it to operate. We do not need to know what genes selection is working on to see how important it might be. Looking at changes in the patterns of birth and death reveals a lot about its actions in the past and in the future.

In affluent countries, the differences between families in how many people survive have decreased. This means that there is less opportunity for natural selection. Ten thousand years ago, the struggle for existence really meant something. Skeletons from cave cemeteries show that few people lived to be more than twenty. If ancient fertility was anything like that found in modern tribal groups each female had about eight children, most of whom died young. For nine tenths of human evolution, society was like a village school, with lots of infants, plenty of teenagers and a few – probably harassed – adult survivors. Almost every death was potential raw material for selection as it involved someone young enough to have had a hope of passing on their genes. Nowadays, things have changed. Ninety-eight out of every hundred new-born British babies live to the age of fifteen, so that selection acting through childhood deaths (once its main mode of operation) has almost disappeared.

There have been changes in the balance of birth and death which have other effects on the opportunity for natural selection. Few modern peoples are as fertile as they once were. The Hutterites in North America wish for the largest possible family for religious reasons but even they, living in a healthy society, rarely have more than ten children. For most of human history it seems that people had as many children as is biologically possible. Only recently has that number begun to decrease.

Only in the past few years have humans lived as long as they are able. In the West, average life expectancy has nearly doubled over the past century. For the first time in history, most people die old; perhaps as old as biology allows. Life expectancy has risen from forty-seven to seventy-five years since 1900. Progress has now stopped, for some social classes at least. In the USA in 1979, a white woman of sixty-five could expect to live for another eighteen and a half years. In 1991 the figure was exactly the same. Even if all infectious diseases and all accidental deaths could be eliminated, average life expectancy in the western world would now go up by only a couple of years. There is still room for progress in the average length of life because of class differences in health. A baby born to an unskilled worker in Britain can expect to live for eight years less than one born to a professional person, a difference which, to our national shame, is actually increasing. However, the prospects for any dramatic improvement in longevity are dim.

This is important for the evolutionary future. The increase in the number of old people means that more people die for genetical reasons than in earlier times (largely because fewer are killed violently or by infection). Paradoxically, it also means that selection is weaker. The genes that kill are now those for cancer or heart disease, which act late in life. Those who die have already reproduced, passing on their fatal inheritance. Natural selection is much less powerful when acting on genes such as these than it is on those which alter the chances of survival before their carriers have children.

The new pattern of human existence (with fewer children than ever before but most people lasting until the biological clock runs down) emerged only about twenty human generations ago, compared to the six thousand or so since we first appeared on earth. It means that natural selection has changed the way it works. What there is nowadays acts more on fertility than on survival.

Differences in fertility among families, and the opportunity which they give for selection, shot up as birth control became popular. The upper classes adopted the idea well before the lower orders. Now that birth control is widespread the differences between families have dropped again, but selection working through variation in the number of children born is still, for the first time in history, greater than that working on the number that survive. The evolutionary fate of our genes depends more on the number of children we choose to have than on their chances of staying alive.

Nearly all the best understood forces of selection – disease, climate or starvation – act on survival rather than on fertility. The shift in the balance of the two may bring in new and unpredictable evolutionary forces. Perhaps the age of reproduction will become important, as those who mature young can have more children. There has been a drop in the age at which girls become sexually mature. In opposition to this trend, western women now marry five years later than they did half a century ago. Any inherited tendency to marry earlier or later (or to limit family size) could become a potent agent of evolution.

What this will do to the biological future is hard to say. A good general rule in evolution is that nobody gets a free lunch: success in one walk of life must be paid for by failure in another. History gives little reason to hope that selection will act as the agent of human perfectibility. It may direct the future, but will never make humanity superhuman.

The number of new mutations and the intensity of natural selection are both declining. This certainly does not mean that evolution is over. There is another change in modern society which is bound to influence our biological prospects. It is one which most people scarcely consider. It has to do with the geography of mating.

For most of history, everyone more or less had to marry the girl (or the boy) next door, because they had no choice. Society was based on small bands or isolated villages and marriages were within the group. In many places, populations were stable and quite inbred. Almost nobody moved. The genes of American Indians, drowned in a peat bog in Florida, display the effect clearly. The DNA in the preserved brains of people who died a thousand years apart shows that their genes are almost the same. There was little migration and the Indians had no option but to marry their relatives.

This pattern persisted in the West until recently and still exists in many parts of the world. In some places it is changing quickly. An increase in mating outside the local group is the most dramatic change in the developed world's evolutionary history. The effect is getting stronger and stronger. The influence of outbreeding on genetical health will outweigh anything that medicine is able to do.

One way of illustrating changes in breeding pattern is to use a crude but effective measure of how closely related our ancestors may have been. All that one needs to know is how far apart they were born. If they come from the same village they may well be relatives, but if they were born hundreds of miles apart this is much less likely. For nearly everyone reading this the distance between the places where they and their own partner were born is greater than that separating their parents' birthplaces. In turn, today's fathers and mothers were almost certainly born further apart than were their own parents. In nineteenth-century Oxfordshire the distance between the birthplaces of marriage partners was less than ten miles. Now it is more than fifty. In the United States it is several hundred, so that most American couples are completely unrelated. All this shows how quickly the world's populations are beginning to mix together.

It will take a long time before the mixing is complete. One estimate is that it will take as much as five hundred years to even out the genetic differences between England and Scotland – and perhaps even longer to get rid of their cultural contrasts.

Even if global homogeneity is a long way away, increased movement will certainly have a biological effect. No longer will large numbers of children be born who have two copies of defective genes because their parents are related. The most common damaged gene in whites is the one for cystic fibrosis, in blacks that for sickle-cell anaemia. Only if a child inherits two copies of either of these will it suffer from an inborn disease. Because cystic fibrosis is unknown in Africans and sickle cell in whites the child of a black–white mating is safe from both illnesses.

This effect can be a strong one. In many societies in the modern world there are immigrant communities which are beginning to merge with the people already there. Imagine that ten per cent of the population of Britain were to immigrate from West Africa (where about one person in fifteen is a carrier of the gene for sickle-cell anaemia) and to mate freely with the locals. The number of sickle-cell carriers in the new mixed British population would go up by seven times. However, the incidence of sickle-cell disease – which demands two copies of the damaged gene, one from each parent – would drop by ninety per cent compared to the previous situation in the two groups considered together. This is because many children would be born to parents from the two different peoples, one of whom – the native British partner – does not carry the sickle-cell gene. There would also be an effect on the indigenous British disease, cystic fibrosis, whose incidence would drop by about a sixth. Although this model of race mixing is simplistic it is not completely unreasonable. In Britain now, about one marriage in thirty is between two people of non-European origin; but a third as many are between a non-European and someone whose ancestors were born in the British Isles.

This change in mating patterns may mark the beginning of a new age of genetic well-being. Increased outbreeding inevitably means that recessive genes will be partnered by a normal copy which masks their effects. This is enough to dwarf the efforts of scientists to improve genetic health.

Most social changes seem to be conspiring to slow down human evolution. Mutation, selection, and random change have all lost some of their effectiveness in the past few centuries. All this means that the biology of the future will not be very different from that of the past. It may even be that economic advance and medical progress mean that humans are almost at the end of their evolutionary road, that we are as near to our biological Utopia as we are ever likely to get. Fortunately, no one reading this will be around to see if I am right.

Steve Jones is Professor of Genetics at University College London. This is an edited version of Chapter 16 of his award-winning book *The Language of the Genes*, which was originally published in 1993 by HarperCollins, London. The order of two paragraphs has been changed.

# 62
# The last well person

## CLIFTON K. MEADOR

'A well person is a patient who has not been completely worked up.' – a resident's answer to the question, 'What is a well person?' (Freymann J: personal communication).

There must be something the matter with someone who goes to see a doctor when there is nothing the matter.[1]

Well people are disappearing. I should have known it was coming when the invalids became extinct. (Invalids disappeared shortly after the advent of Medicare, which demanded specific diagnostic labels even though none applied.)[2] However, I began to realize what was happening only a year ago, at a dinner party. Everyone there had something. Several had high cholesterol levels. One had 'borderline anemia.' Another had a suspicious Pap smear. Two others had abnormal treadmill-test results, and several were concerned about codependency. There were no well people. After that, I began to look more carefully. I have not met a completely well person in months. At this rate, well people will vanish. As with the extinction of any species, there will be one last survivor. My guess is that the extinction will occur sometime in late 1998. Before we can speculate about the last well person, we need to understand what is happening. Why are they vanishing?

The demands of the public for definitive wellness are colliding with the public's belief in a diagnostic system that can find only disease. A public in dogged pursuit of the unobtainable, combined with clinicians whose tools are powerful enough to find very small lesions, is a setup for diagnostic excess.[2] And false positives are the arithmetically certain result of applying a disease-defining system to a population that is mostly well.

What is paradoxical about our awesome diagnostic power is that we do not have a test to distinguish a well person from a sick one. Wellness cannot be screened for. There is no substance in blood or urine whose level is reliably high or low in well people. No radiologic shadows or images indicate wellness. There is no tissue that can undergo biopsy to prove a person is well. Wellness cannot be measured, yet we seek it with analytic methods.

In the final definition, wellness can be distinguished from sickness only by the person involved, sometimes with the help of another person who cares and listens. About all any of us can expect is to know that if we feel good, stay active, and are comfortable, then we are probably well – at least for the time being. Clinical medicine can only say, 'With the methods we used, we found none of the diseases we looked for.' No one can measure the absence of all disease.

If the behaviour of doctors and the public continues unabated, eventually every well person will be labeled sick. Like the invalids, we will all be assigned to one diagnosis-related group or another. How long will it take to find every single lesion in every person? Who will be the last person? How will that person avoid diagnostic labels? From my experience with those who pursue wellness compulsively, I imagine that the last well person will be something like this:

## A composite case presentation

TIME: late 1998.
PLACE: A shopping mall near Kansas.
OCCASION: The Mid-America Health Fair, offering screening for all known human diseases.

The last well person is a 53-year-old professor of freshman algebra at a small college in a fictitious town. Once a successful stockbroker, he quit that job after attending a weekend workshop on stress-reduction and codependency conducted by a local church. He mistakenly thought he was sexually addicted. He has taken countless aptitude tests. By combining his Myers-Briggs profile with his scores on the Minnesota Multiphasic Personality Inventory, he found that his level of stress would be reduced if he taught introductory mathematics at a small coeducational college. He chose one in a temperate location with a median yearly temperature of about 15°. After checking into the average pollen count and the mean wind-chill factor in January, he selected the college. The new occupation gave him the free time he needed to devote to staying healthy – about 7 hours and 13 minutes a day.

Along with annual diagnostic workups, the man regularly has himself tested for a variety of conditions at assorted health fairs in the area. These screening tests include determinations of blood sugar, cholesterol (high-density and low-density lipoprotein), hematocrit, serum ferritin, carcinoembryonic antigen, and prostate-specific antigen and an occasional stool test for parasites after he visits relatives in Florida. All the tests to date have been negative. After undergoing two unnecessary colonoscopies because of false positive tests for blood in his stool, he now tests his own stool monthly for blood. Naturally, he abstains from meat for a full week beforehand.

The patient regularly watches the health reports on morning television, simultaneously videotaping those on all three major channels for delayed viewing. With each report of a new potential toxin or food additive or any of the myriad newly discovered health hazards, he narrows his diet, adjusts the humidity in this home, adds extra filters to his heating system, or makes yet another change in his lifestyle. On one occasion he tore out the floor of his basement to install a radon shield. He subscribes to several magazines offering tips on wellness and health, attaching the latest advice to his bathroom mirror to review while he shaves with his well-grounded electric razor. Of course, he has smoke detectors in every room and a rope ladder from his upstairs study. He installed an elaborate reverse-osmosis water-filtering system that also checks the fluoride level.

According to his best calculation, he consumes 15 per cent of his calories as fat, with the remainder split between protein and carbohydrate ('complex carbos', he calls them). He completely avoids saturated fat, salt, sugar, red meat, and all but trace amounts of vegetable oil, which he uses in his wok when he stir-fries his vegetables. He fortifies the vegetable fat with n-3 fatty acids. He initially discovered that animal crackers were the only commercially available bread low enough in fat to permit him to eat bread and remain on his fat-restricted diet. He was ecstatic when low-fat bread appeared on the market. However, the additives began to worry him. Therefore, he still limits himself to animal crackers.

He was a regular eater of tofu until he heard Garrison Keillor say on the radio that tofu did not extend one's useful life, but only the last few weeks of one's terminal coma. He saw no point in continuing anything that foolish. He does not smoke or chew tobacco, of course, or drink tea, coffee, or anything alcoholic. Recently he abandoned decaffeinated coffee because of reports about its harmfulness.

Every day he takes vitamins C, E, B6, and small amounts of D; several doses of kelp; and a concoction of dried seaweed mixed with desalinated sea water, along with a baby aspirin. He takes three doses of bulk laxatives, eats a bowl of bran, and drinks eight glasses of water daily after having heard of 'occasional irregularity' on television.

He is an aerobic wonder. He can run just about forever without getting winded. He rides his bike every weekend and uses his rowing machine on rainy days. He has installed a pulse-rate analyzer, a blood-pressure monitor, and an ear oximeter on his stationary bike and rowing machine. Both have alarms set at the prescribed maximal levels, which he readjusts every birthday.

He sees his dentist twice a year, flosses three times a day after brushing, and paints his teeth with a specially mixed solution of fluoride and calcium with a trace of vitamin D. He gargles with a weak solution of hydrogen peroxide and plaque remover before bed. He has learned to examine his own vocal cords with a hand-held mirror.

He wears a prescription wavelength-adjusted set of dark glasses whenever he goes outside. The wave-length is calculated precisely to filter out those ultraviolet waves of the sun known to cause cataracts (I forget the wavelengths, but I am sure the glasses are available at any local House of Eyes and Glasses). If he is in the sun more than five minutes, he applies number 15 sunscreen. There is a space marked out on his den wall so that he can check his visual fields monthly and simultaneously calculate his visual acuity.

Every year he and his significant other stand naked in front of a full-length mirror. They record all nevi [moles] and measure each one with a millimeter ruler. If any look suspicious, they photograph them with a Polaroid camera. The significant other is needed to help in examining those areas of the body inaccessible to ordinary viewing. To date the man has found 113 nevi, and biopsies have been performed on 9 of them. All have been benign.

The patient has made many efforts to be screened for every known psychopathological disorder. Because there are many psychological schools of thought, this pursuit has consumed a large amount of time. The patient even spent several months of his quest for psychological health in southern California, the bastion of new schools of psychology. He tried Rolfing, client-centered therapy, transactional analysis, primal-scream therapy, gestalt therapy, and neurolinguistic reprogramming – all with no success. Each school rejected him as utterly normal.

On two occasions he was asked to a leave a group – once an encounter group and the other time an experiential-learning group – after making his first utterances. Finally, to his embarrassment, he was thrown out of a psychic-channeling session at a New Age harmonic conversion in the Mojave Desert. He had failed to channel anything except vague memories of his high-school janitor.

In summary, all extant psychiatric and psychological schools of clinical thought have rejected him. From the patient's experience, it is fair to say that all psychiatric and psychological diseases defined by these schools have been ruled out.

[*Editorial note*: In earlier times the man would have been considered to have an obsessive-compulsive neurosis, but that diagnosis has had to be dropped. Obsession is no longer a disease, but an essential attribute of staying healthy.]

His medical workups are lengthy. Every orifice has been subjected to endoscopy at least once, and most of them annually. He has had countless computed tomographic scans, magnetic resonance imaging scans and one scan by positron-emission tomography – all of which were normal. He has had one biopsy of his thyroid and two of his prostate. He regularly gets profiles of his blood and urine chemistry. At no time has any test or procedure yielded a positive or abnormal result that remained abnormal when the test was repeated.

That is how I suppose the last well person might appear. It is miraculous that he escaped being labeled with a disease for so long, and incredible that he missed being given a false diagnosis. In my imagined meeting with the last well person I can hear myself saying, 'Doing all those boring things you do to stay healthy may or may not make you live longer. However, I am sure of one thing; it will make your life seem longer.'

The last well person would not smile. Escaping disease in the 1990s is very serious business.


## References

1. Barsky, A. J. *Worried Sick: Our Troubled Quest for Wellness*. Little, Brown, Boston (1988).
2. Meador, C. K. 'A lament for invalids', *J. Amer. Med. Assoc.* **265**, 1374–5 (1991).

This article has been reproduced in its entirety from *The New England Journal of Medicine*, 330(6) 440–1 (1994). Clifton K. Meador is a medical doctor working at Saint Thomas Hospital, Nashville, Tennessee, and a member of the teaching staff of Vanderbilt University in the same town.

# Author index[1]

---

[1] Several (unfamiliar) authors' names come from the collection of articles listed under 'Ethical dilemmas in evaluation — a correspondence'; others are second /third/etc. authors of multiply-authored articles.

# Subject index

abortion: access to 369; spontaneous, and neural tube defects (NTD) 210, 211

accidents: in childhood 127, 170–7, 240; in hospitals 240; inequalities in 368; preventive measures 174–5, 176–7; responsibility for safety 173–4

Acheson report 384–5, 387

acupuncture 39, 391

Addison, Thomas, and pernicious anaemia 11–12, 14

adolescence, growth spurt in 161–5

advocacy schemes 281

Africa: famine in sub-Saharan 148, 151–2; 'food insecure' numbers in 397

age: and definitions of health 27, 28, 31, 32; of marriage and childbirth 419, 421; of onset of pernicious anaemia 14

ageing: and the division of the life course 127, 166–9; and the greening of medicine 390, 391; and work satisfaction 244

agoraphobia, and migraine 91

AIDS (Acquired Immune Deficiency Syndrome): and HIV 103–4; living with 70, 100–6; and NHS spending 270; public and private world of 100–2; social factors 103, 105

airborne diseases: death rates 183–7, 188, 192, 193–6; and global warming 397

alcohol consumption: deaths through excessive 154; of workers in 1844 131

allocative intervention policies, of state intervention 245

alternative medicine: as alternative to surgery 39–40; and the greening of medicine 388; ideological commitment to 43; information sources on 40–1; and personal support in illness 40; and spiritual healers 391; and use of orthodox medicine 40, 42, 43; users of 38–44; whole family involvement in 41–2, *see also* holistic medicine

Alzheimer's disease: caring for wife with 70, 79–82; genes causing 413, 414; stages of 80, 81, 82

Amiel, Henri 35

amniocentesis, and neural tube defects (NTD) 209

anaemia: history of pernicious anaemia 1, 11–17; megaloblastic anaemias 14

anencephaly 221

animals, asthma triggered by 83, 84

anorexia nervosa 158, 159

ante-natal clinics, personal experiences of 115, 116

antibiotics: and alternative medicine 39; in medical folklore 23, 24; overprescribing of 24; potential hazards of 240

apothecaries 264

appendicitis, death rates from 189

Armstrong, D. 66

Asclepius (healing god) 1, 7, 8

Asians, and psychiatric illness 53

asthma, childhood 70, 83–8

attendance allowance 318

authority, symbols of, abandonment of by psychiatrists 2, 51

auto-immune diseases, and pernicious anaemia 15–16

Ayurveda system of medicine 293, 294, 297

'back to nature' movement 389

Bacon, Francis 390

bacteria, and viruses 24

bacterial toxins, as cause of pernicious anaemia 13, 15

Bangladesh: effects of global warming 394; famine and floods 148, 150–1; smallpox 234

Bashkirtsev, Marie 34

Belgiojoso, Princess 34

Bergstedt, Kenneth 107, 108–9

Bernard, Claude 6–7

Bible, the, and mirages of health 4

biomedical model of health 26

black patients, and psychiatrists 50–4

Black Report 125–6, 135–9

Bland, Anthony 408, 409

Bliss, Dr Mary 410

BMA (British Medical Association) 274; and euthanasia 407

body: replacement by artificial structure 359, 362–6; separation of the mouth from in dentistry 2–3, 62–8

Bourneville, D. M. 58, 59

Bouvia, Elizabeth 107

Boyd, M. F. 64

Boyes, Mrs Lilian 407–8

boys: adolescent 127, 161, 164–5; pre-pubescent 162–3

Brackenbury, H. B. 48

Bradshaw, Steven 109

breast biopsy, as day surgery 304

breast cancer: effectiveness of treatment 202, 203; screening for 225, 229–30

British Dental Association 62

British Diabetic Association 99

British Medical Association, and child poverty 138

British Tuberculosis Association 205